AF790715

Advances in Image-Guided Cancer Nanomedicine

Online at: https://doi.org/10.1088/978-0-7503-3675-8

IPEM–IOP Series in Physics and Engineering in Medicine and Biology

Editorial Advisory Board Members

Frank Verhaegen
Maastro Clinic, The Netherlands

Carmel Caruana
University of Malta, Malta

Penelope Allisy-Roberts
formerly of BIPM, Sèvres, France

Rory Cooper
University of Pittsburgh, PA, USA

Alicia El Haj
University of Birmingham, UK

Kwan Hoong Ng
University of Malaya, Malaysia

John Hossack
University of Virginia, USA

Tingting Zhu
University of Oxford, UK

Dennis Schaart
TU Delft, The Netherlands

Indra J Das
Northwestern University Feinberg School of Medicine, USA

About the Series

The series in Physics and Engineering in Medicine and Biology will allow the Institute of Physics and Engineering in Medicine (IPEM) to progress its mission to 'advance physics and engineering applied to medicine and biology for the public good'.

It is focused on key areas including, but not limited to:

- clinical engineering
- diagnostic radiology
- informatics and computing
- magnetic resonance imaging
- nuclear medicine
- physiological measurement
- radiation protection
- radiotherapy
- rehabilitation engineering
- ultrasound and non-ionising radiation.

A number of IPEM–IOP titles are being published as part of the EUTEMPE Network Series for Medical Physics Experts.

A full list of titles published in this series can be found here: https://iopscience.iop.org/bookListInfo/physics-engineering-medicine-biology-series.

Advances in Image-Guided Cancer Nanomedicine

Edited by
Nanasaheb D Thorat
Nuffield Department of Women's & Reproductive Health, John Radcliffe Hospital, Medical Sciences Division, University of Oxford, Oxford, UK

IOP Publishing, Bristol, UK

© IOP Publishing Ltd 2022

All rights reserved. No part of this publication may be reproduced, stored in a retrieval system or transmitted in any form or by any means, electronic, mechanical, photocopying, recording or otherwise, without the prior permission of the publisher, or as expressly permitted by law or under terms agreed with the appropriate rights organization. Multiple copying is permitted in accordance with the terms of licences issued by the Copyright Licensing Agency, the Copyright Clearance Centre and other reproduction rights organizations.

Permission to make use of IOP Publishing content other than as set out above may be sought at permissions@ioppublishing.org.

Nanasaheb D Thorat has asserted their right to be identified as the editor of this work in accordance with sections 77 and 78 of the Copyright, Designs and Patents Act 1988.

ISBN 978-0-7503-3675-8 (ebook)
ISBN 978-0-7503-3673-4 (print)
ISBN 978-0-7503-3676-5 (myPrint)
ISBN 978-0-7503-3674-1 (mobi)

DOI 10.1088/978-0-7503-3675-8

Version: 20221101

IOP ebooks

British Library Cataloguing-in-Publication Data: A catalogue record for this book is available from the British Library.

Published by IOP Publishing, wholly owned by The Institute of Physics, London

IOP Publishing, No.2 The Distillery, Glassfields, Avon Street, Bristol, BS2 0GR, UK

US Office: IOP Publishing, Inc., 190 North Independence Mall West, Suite 601, Philadelphia, PA 19106, USA

Contents

Preface

Nanomedicine has been one of the key research areas for diagnosis and curing of cancer for about 30 years. Cancer nanomedicine using functional hybrid nanomaterials has been expected to provide new opportunities in early diagnosis, imaging and treatment of cancerous tumors. In preclinical settings, nanomedicine demonstrates very promising applications for cancer imaging and therapeutics. Currently used imaging techniques in combination with nanomedicine show some important properties to address key challenges in modern cancer therapy: (i) monitoring an active tumor targeting mechanism of therapeutic drugs driven by a physical force; (ii) providing guidance for on-demand drug release mechanism; and (iii) a capability for next generation image-guided cancer therapy and therapy monitoring.

The oncological branch that performs the diagnosis and treatment of cancer using non-invasive imaging techniques 'interventional oncology' employs x-ray, ultrasound, computed tomography (CT), positron emission tomography (PET) or magnetic resonance imaging (MRI) techniques for image-guided cancer therapies. The radio imaging techniques are helping to guide targeted and precise treatment of solid tumors located in various organs of the human body. On the other hand, advances in nanomedicine provided functional nanomaterials that enable high tumor tissue imaging contrast effects during image-guided therapeutic procedures. Thus, the unique combination of imaging techniques and nanomedicine offer a new opportunity of image-guided cancer nanomedicine approach which can bypass the low tumor targeting and toxicity issues in advanced clinical settings. The book address the advances of next generation medical imaging techniques coupled with nanomedicine, for image guidance, for tumor detection, tumor tissue characterization, monitoring of drug targeting, pre- and post-therapy monitoring of solid tumors. Furthermore, the book outlines the latest advances in detail by the ground of currently used cancer therapies and nanomedicine synergy, for patient-specific therapeutic dosimetry and tumor-specific treatment of cancers. Eventually, this new generation image-guided cancer nanomedicine has shown to be a superior therapeutic effect in a personalized manner without major complications, with faster recoveries, and low treatment cost.

The book is designed to promote scientific knowledge exchanges, technological implementation and innovative solutions in new generation imaging modalities coupled with nanomedicine within both the academic and industrial level. Understanding the fundamentals of nanomedicine driven imaging is a long pathway and requires inherently multidisciplinary expertise, intertwined with the contribution of highly qualified scientists, regulatory entities, enterprises and medical practitioners. The current book is a prominent platform of required highly qualified expertise for preparing an up-to-date status document for reference. Therefore, this book gathers together experts with the eventual aim of removing at least some of the major obstacles that hamper the translational aspects of cancer imaging.

Different from current and previous reviews or literature available, this book update provides a review of the most recent advances of imaging techniques coupled with nanomedicine for disease management with high efficiency and safety by taking advantage of each composition and imaging along with therapeutic effect, which have never been documented in such a systematic way for cancer disease management. The book outlines the latest advances in detail by the analysis of imaging techniques used to treat, to diagnose and to monitor cancer. Furthermore, synergy of these imaging techniques with nanomedicine is presented. Detailed in the book is not only basic physics or nanoscience of image-guided cancer nanomedicine, but also clinical relevance and the clinical progress beyond the current state of the art.

The key features of the book are.

1. An overview of the synergy between imaging techniques and nanomedicine.
2. Newly developed imaging modalities for cancer management.
3. Nanomedicine standardization in advanced clinical settings for monitoring and treating cancer.
4. Synergy of next generation cancer therapy modalities and nanomedicine for cancer treatment, diagnostic and treatment monitoring.
5. All-in-one comprehensive underlying physics of imaging and its combination with nanomedicine, in cancer disease management and designing the roadmap of future clinical translation.

Acknowledgements

The project leading to this work has received funding from the European Union's Horizon 2020 research and innovation program under the Marie Sklodowska-Curie grant agreement 'SUPERBRAIN' 840964. The book is the scientific dissemination activity of 'SUPERBRAIN' project.

Editor biography

Lead editor Dr Nanasaheb Thorat, MSc, PhD (Gold Medal), MRSC

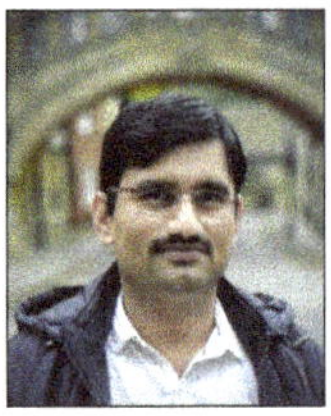

Dr Thorat is an outstanding researcher currently working as Research Scientist and Marie-Curie Fellow at the University of Oxford, Oxford, UK. Dr Thorat has published 7 books, ~65 peer reviewed journal articles and 20 book chapters (total citations ~3100, H-index: 34), presented 5 keynote speeches, 25 invited talks at prestigious scientific peer-conferences, received international acclaim and awards for research contribution, supervised students/junior researchers and actively participated in outreach and scientific dissemination for the service of the wider community. He is also a recipient of various prestigious fellowships including Marie Skłodowska-Curie Fellowship (IF) in Poland/Switzerland 2018, Japanese Society for the Promotion of Science (JSPS) Fellowship in Japan 2017, Government of Ireland IRC fellowship Ireland 2015. In addition to his current research, he has been deeply engaged in collaborative work with many eminent scientists from Japan, USA, Germany, Korea, Ireland, India, Poland, Saudi Arabia and Australia. He also has excellent collaboration and interactions with over 30 junior and senior colleagues in India, South Korea, Japan, Taiwan and Ireland with whom he has co-authored his publications.

Dr Thorat is the awardee of the European Commission's innovation Radar 'Grand Prix of the Innovation Radar Prize 2020' for developing ground-breaking technology for breast cancer theranostics, funded under EU's Marie Curie IF Project 'NANOCARGO' He is a recipient of many prestigious awards such as, Young Scientist Awardee through open competition by Lindau Nobel Laureate Foundation in the 67th Lindau Nobel Laureate Meeting 25th to 30th June 2017 in Lindau, Germany, European Materials Research Society (EMRS) Young Investigator Award in Biomaterials field. Dr Thorat's contribution in the area of nano-biotechnology and theranostics has been recognised by Royal Society of Chemistry (RSC, UK) and he was admitted as a Member of The RSC and entitled the designation MRSC in the year October 2017. Dr Thorat is a Management Committee member of three European Cooperation in Science and Technology (COST) actions such as COST Action CA17140, Cancer Nanomedicine-From the Bench To The Bedside (NANO2CLINIC), CA17104, New Diagnostic And Therapeutic Tools Against Multidrug Resistant Tumors and CA17115, European network for advancing Electromagnetic hyperthermic medical technologies. Dr Thorat was also involved in an Enterprise Ireland innovation partnership research project that involved four world leading pharmaceutical companies Jansen, GSK, Pfizer and MSD (year 2017–2018) at pharmaceutical manufacturing technology centre (PMTC) University of Limerick. His work involved upskilling to spectroscopic techniques such as x-ray photoelectron spectroscopy and Raman spectroscopy to probe the drug/material interface. Dr Thorat has established his own educational start-up REINSPIRE Research and Education LLP in India (http://reinspire.in/). The REINSPIRE provides a conceptual framework as a starting point for implementation and evaluation of effective consulting for systemic improvement in research, education and institutional human resource (HR) policies to Indian institutes.

List of contributors

R K Chandunika
Centre for Nanotechnology Research, Vellore Institute of Technology, Vellore, India

Ahmaduddin Khan
Centre for Nanotechnology Research, Vellore Institute of Technology, Vellore, India

Professor Niroj Sahu

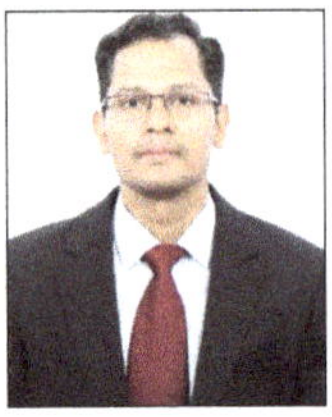

Centre for Nanotechnology Research, Vellore Institute of Technology, Vellore, India

Dr Sahu is currently working as an Associate Professor at the Centre for Nanotechnology Research at the Vellore Institute of Technology, India. His areas of research are focused on the development of functionalized nanomaterials, study of the physical and chemical properties of nanomaterials and applications of nanomaterials in cancer therapy as well as energy storage. He is the author of 45 peer reviewed journal articles, eight conference proceedings, 10 book chapters and one book.

Dr Sandeep B Somvanshi

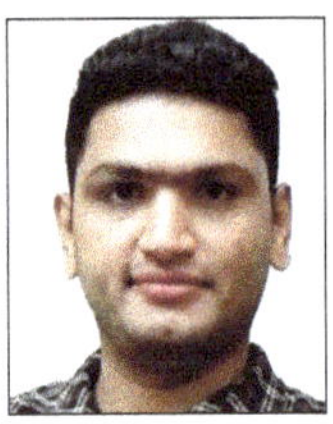

School of Materials Engineering, Purdue University, 47907 West Lafayette, USA

Sandeep B Somvanshi, is working as a visiting fellow at Department of Materials Engineering, Purdue University, USA. He has published more than 45 research papers in peer reviewed journals and 5 book chapters. His major research interests include magnetism and magnetic nanomaterials, magnetic fluid hyperthermia for cancer treatment, magnetic resonance imaging, drug delivery system, silica aerogels, nanocatalyst and photocatalyst etc. He is a recipient of many prestigious awards such as, Young Scientist Award by DST, Govt. of India for participation in 5th BRICS Young Scientist Conclave, DST-Inspire Fellowship by Govt. of India, Overseas Doctoral Fellowship by Government of India and Several Merit Scholarships.

IOP Publishing

Advances in Image-Guided Cancer Nanomedicine

Nanasaheb D Thorat

Chapter 1

Introduction to cancer nanomedicine and nanotheranostics

R K Chandunika, Ahmaduddin Khan, Nanasaheb D Thorat and Niroj Kumar Sahu

1.1 Introduction

Cancer is recognized as the most complex, challenging and aggressive disease globally in terms of clinical management. In 2018, GLOBOCAN estimated 18.1 million new cases worldwide and 9.6 million deaths were due to cancer. Despite the diverse existence of the disease, there are key cell elements involved in proliferation, differentiation, and immortalization, and ultimately the capability to evade treatment strategies. Thus, understanding the complexity of the tumor environment will provide an opportunity to improve clinical outcomes. Unfortunately, to date, conventional theranostics strategies against cancer have failed to tackle the detailed information of the tumor environment. However, optimized cancer theranostics would help to deliver the correct type of therapy with minimal systemic toxicity. This task is daunting because there is considerable variation among tumors and individual patients. In this context, recent advancements in nanomedicine have been proposing novel strategies by combining biomaterials and nanotechnology to provide complex multipurpose nanosystems for cancer treatment. These nanosystems are providing both therapeutic and diagnostic functions that are often referred to as 'nanotheranostics'. In addition, these systems usually can carry and deliver drugs to the tumor site, enabling early detection of cancer, and therapy can be monitored non-invasively and in real-time.

1.2 Nanotheranostics and nanomedicine

A few decades ago, nanosized materials were first proposed for their unique physicochemical properties in biomedical and sensing applications. Later on, nanoplatform took precedence over other materials in the field of biomedicine for various reasons such as tunable property, easy functionalization, high surface area, multifunctionality and better accumulation and binding on specific sites. In terms of

doi:10.1088/978-0-7503-3675-8ch1 © IOP Publishing Ltd 2022

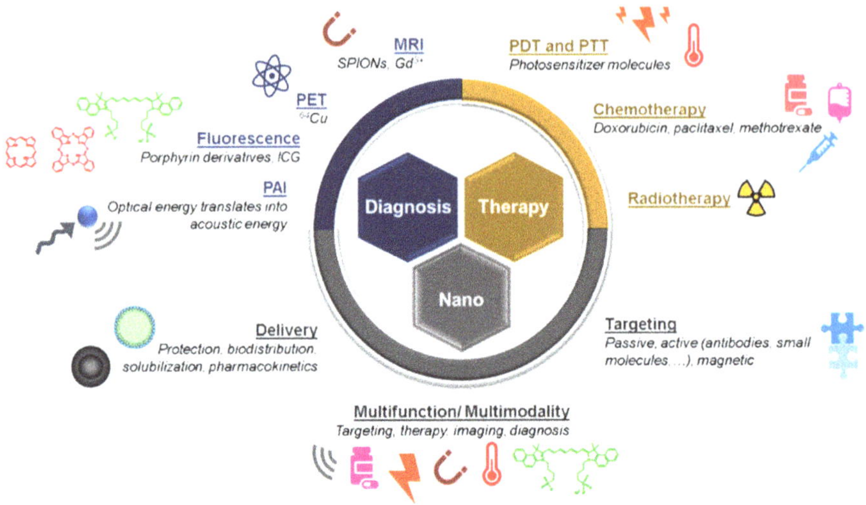

Figure 1.1. Schematic illustration of triple feature single entity nanotheranostic agent with characteristics of nanosized particle, diagnostic and therapeutic agent. Adapted from [2], with permission from MDPI. Copyright 2019 by the authors.

design, nanosized materials in a size range of 5–100 nm are suitable for tumor targeting [1]. Nanosized materials called nanomedicine show versatile medical properties by playing significant roles in diagnostic and therapeutic fields of healthcare. These nanomedicines are primarily classified into three groups metallic, non-metallic and biological. Indeed, nanomedicines show remarkable growth in the field of cancer studies due to their easy uptake and homogeneous distribution in the heterogeneous tumor microenvironment. However, they have certain limitations such as, non-specific distribution, size effect (sometimes too large particle size makes entering the tumor site difficult or too small in size allows easy uptake by the reticuloendothelial system (RES)), high concentrations required, aggregation, too long circulation time that may cause side effects and time-consuming diagnostic or therapeutic procedures. To address these concerns, integrating diagnostic and therapeutic properties into a single nanosized platform known as nanotheranostics is necessary (figure 1.1).

John Funkhouser the president of PharmaNetics, in 2002, demonstrated nanotheranostics as one platform by integrating targeting ligand, imaging and therapeutic probes together [3]. Nanotheranostics agents have a significant advantage for site-specific image-guided therapy with minimum dose requirement but maintaining its effectiveness and efficiency has been a major challenge. On the other hand, theranostic nanomedicines have become a trend in biomedical applications for their reduced side effects, treatment time, expense, etc [4]. Hence, for improved clinical cancer diagnostic and therapeutic applications, this all-in-one multifunctionality model with immense potential for better contrast, controlled delivery, and being target specific with improved transport efficiency must be adapted for clinical usage. Thus, researchers have been trying to design clinically suitable nanotheranostic agents by improving the synthesis procedures without losing the efficacy of the fabricated platforms. Some of the critical challenges faced by multifunctional nanotheranostics at *in vivo* and *in vitro* testing level are site-specific targeting, premature release of loaded drug, toxicity, slow degradation and rapid clearance.

1.3 Nanomedicine as contrast agents for localized imaging

In cancer research, site-specific and early-stage detection are major challenges in diagnostic techniques. In the past few decades, conventional contrast agents based on small inorganic molecules have been widely used even though they possess severe side effects. Some of the potential drawbacks of current contrast agents are rapid clearance, poor uptake by tumor cells, non-specific distribution, nephrotoxicity, low biocompatibility and poor image resolution [5–7]. The elements that are in use as imaging agents for bioimaging applications are organic dyes, Au, Ba, Bi, Cu, Dy, Gd, Lu, Pb, Ta, U, W, and Yb because of their high atomic number, density and radio contrasting. However, they have drawbacks such as high toxicity and poor uptake by the tumor microenvironment [5]. To overcome these limitations and for better and higher resolution images, engineering the aforementioned contrast agents into nanosized materials or integrating them into nanoscale matrices has been proposed.

Initially, nanomaterials are used as contrast for magnetic resonance imaging (MRI) to enhance the image contrast in *in vivo* studies. It became a natural fit because since the 1960s, iron oxide nanoparticles (NPs) have been used clinically to treat anemia [8]. Iron oxides in clinical MRI had much promise due to their high magnetic moment affecting nearby water molecules by reducing their relaxation times. In 1978, Ohgushi and colleagues showed the application of iron oxides in MR imaging by the simple mixture of dextran and tri-iron tetroxide coating [9]. Later on, fabrication techniques emerged to control the properties of iron-based agents to make them more likely in the clinical standard for imaging. This paved the way for the major breakthrough for the broad assortment of NPs available today preclinically. These include computed tomography (CT), nanomaterial-based contrast agent for imaging the blood pool, liver, and spleen and optical nanomaterials for use in cancer diagnostics/cell tracking, sentinel lymph node imaging during surgery etc [10–13]. Some of the clinically used contrast agents and their advantages and disadvantages are listed in table 1.1.

Nanotechnology-based contrast agents have been chosen to be better candidates for bioimaging for several reasons. Firstly, they are in very small dimensions that provide high loading capacity, easily controllable physicochemical properties (size, shape, material, density, and surface charge), target specific, and possible multiplex imaging. Nanomaterial sized contrast agent is advantageous in bioimaging compared to small molecules due to its ability to carry much more contrast in a single structure and easy travel through the bloodstream [14]. Moreover, selective entry into the desired tumor site is more possible than for molecularly sized agents because of the enhanced permeability and retention effect (EPR effect) [15]. The control of physicochemical properties like size, shape, and surface charge of a nanomaterial

Table 1.1. Contrast agents with their advantages and disadvantages [3, 4, 22, 23]. Reprinted from [3], copyright 2020 The Author(s). Published by Elsevier Ltd.

Contrast agent	Imaging modality	Advantages	Disadvantages
Iohexol, iodixanol, iothalamate etc (iodinated contrast agents)	X-ray and CT imaging	• Higher signal-to-noise and contrast-to-noise ratios • Better image resolution • Cost-effective	• Nephrotoxicity • Multiple- and high-dose requirement • Non-specific interactions • High viscosity and rapid clearance
Plasmonic NPs (Au, Ag, Pt)	X-ray and CT imaging	• Easy synthesis and large production • Surface engineering • Good stability and biocompatibility • High image resolution and deep penetration due to high x-ray attenuation and atomic number • Specific distribution and prolonged circulation time	• Expensive to synthesis • Long-time retention in the body and slow degradation • Inflammation of major organs • High accumulation in the liver and spleen
Carbon nanotubes, gold nanorods, gold–silica nanohybrids, organic dyes, porphyrin-phospholipid coated upconversion NPs, silicon NPs	Photoacoustic imaging	• Simple design and high photostability • Enhanced surface plasmon resonance • Good biocompatibility • Deep tissue penetration ability	• High accumulation of NPs in the liver (30%–99%) • Low tumor accumulation and binding abilitySlow degradation in the case of inorganic hybridsLow sensitivity
Cyanine 5.5, fluorescein isothiocyanate, indocyanine green	Optical and fluorescent imaging	• Biocompatible, easily soluble and deep tissue penetration	• Poor circulation and photostability • Rapid excretion • Non-specific distribution

^{124}I-labeled cRGDY silica	PET imaging	• Better photostability and biocompatibility • Specific binding ability and prolonged circulation time • High resolution	• Difficult to synthesize and low yield • Slow biodegradation • Long-term retention in the body • Low tumor accumulation
Superparamagnetic iron oxide NPs, macrocyclic compounds chelated with paramagnetic metal ions like gadolinium (Gd^{3+}) and manganese (Mn^{2+}), MnO NPs	MR imaging	• Better image contrast due to high rotational correlation time and low relaxivity • Biocompatible • Strong and better tumor accumulation ability • Better dispersibility • High surface-to-volume ratio	• Complicated synthesis and low product yield • Non-specific biodistribution • High concentration needed for high image resolution • Requirement of high magnetic field • Low circulation and slow degradation

sized contrast agent for different types of cancer is essential. More importantly, these properties can often dictate their utility as contrast agents and determine their efficacy [16]. The particle size determines the surface area-to-volume ratio. The higher surface area of nanomaterials facilitates the presence of numerous targeting ligands, making contrast agents more target specific and more stable. Moreover, recently they have become more important for multimodality imaging with contrast for multiple imaging modalities all on a single nanosized particle (e.g., multiple contrast types such as MRI, fluorescence, and Raman contrast) [17]. These are the key reasons for the potential revolution in the field of bioimaging using nanotechnology.

Nanosized agents intended for clinical imaging should display the key feature of lack of toxicity as coating NPs with functional linkage is essential. Since the contrast agent is generally injected to the healthy population of cells to diagnose diseases, the coating is essential for diagnostic nanomaterials more than therapeutic nanomaterials. For example, gadolinium-based nanomaterials can cause nephrogenic systemic fibrosis (NSF), particularly in patients with advanced kidney disease, which can be fatal under some circumstances [18]. Even though it affects only a very small portion of the population, it still remains as an imaging agent. Hence, it must maintain a higher bar of safety than typical therapeutic agents. Another key feature for better imaging is the polydispersity of the contrast agent. This can affect the imaging property such as signal strength by aggregating. It can be controlled by modifying physicochemical properties such as surface charge, shape, and coating during fabrication. Intriguingly, it has either positive or negative effects on imaging. For example, on the positive side, research shows aggregation of quantum dots displays better targeting and circulation behavior with improved images than the individual NPs [19]. Aggregation also positively affects Raman imaging by boosting the image signal into tiny 'hot spots' at interfaces due to plasmon resonance coupling [20]. On the negative side, aggregated NPs disturb the pharmacokinetic biodistribution of nanomaterials, reduced circulation half-life, and capillary blockage. For example, nanomaterial aggregation diminishes image quality in iron oxide material for magnetic resonance imaging (MRI) due to the variation in magnetic behavior [21].

1.4 Nanomedicines for imaging-guided cancer therapy

Traditionally, cancer is treated by chemotherapy with the help of anticancer drugs like doxorubicin. However, these chemotherapeutic drugs have high toxicity and adverse side effects due to their non-specific distribution. In addition, they are unable to differentiate between healthy and cancer cells and easy penetration into the cellular regions occurs. To overcome this, the nanocarrier idea was proposed to make them target specific delivery by carrying drugs through easy functionalization. To promote high accumulation at the tumor site, identification of receptors on the cell membrane is essential to engineer surface-modified nanocarriers. The surface modification will also enhance blood circulation and drug loading and also make nanocarriers biocompatible. Importantly, surface-modified nanocarriers have a strong binding ability toward cancer cells. Furthermore, the accumulation of nanocarriers in the tumor environment by the EPR effect has also been widely studied for localized therapy. Some of the major concerns in delivering drugs are: (1) poor uptake and non-specific distribution of anticancer drugs to various side effects on major organs; (2) entry of nanocarriers/drug molecules are restricted in low vascularized areas in tumors resulting in the recurrence of cancer after treatment; (3) cancer cells often resist and prevent the movement of chemotherapeutic drugs due to the acid environment [24]. To resolve these issues, current research is focused on developing nanosystems called nanotheranostics for targeted treatment. Some of the recently developed nanotheranostic agents for cancer therapy are listed in table 1.2.

In recent years, studies have shown the effective interaction between nanosystem and tumor microenvironment is achieved by material with a size less than 500 nm compared with larger particles [25]. After entering into cancer cells, these particles produce reactive oxygen species (ROS), sound and heat upon exposure to external stimuli. This property of generation heat and sound waves from light is used to treat targeted cancer cells. On the other hand, the irradiation of external stimuli can also be used to induce the triggered release of loaded anticancer drugs [26]. Moreover, according to the need for internal (H_2O_2, pH, etc) or external (light, ultrasound, heat, magnetic field etc) stimulus nanosystems can be engineered for safe and better treatment, shown in figure 1.2. Some nanosystems have even already been tested at the clinical level, showing promising response without any side effects.

Some of the nanomedicine proposed cancer therapies are photothermal therapy (PTT), photodynamic therapy (PDT) and chemotherapy. PTT uses photothermal active nanomedicine for treating selective and deep-seated tumor by exposure to high power near-infrared (NIR) light. Recently, it attracted the attention of researchers for its high photothermal conversion efficiency and low absorption ability by healthy tissue. Upon NIR light exposure to the area where photothermal agents accumulate, this generates photothermal heat to the selective tumor regions without affecting the surrounding healthy cells [28]. So far, many NPs have been studied for PTT, like organic dyes, gold-based nanostructures, gold-liposome, gold–silica, $CuS@MnO_2$ hybrids, 2D nanosheets (graphene oxide, MoS_2, WS_2, MXene), plasmonic nanoshell etc [29]. Notably, different types of gold NPs have been validated as PTT agents due to their surface plasmon resonance and photo-transduction property. For example, functionalized gold nanorods have been studied for localized PTT by Pan *et al* [30]. The study showed homogeneous distribution of nanorods in the tumor microenvironment and obtained a promising photothermal response during NIR light exposure. Animal studies also validated that the generated heat enhances the photothermal damage of tumor cells. PDT is another NIR light-mediated therapy with a promising approach for selective tumor therapy. In PDT, during light exposure, the cancer cell produces toxic oxygen species ROS generation, which helps kill cancer cells. For example, recently, Yang *et al* proposed liposomal nanostructures for PDT applications [27]. They fabricated PEGylated liposomal nanohybrids named DSPE-PEG liposomes with folic acid as a targeting ligand. They have validated this nanostructure as an effective PDT agent by conducting *in vivo* and *in vitro* studies. The results show a significant tumor

Table 1.2. Therapeutic agents with their advantages and disadvantages [3, 25, 33, 34]. Reprinted from [3], copyright 2020 The Authors. Published by Elsevier Ltd.

Therapeutic agent	Therapeutic technique	Advantages	Disadvantages
Gold NPs (nanorods, nanocages, gold-liposomes, gold–silica, PEGylated silica-gold nanoshells etc)	Photothermal therapy	• Easy preparation • Biocompatible, biodegradation and smooth circulation • Good optical property, photothermal response and enhanced surface plasmonic property	• Easy aggregation • Low binding efficiency and slow clearance • Uncontrolled photothermal damage of surrounding healthy tissues • Need long-term exposure time and high power of near-infrared (NIR) light
Quantum dots, organic dye-based photosensitizer (indocyanine green toluidine blue, methylene blue, hypericin), porphyrin, chlorine 6, dye-conjugated gold nanorods and 2D Mxene, dye-loaded liposomes, NaYF4: Yb3þ, Er3, metal-organic framework, copper bismuth sulfide	Photodynamic therapy	• Easy synthesis, high production and product yield is possible • Effective reactive oxygen species (ROS) generation and better optical property • Specific tumor-binding ability, biocompatibility and good circulation time	• High cost and low stability • Controlling particle size and shape is difficult • Uncontrolled oxidative stress due to non-specific ROS distribution • High power NIR light required
Doxorubicin (DOX), Sorafenib (SF), Paclitaxel etc, drug-loaded nanocarries	Chemotherapy	• Easy preparation and reproducibility • Easy surface modification, large surface area • Better stability and good circulation time	• Poor accumulation at tumor site • Non-specific or premature drug release • Slow degradation results in long-term toxicity

Drug-loaded plasmonic nanoshell, DOX-loaded graphene oxide wrapped liposome, DOX@single-wall carbon nanotubes@BSA@AueS-PEGFA, DOX@GNR-mSilica, DOX-graphene oxide, DOX-AuNRs@liposomal nanohybrids	Combined chemo-photothermal therapy	• Easy preparation with high reproducibility • Large loading capacity and good biocompatibility • Good controlled release and thermal conversion efficiency • Significant tumor reduction and easy degradation • Low power NIR light	• Side effects due to chemotherapeutic drugs on healthy tissues/cells • Poor blood circulation • Expensive process and has some long-term side effects

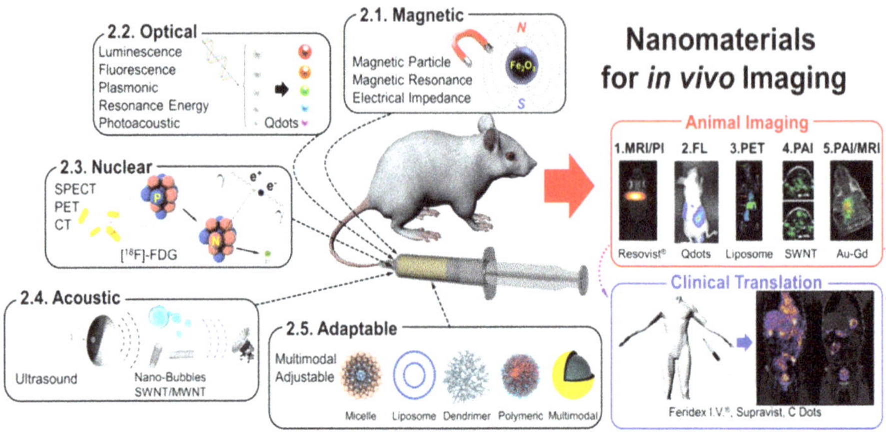

Figure 1.2. The framework of bioimaging with magnetic, optical, nuclear, acoustic, and adaptable nanomaterials. Reprinted with permission from [6], copyright 2017 American Chemical Society.

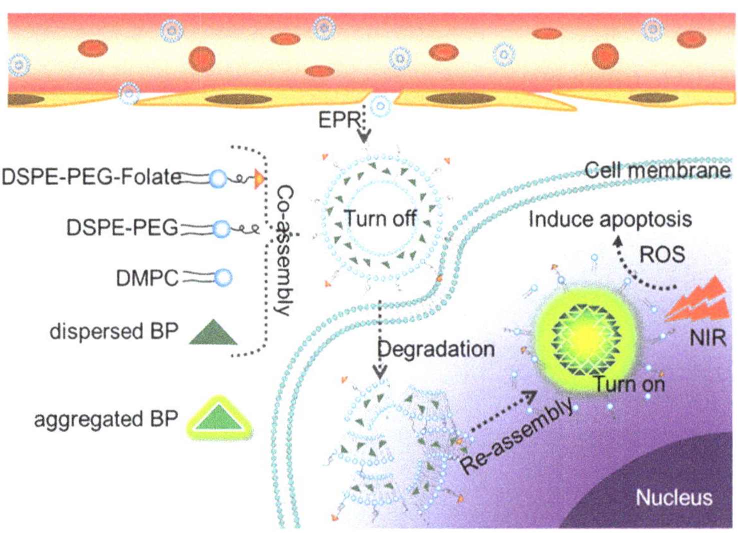

Figure 1.3. Schematic of NIR light-activated PDT agent in *in vivo* tumor model. Reprinted with permission from [27], copyright 2019 American Chemical Society.

reduction (more than 64%) is on NIR light exposure, indicating the site-specific delivery of the produced ROS and their oxidative stress on the tumor microenvironment, shown in figure 1.3. Up until now, individual treatments like phototherapy, chemotherapy, and radiation therapy remain popular treatments for various cancers. They have become promising cancer therapy approaches and are as a popular research topic. However, they have a limitation of being unable to eliminate or reduce the tumor completely at the clinical level. Hence, combining these strategies emerges as an effective way for significant tumor regression [31]. For

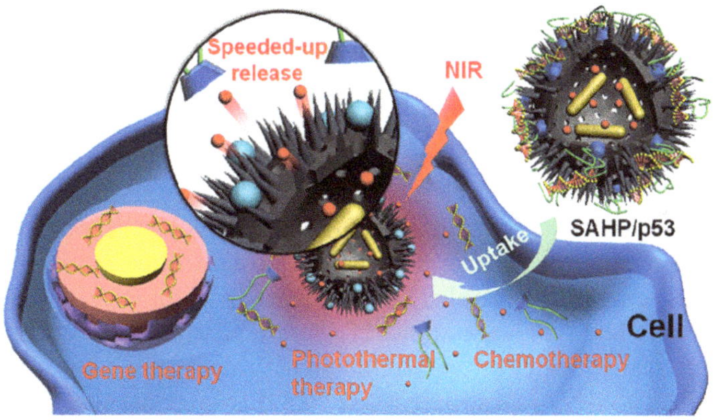

Figure 1.4. Schematic illustration proposed gold nanorods for combination therapies. Reprinted with permission from [32], copyright 2018 American Chemical Society.

example, Chen *et al* successfully designed a novel structure of silica coated gold nanorod loaded with anticancer drug Sorafenib(SF hydrophobic antiangiogenic drug) that has been proposed for synergistic Gene-chemo-photothermal therapy, shown in figure 1.4 [32]. The nanorods exhibit strong absorption upon NIR exposure, enhancing cell death by induced heat. They aslo validated the effective photothermal responses of prepared nanostructures in *in vivo* and *in vitro* studies.

1.5 Nanotheranostics in cancer treatments

1.5.1 Gold nanoparticles

Gold NPs are small colloidal gold particles having size in the range of 1–100 nm. They are extensively used in nanotechnology and biomedical fields because of their lower toxicity and biocompatibility which are necessary attributes for their application in the biomedical field [35]. The most common method for the synthesis of gold NPs was developed by Turkevich *et al* which infers chloroauric reduction by trisodium citrate which also acts as a ligand for the formed gold NPs at 100 °C. Depending upon the sodium citrate initial concentration, the reaction led to the formation of nearly monodisperse NPs which are spherical in shape having size in the range of 15–150 nm [36–38]. Gold NPs multifunctional design produces heat in a localised manner nearby cancer tissues as well as the delivery of various required drugs specifically in a controlled way. There are various advantages of using gold NPs which makes them appropriate for PTT: they can penetrate deeply into the tissues with the help of near infrared laser light, they can be injected into the tumor area locally, therefore, reducing its non-targeted distribution and they can be engineered in such a way to form a complex drug delivery and photothermal agent for cancer therapy [37, 39]. Advancement of nanotechnology in medicinal research bids to targeting the metal NPs specifically towards the tumor cells. When non-ionizing electromagnetic radiation such as laser is applied, excitation and relaxation of electrons lead to the conversion in heat energy in metal NPs [40, 41]. Additionally, according to the surface plasmon resonance frequency of NPs which differs with shape, size and composition of NPs, a laser can be tuned precisely [41, 42]. Gold NPs have some distinctive properties such as scattering and absorption of electromagnetic radiation which makes them valuable for its specific use in photothermal therapy. Cancer cells are killed thermally by heat produced by electromagnetic radiation [38, 43]. Use of photothermal agents can enhance the efficiency of photothermal therapy by enhancing the conversion of light to heat. Gold NPs can also produce heat under radiofrequency irradiation [44]. In a report by Costantini *et al* branched gold NPs (BGNPs) were synthesized and utilized as an efficient tool for PTT for the treatment of colorectal cancer. The NPs were stable at room temperature and showed effectual light-to-heat conversion after getting irradiated with an 808 nm laser. After irradiation by laser branched gold NPs cause necrosis in DLD1 colorectal cancer cells mainly due to the thermal stress instigated on the cells [45]. Park *et al* reported pH-responsive gold NPs which get aggregated at low pH values and gets disassembled at higher pH values or at physiological pH (figure 1.5). The aggregation of gold NPs at acidic pH results in more efficient PTT than at normal physiological pH. By changing the relative quantity of cytochrome c and ssDNA on gold NPs, the pH value of aggregation of particles can be controlled [46]. To improve the pharmacokinetic ability of drugs, reduction of unwanted side effects due to non-specific distribution and to deliver more quantity to the tumor tissues, gold NPs were considered for drug delivery purpose too. Elbialy *et al* reported novel magnetic gold NPs (MGNPs) which can serve various purposes. The

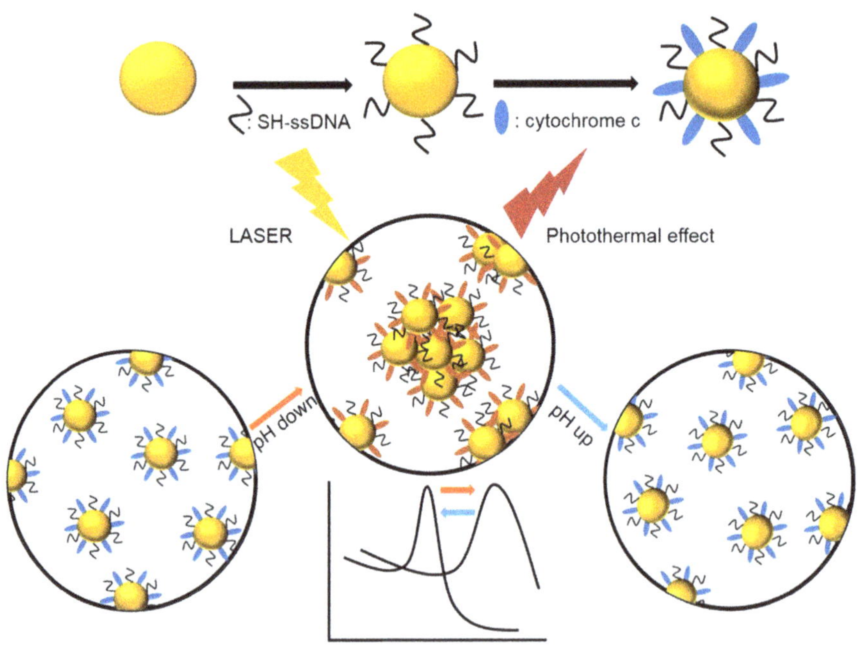

Figure 1.5. Surface modification of gold NPs with cytochrome c and ssDNA (top) and pH effect on CytC/ ssDNA-AuNPs. Reprinted from [46] by permission of Springer Nature.

NPs consist of magnetic core with a plasmonic gold shell. The inner core made up of iron oxide acts as a targeted drug delivery system. The gold shell upon exposure to NIR laser elevates the temperature in proximity of the cancerous tissue. Elevation in temperature also helps in the release of doxorubicin (DOX) drug from the NPs [47].

1.5.2 Magnetic nanoparticles

The application of magnetic NPs in cancer therapeutics relies on some exclusive features. It acts as a nanoscale heat source, it gets manipulated by the magnetic field, and target specific delivery of therapeutics [48]. Upon exposure to the alternating magnetic field (AMF), heat can be generated by frequent Brownian relaxation and Néel relaxation of the magnetic NPs [48, 49]. Therefore, magnetic NPs can be utilized for confined heat generation for cancer therapy through magnetic hyperthermia [48, 50, 51]. Conventionally, magnetic NPs synthesis includes various techniques such as solvothermal, hydrothermal, reverse microemulsion, thermal decomposition, sonochemical or co-precipitation of salts with any biocompatible polymer which act as a capping agent [52, 53]. The functionalization and surface coating of magnetic NPs increases its colloidal stability, facilitates electrostatic or covalent attachment with the drugs, imaging and targeting modalities. They also modify various properties of the magnetic NPs such as toxicity, pharmacokinetics, drug release, cell interactions or adsorption of protein, clearance rate etc [53, 54]. Various parameters such as shape, size, magnetic activity, chemical composition and morphology are significant in defining the biomedical applications of magnetic NPs [55, 56]. The magnetic NPs have to be engineered in such a way to increase their acceptability for a particular target *in vivo* [56, 57]. Dutta *et al* reported malic acid coated Fe_3O_4 magnetic nanocarriers (MMNCs). Malic acid an α-hydroxy acid provide hydrophilicity to the nanocarriers due to the presence of free carboxyl and hydroxyl groups as well as facilitating DOX binding. 79% of DOX got released at pH 6.5 and 22% of DOX got released at pH 7.4 which is physiological pH in an interval of 50 h. At all the concentrations, DOX-loaded MMNCs showed significant cytotoxicity. DOX-loaded MMNCs showed less cytotoxicity in comparison to pure DOX because of constant DOX release. Aqueous suspension of MMNCs at a concentration of 2.5 mg ml^{-1} generates SAR value of 164.2 W g^{-1} at an applied AMF of 336 Oe [58]. In another report, chitosan was utilised to stabilize the magnetic NPs (Fe_3O_4-CHI) synthesized at room temperature by the aqueous hydrolysis method. DOX was used as a model drug and was conjugated to the Fe_3O_4-CHI by glutaraldehyde cross-linker with imine bond which is pH sensitive (figure 1.6). 90% DOX released at pH 4.6 after 8 h. IC_{50} value of DOX-loaded NPs on MCF-7 breast cancer cells is 1.4 μM in comparison to 4.8 μM of free DOX which represents DOX-loaded NPs showing higher cytotoxicity. A similar trend was also observed for SKOV-3 ovarian cancer cell lines [59]. Afzalipour *et al* reported temozolomide (TMZ) loaded folic acid attached magnetic NPs (TMZ/MNPs-FA) for the treatment of C6 glioma in rats in the presence of an alternating field. TMZ/MNPs-FA are thermosensitive and are stable at body temperature (37 °C). Upon exposure to AMF, subsequent heat enhances the release of TMZ by disrupting the

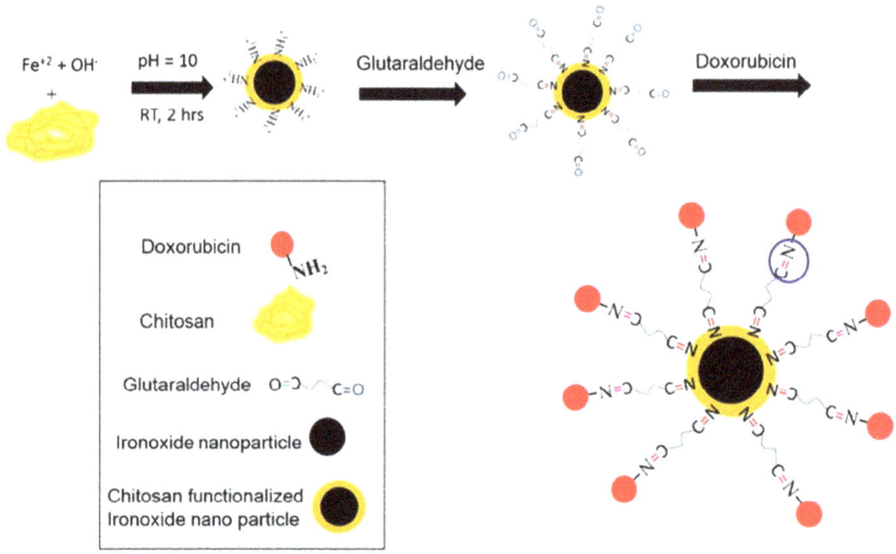

Figure 1.6. Formation and functionalization of Fe_3O_4-DOX NPs. Reprinted from [59], copyright 2017 Elsevier B.V. All rights reserved.

polymer. Drug release decrease as soon as the AMF switches off specifying sustained release. Combinatorial therapy consists of TMZ/MNPs-FA along with hyperthermia showing potent anticancer effect in the glioma treatment [60].

1.5.3 Mesoporous silica nanoparticles

Mesoporous silica NPs are materials that have been explored by various researchers widely; the reason behind this is large pore volume, surface area, even pore size and simple mass production. These characteristics make mesoporous silica NPs a better drug cargo due to high drug loading efficiency and delivery [61–63]. Because of their distinctive mesopores and nanochannels, the particles are able to carry high drug payloads and stimuli responsible drug release thus making mesoporous silica NPs useful for drug and gene delivery [64–66]. Pore size and particle size of mesoporous silica NPs can be adjusted thereby easily conjugating guest moieties with varying sizes into the mesopores [67]. There are plenty of silanol groups present on the surface of mesoporous silica NPs, which are helpful in conjugating with most of the functional groups like targeting ligands, polymers, metals and metal oxides. This type of functionalization endows the NPs with several properties such as specific tumor targeting, drug release etc [67]. To utilize the specific tumor targeting and to enhance drug utilization, a strategy called tumor triggered targeting was presented by Liao *et al* for the fabrication of dual-pH sensitive chitosan/mesoporous silica NPs as a drug delivery system. In this work, mesoporous silica NPs were loaded with DOX and then modified with benzimidazole (Bz) group. Chitosan was attached with β-cyclodextrin (CHI-g-CD) and attached further with benzimidazole (Bz) group by host–guest interaction to act as a gatekeeper. Further, a targeting peptide adamantane-glycine-arginine-glycine-aspartic acid-serine (Ad-GRGDS) was conjugated to β-cyclodextrin with adamantane moiety. Lastly, methoxy-PEG benzaldehyde was attached to chitosan by benzoic imine bond. The aforementioned drug delivery system has the ability for tumor triggered targeting. DOX gets released due to the destruction of host–guest interaction between β-CD and Bz [68]. In a report by porrang *et al* biogenic mesoporous silica NPs were synthesised by sol–gel method from rice and wheat husk. NPs prepared from the rice husk had slit type pores while the NPs prepared from wheat husk have cylindrical type pores. DOX was used as the model drug for anticancerous activity. The NPs showed pH responsive drug release as well as higher toxicity on MFC-7 breast cancer cells [69]. Higher drug loading efficiency is an integral property of mesoporous silica NPs. In this direction, Amin *et al* have reported lipid coated mesoporous silica NPs with higher drug loading which can deliver higher drug payloads towards the tumor site. Porous structure of the NPs plays a major part in higher DOX loading efficiency. The lipid layer acts as a gatekeeper for the drug, increases cellular uptake and helps in sustained drug release [70].

1.5.4 Dendrimers

For targeted cancer therapy, advancement in the area of nanomedicines is one of the most significant applications in the area of nanotechnology. Dendrimer, a synthetic globular macromolecule having size in the range of 1–100 nm has been widely researched as cargo for the delivery of anticancer drugs. Dendrimers can be defined by a tree-like structure having a central core, branches also known as generations with repeating units and various functional groups attached on the periphery [71, 72]. For the applications in drug delivery, dendrimer shows generation dependent drug encapsulation efficiency, cytotoxicity, cell internalization, pharmacokinetics and biodistribution [73]. They have been researched widely as a drug cargo for anticancerous drugs along with their diagnostic applications for cancer therapy. Conjugates of anticancer drugs with dendrimer have represented the capability to intracellularly deliver the drugs, avoid efflux transporter and improve the bioavailability of the loaded drugs [74]. In a report by Karimi and Namazi, triazine dendrimer grafted on the graphene oxide and further grafted graphene oxide was modified with Fe_3O_4@PEG as a DOX delivery system for MCF-7 breast cancer cells. The encapsulation efficiency and drug loading content for the nanocomposites were 92.6% and 9.26%. The nanocomposite shows pH sensitive release as at pH 5, 97.3% drug gets released as compared to 69% at pH 6.8 and 66.1% at pH 7.4. IC50 values of DOX and nanocomposite are 5.6 $\mu g\ ml^{-1}$ and 3 $\mu g\ ml^{-1}$, respectively, in MCF-7 cells [75]. In another report, a generation 3.5 anionic poly (amidoamine) (PAMAM) dendrimer modified with N-acetyl-D-glucosamine loaded with camptothecin was utilized as a drug delivery cargo for the treatment of lung cancer. The dendrimer showed drug encapsulation efficiency of ~66%. A549 human lung adenocarcinoma cells showed overexpression of glucose transporter and the results showed that NAG labeled dendrimer is 5.7 times more cytotoxic towards A549 cells after 72 h in comparison to free camptothecin [76]. In a report, pH sensitive charge conversion micelle was fabricated using poly(lactide) PLA and hyaluronic acid (HA) with a PAMAM 4.5G for docetaxel (DTX) delivery. Poly(lactide) was used to increase the drug loading. In order to improve biocompatibility, hyaluronic acid was used to armor the positive charges. The material shows 92.2% of drug loading efficiency. 93.72% of drug gets released at pH 5.0 in the presence of hyaluronidase (HAse). The micelle shows enhanced cytotoxicity over the free DTX and Taxotere [77].

1.5.5 Polymeric nanoparticles

Polymeric NPs are colloidal particles having size in the range of 1–100 nm and are made up of biodegradable or non-biodegradable polymer derived from synthetic, semisynthetic or natural sources [78, 79]. They can carry DNA, protein or drug for particular targeting towards an organ or cell [79, 80]. Polymeric NPs are getting substantial attention regarding cancer therapy because of their core–shell structure for chemical conjugation or physical encapsulation of drugs into the core [81, 82]. Such nano cargos are intended to be stimuli responsive and are widely used as drug delivery cargos. With enhanced permeability and retention, these delivery systems enhance the accumulation of drugs in tumors, advance the pharmacokinetics, and upsurge drug solubility [15, 82, 83].

In a report, indocyanine green was used as a photothermal agent for improvement in cancer therapy. Using Schiff base reaction, 1-octadecanamine (C18) having an acid labile bond and methoxy-PEG (mPEG) was prepared. As-prepared mPEG-benzoic-imine-C18 (mPEG-b-C18) and tocopheryl polyethylene glycol succinate (TPGS) were inserted on the indocyanine green (ICG) loaded poly(lactic-co-glycolic acid) PLGA cores by hydrophobic anchoring. At pH 7.4, the zeta potential of ICG loaded NPs was lower due to the partial shielding of the negative charges of ICG by mPEG rich surface. As the pH gets reduced from 7.4 to 5.5, the zeta potential of the ICG loaded NPs gets slightly positive, thus mPEG-CHO segments start segregating and releasing ICG [84]. In another report, hybrid NPs were designed in which polylactic-co-glycolic acid (PLGA) core was wrapped with bovine serum albumin (BSA) shell and functionalized with acid triggered rational membrane peptide (ATRAM). ATRAM-BSA-PLGA NPs did not show any cytotoxic effect on MCF-7 cells probably because of the biocompatible nature of PLGA. Exposure of the drug (DOX-triphenyl phosphonium) loaded NPs on various cancer cell lines such as MCF-7, HeLa cells and pancreatic carcinoma MIA PaCa-2 showed significant viability loss at lower pH (6.5) than at higher normal physiological pH (7.4) at higher drug concentrations [85].

1.6 Nanomedicine interaction with tumor environment and its clearance pathways

To determine the exact nanomedicine for treating cancer, understanding of effective penetration and delivery of diagnostic and therapeutic nanomedicines into tumor sites is essential [86]. Research shows that the tumor vasculature and the morphology of blood vessels exhibit extensive permeability of nanomedicines effectively into the tumor environment [59, 87]. The major challenge in cancer theranostics to be considered is the ineffective delivery of nanomedicines to specific sites [88]. The utilization of nanomedicine in cancer theranostics has significant effects on targeting, treatment efficiency, and biodistribution due to its physicochemical properties. The passive targeting of nanomedicine in cancer theranostics through tumor vasculature occuring by the EPR effect is the easiest known pathway for solid tumor targeting [89]. Prasad *et al* show biotin-PEGylated gold NPs biodistribution and accumulation in the tumor environment through the EPR effect [3]. In general, the tumor environment appears to have a more dense extracellular matrix with slow diffusion within the tumor. Moreover, the nanocarriers do not travel in slow diffusion within the tumor through the EPR effect [22]. Due to this, the transportation of nanocarriers into the tumor environment is often regulated by the perivascular regions. In addition, research shows heterogeneous vasculature perfusion in tumors that have several areas with poor vessel perfusion and necrosis. However, the precise mechanism of transportation of nanocarriers into the tumor microenvironment is less explored. So far, clinically reduced size nanocarriers and external stimulus-based approaches have been used to improve diffusion in the tumor site. It has been validated from its treatment outcome that the properly designed nanocarriers have a long circulation time, which helps for their tumor uptake [90]. At the same time, only a few studies showed that the biodistribution, targeting, blood circulation time, and easy clearance of nanocarriers are affected by their physicochemical properties. Recently, studies show that 97% of NPs pass through the gaps between endothelial cells in the blood vessel inside the tumor environment, followed by active uptake process. Pharmacokinetics and clearance pathways of tumor targeting small-molecule or inorganic NPs are schematically shown in figure 1.7 [91]. Pharmacokinetics describes a processes of absorption, distribution, metabolism and excretion of inorganic NPs. The excretion of NPs takes place through the RES and the NPs that escape the RES are rapidly eliminated by kidneys. Also, the NPs that escape RES can passively target the tumor with high efficiency through the EPR effect.

So far, several nanosized systems like metal oxides, gold, silica, liposomes etc have been used successfully as nanotheranostics agents in versatile nanomedicine applications. As a result, they have attracted a major breakthrough in the field of cancer nanomedicine, demonstrating their potential role in preclinical/clinical diagnostic and therapeutic applications. However, for clinical translation, nanomedicine has some major concerns like biological response, circulation time, degradation, and retention [4]. For example, when the nanocarriers show long-term retention after being taken by the reticuloendothelial system this leads to toxicity [92]. Therefore, the Food and Drug Administration (FDA) has guidelines that the theranostic agents must be completely cleared within a reasonable time period after the mode of action. Thus, renal clearance and degradation have become a priority for designing nanomedicine. So far, to understand the degradation of injected nanomedicines, the internal parameters such as pH, glutathione(GSH), H_2O_2 and ROS, and external stimulus like radiofrequency, heat, NIR light, external fields etc have been widely evaluated before their application in *in vivo* studies, as

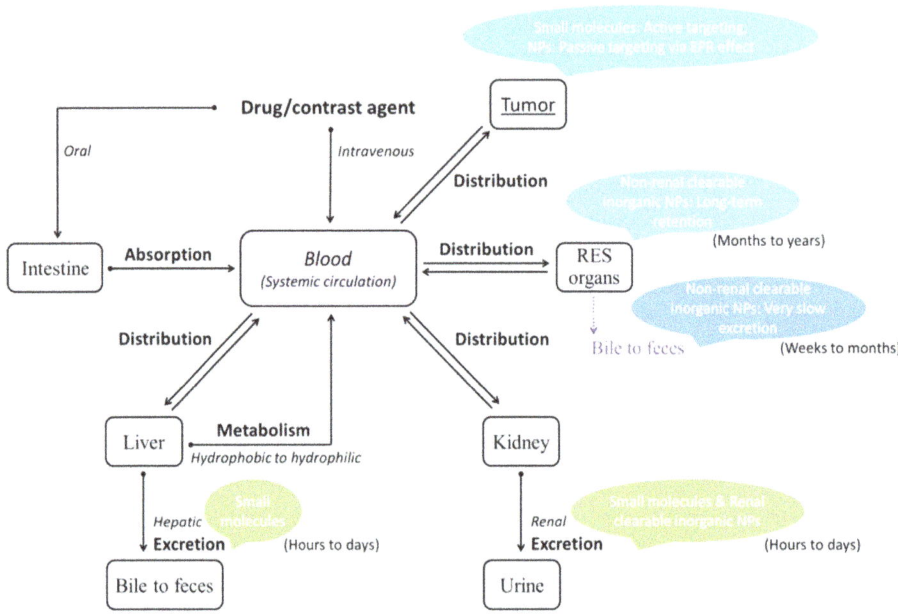

Figure 1.7. Schematic pharmacokinetics includes absorption, distribution, metabolism, and excretion of a nanocarrier. Reproduced with permission from [91], copyright 2015 American Chemical Society.

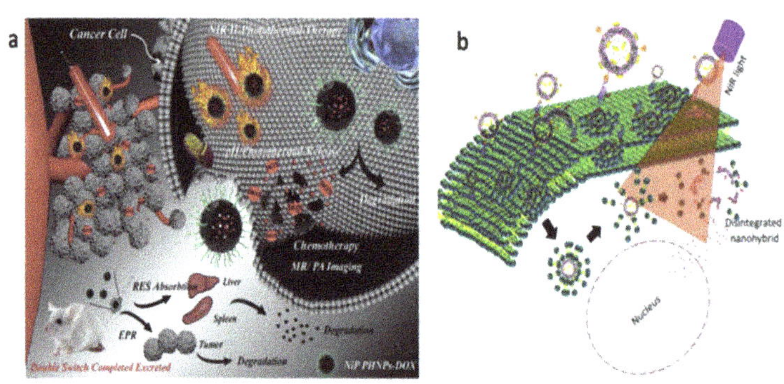

Figure 1.8. Schematic design of degradation/disintegration of inorganic and bioinorganic nanohybrids during therapeutic conditions. (a) Reprinted with permission from [97], copyright 2019 American Chemical Society. (b) Reprinted with permission from [93], copyright 2018 American Chemical Society.

shown in figure 1.8(a). For example, a study by Chauhan and co-workers demonstrates the degradation/disintegration of gold nanorod decorated liposomal nanohybrids during NIR light irradiation for cancer theranostics application, as shown in figure 1.8(b) [93]. They also showed that the disintegrated nanohybrids are easily cleared from the tested animal body after localised treatment, ensuring a high survival rate, which is a major factor of safe nanomedicine. Additionally, studies also showed that ultrasmall particles with a size less than 5 nm could be easily cleared through the renal pathway [94]. Moreover, ultrasmall particles show rapid clearance with a very short circulation time, reducing the efficiency of diagnosis or treatment and demonstrating non-specific biodistribution [95]. In contrast, large-sized particles with a size larger than 25 nm have a longer circulation time with high loading and site-selective targeting property, but they also have high retention time in RES leading to potential toxicity for the biological system [96]. Therefore, degradation of larger particles is a promising approach to develop safe nano-medicines by having sufficient time to perform precise diagnosis and treatment.

1.7 Clinical status of nanomedicines

Nowadays, cancer treatment utilizes a wide range of nanosized materials for localized imaging and targeted therapy, especially for chemotherapy, PTT and PDT. For imaging and treatments, various nanosystems such as gold, PEGylated NPs, silica-based NPs, magneticNPs, ruthenium NPs, liposome-based NPs etc have been developed through to the clinical level due to their selective binding, high biocompatibility, high circulation time, and easy clearance. Some of the clinically studied nanosystems are listed in table 1.3. In addition to the aforementioned particles, biocompatible molecules such as doxorubicin, folic acid, and ICG have also been used at the clinical level. Importantly, for targeted treatment, light-based therapies like photothermal and photodynamic cancer therapy show promising results by using NIR-responsive nanomedicine for targeted triggerable drug delivery

Table 1.3. Nanosystems at clinical studies [3, 4, 105]. Reprinted from [3], copyright 2020 The Authors. Published by Elsevier Ltd.

Nanohybrids	Status of the clinical trial	Type of cancer	Diagnostics and therapeutic modality
Aminosilane-coated SPIO	Phase I	Pancreatic and prostate cancer	Therapy
Carboxydextran-coated SPIO	Approved	Hepatocellular carcinoma	Imaging
CdS/ZnS quantum dots	Phase I started	Breast cancer	Diagnosis and therapy
cRGDY-PEGCy5.5-C dots	Phase II ongoing	Head and neck, and breast cancer	Imaging
DOX@Liposomal	Phase II/III	Breast cancer	Targeted therapy
Hafnium oxide NPs	Phase I and II ongoing	Prostate cancer	Targeted radiotherapy
Liposomal vincristine sulfate	Approved	Leukemia	Targeted therapy
NIR active gold nanoshell	Phase 0	Head and neck cancer	Photothermal therapy
PEGylated gold NPs	Phase I (2012)	Solid tumor	Targeted therapy
Poly-L-glutamic acid (poliglumex) conjugate with paclitaxel	Phase III	Ovarian cancer	Therapy
Ruthenium NPs (NKP-1339)	Phase I (2012)	Solid tumor	Targeted therapy

[98, 99]. One of the most studied nanomedicines in clinical level testing is a gold–silica NP. Recently, Ardeshir and his co-workers developed silica core and gold shell NPes (GSNs or AuroShells) with a size of ~150 nm [100]. GSN particles have gained significant interest in biomedical application due to their maximum absorption of NIR light and conversion of it to significant heat with high tissue transparency. The induced amount of heat was used as highly localized hyperthermia for effective PTT of cancer. These GSNs were employed in the clinical trial to ablate low-grade tumor using multiplex imaging by magnetic resonance (MRI)–ultrasound (US) technique. In this pilot study, 16 patients diagnosed with localized prostate cancer were examined, and the overall outcome of the study was 94% success. Another example, the anticancer drug doxorubicin-loaded nanosystem, has been recognized as the first FDA-approved nanomedicine [101]. Currently, doxorubicin liposomal (Doxil) nanomedicine and other 30 lipid or liposomal based biotherapeutic agents are presently being considered in clinical investigation [102]. These formulations have been tested at the clinical level for different types of cancers like breast, gastric, ovarian etc. In the first clinical trial of Doxil, the particle with 300–500 nm size was injected into 32 liver cancer patients. It is noted that they have slow clearance compared with free doxorubicin. Afterward different doses and various formulations of liposomes have been studied, and it has been noticed that at the dosage level of 60 and 90 mg m^{-2}, hematologic toxicity occurs. In this regard, to reduce the toxicity due to non-specific delivery, the binding of targeting ligand on the drug and nanocarriers has been exploited. These ligands can simply deliver the therapeutic agent precisely into the localized tumor cells, thereby preventing unsolicited damage to the normal tissues/cells. For example, folic acid used as a targeting ligand has been recently examined in clinical trials [103]. It is a vitamin that is widely explored as a targeting ligand for folate receptor overexpressed cancer cells, and it has a significant impact on targeted imaging and therapy. Other NPs such as gold nanorods, gold-liposome NPs and gold nanocages have also been tested at the *in vitro* and *in vivo* level and are expected to be tested soon in clinical trials [104]. Based on the research, gaining confidence and trust in nanomedicine for cancer therapy will require several years of clinical trials.

1.8 Conclusion

Cancer nanomedicine has been discussed in this chapter. Due to time-consuming, expensive, poor imaging resolution, high dose requirement and rapid clearance in the traditional methods need a better replacement for safe and effective cancer imaging and treatment. Therefore, nanomedicine-based multifunctional localized imaging and therapy of cancer have gained much attention in the past few years. The localized therapy with precise and deep imaging and potential treatment reduces the prolonged procedure time and high-dose requirement. Thus, the nanomedicine concept is noticed to be a promising alternative in cancer theranostics for localized therapy. Moreover, the intrinsic property of fabricated nanomedicine shows multifunctionality behavior in terms of multimode imaging and therapy. Hence, the term nanotheranostics emerged, where a single nanoscale entity has the capability for imaging and therapy. However, integrating imaging and targeted therapeutic agents without losing their individual functionality has been a major challenge. Nevertheless, many individual imaging and therapeutic agents have been successfully tested at the preclinical level for cancer treatment. For further translation to clinical studies for better diagnosis and treatment, various nanosystems are currently in the developing phase. To summarize, major concerns in translating nanomedicines into clinical application for cancer theranostics are as follows: (1) nanotechnology-based theranostic materials are still in the early stages of preclinical and clinical development; (2) the interaction between the theranostics agent and tumor environment is still unclear;(3) long-term toxicity and non-specific distribution; (4) localized imaging, clearance and complete elimination of tumor are the critical issues faced by current nanomedicines; (5) safe clearance and biodegradation of nanomedicine. So far, many researchers and research projects on targeted cancer theranostics and cancer nanomedicine provide promising and successful nanostructures. However, their success is determined by the clinical outcomes of cancer patients. Thus the future of diagnostics, combination therapies and localized theranostics depends on the engineering of successful nanomedicine for better healthcare.

References

[1] Lammers T *et al* 2010 Nanotheranostics and image-guided drug delivery: current concepts and future directions *Mol. Pharm.* **7** 1899–912

[2] Silva C O *et al* 2019 Current trends in cancer nanotheranostics: metallic, polymeric, and lipid-based systems *Pharmaceutics* **11** 22

[3] Prasad R *et al* 2020 Localized nanotheranostics: recent developments in cancer nanomedicine *Mater. Today Adv.* **8** 100087

[4] Brigger I, Dubernet C and Couvreur P 2012 Nanoparticles in cancer therapy and diagnosis *Adv. Drug Deliv. Rev.* **64** 24–36

[5] Lee N, Choi S H and Hyeon T 2013 Nano-sized CT contrast agents *Adv. Mater.* **25** 2641–60

[6] Smith B R and Gambhir S S 2017 Nanomaterials for *in vivo* imaging *Chem. Rev.* **117** 901–86

[7] Li H, Li H and Wan A 2020 Luminescent gold nanoclusters for *in vivo* tumor imaging *Analyst* **145** 348–63

[8] Stephen Z R, Kievit F M and Zhang M 2011 Magnetite nanoparticles for medical MR imaging *Mater. Today* **14** 330–8

[9] Ohgushi M, Nagayama K and Wada A 1978 Dextran-magnetite: a new relaxation reagent and its application to T2 measurements in gel systems *J. Magn. Reson.* **29** 599–601

[10] Gazelle G S *et al* 1994 Nanoparticulate computed tomography contrast agents for blood pool and liver-spleen imaging *Acad. Radiol.* **1** 373–6

[11] Michalet X *et al* 2005 Quantum dots for live cells, *in vivo* imaging, and diagnostics *Science* **307** 538–44

[12] Harisinghani M G *et al* 2003 Noninvasive detection of clinically occult lymph-node metastases in prostate cancer *N. Engl. J. Med.* **348** 2491–9

[13] Yan J *et al* 2014 A multi-center study of using carbon nanoparticles to track lymph node metastasis in T1–2 colorectal cancer *Surg. Endosc.* **28** 3315–21

[14] Liu Z, Kiessling F and Gätjens J 2010 Advanced nanomaterials in multimodal imaging: design, functionalization, and biomedical applications *J. Nanomater.* **2010** 894303

[15] Prabhakar U *et al* 2013 Challenges and key considerations of the enhanced permeability and retention effect for nanomedicine drug delivery in oncology *Cancer Res.* **73** 2412–7

[16] Cortie M B and McDonagh A M 2011 Synthesis and optical properties of hybrid and alloy plasmonic nanoparticles *Chem. Rev.* **111** 3713–35

[17] Louie A 2010 Multimodality imaging probes: design and challenges *Chem. Rev.* **110** 3146–95

[18] Perazella M A 2009 Current status of gadolinium toxicity in patients with kidney disease *Clin. J. Am. Soc. Nephrol.* **4** 461–9

[19] Smith B R *et al* 2008 Real-time intravital imaging of RGD-quantum dot binding to luminal endothelium in mouse tumor neovasculature *Nano Lett.* **8** 2599–606

[20] Willets K A, Stranahan S M and Weber M L 2012 Shedding light on surface-enhanced raman scattering hot spots through single-molecule super-resolution imaging *J. Phys. Chem. Lett.* **3** 1286–94

[21] Ferguson R M *et al* 2013 Tailoring the magnetic and pharmacokinetic properties of iron oxide magnetic particle imaging tracers *Biomed Tech (Berl)* **58** 493–507

[22] Thakor A S and Gambhir S S 2013 Nanooncology: the future of cancer diagnosis and therapy *CA: Cancer J. Clin.* **63** 395–418

[23] Lim E-K *et al* 2015 Nanomaterials for theranostics: recent advances and future challenges *Chem. Rev.* **115** 327–94

[24] He W *et al* 2019 Self-assembly of therapeutic peptide into stimuli-responsive clustered nanohybrids for cancer-targeted therapy *Adv. Funct. Mater.* **29** 1807736

[25] Yong Y *et al* 2015 Tungsten sulfide quantum dots as multifunctional nanotheranostics for *in vivo* dual-modal image-guided photothermal/radiotherapy synergistic therapy *ACS Nano* **9** 12451–63

[26] Prasad R *et al* 2018 In vivo examination of folic acid-conjugated gold-silica nanohybrids as contrast agents for localized tumor diagnosis and biodistribution *Bioconjugate Chem.* **29** 4012–9

[27] Yang Y *et al* 2019 Photodynamic therapy with liposomes encapsulating photosensitizers with aggregation-induced emission *Nano Lett.* **19** 1821–6

[28] Chen J *et al* 2019 Nanomaterials as photothermal therapeutic agents *Prog. Mater Sci.* **99** 1–26

[29] Liu S, Pan X and Liu H 2020 Two-dimensional nanomaterials for photothermal therapy *Angew. Chem. Int. Ed.* **59** 5890–900

[30] Pan L, Liu J and Shi J 2017 Nuclear-targeting gold nanorods for extremely low NIR activated photothermal therapy *ACS Appl. Mater. Interfaces* **9** 15952–61

[31] Cao Y *et al* 2017 Efficient cancer regression by a thermosensitive liposome for photoacoustic imaging-guided photothermal/chemo combinatorial therapy *Biomacromolecules* **18** 2306–14

[32] Chen X *et al* 2018 Rattle-structured rough nanocapsules with in-situ-formed gold nanorod cores for complementary gene/chemo/photothermal therapy *ACS Nano* **12** 5646–56

[33] Wang R, Zhao N and Xu F-J 2017 Hollow nanostars with photothermal gold caps and their controlled surface functionalization for complementary therapies *Adv. Funct. Mater.* **27** 1700256

[34] Liu X *et al* 2020 Reduced graphene oxide/mesoporous silica nanocarriers for ph-triggered drug release and photothermal therapy *ACS Appl. Bio Mater.* **3** 2577–87

[35] Gupta N and Malviya R 2021 Understanding and advancement in gold nanoparticle targeted photothermal therapy of cancer *Biochim. Biophys. Acta (BBA)—Rev. Cancer* **1875** 188532

[36] Turkevich J, Stevenson P C and Hillier J 1951 A study of the nucleation and growth processes in the synthesis of colloidal gold *Discuss. Faraday Soc.* **11** 55–75

[37] Vines J B *et al* 2019 Gold nanoparticles for photothermal cancer therapy *Fron. Chem.* **7** 167

[38] Sztandera K, Gorzkiewicz M and Klajnert-Maculewicz B 2019 Gold nanoparticles in cancer treatment *Mol. Pharm.* **16** 1–23

[39] Kennedy L C *et al* 2011 A new era for cancer treatment: gold-nanoparticle-mediated thermal therapies *Small* **7** 169–83

[40] Cherukuri P and Curley S A 2010 Use of nanoparticles for targeted, noninvasive thermal destruction of malignant cells *Methods Mol. Biol.* **624** 359–73

[41] Jain S, Hirst D G and O'Sullivan J M 2012 Gold nanoparticles as novel agents for cancer therapy *Br. J. Radiol.* **85** 101–13

[42] El-Sayed I H, Huang X and El-Sayed M A 2005 Surface plasmon resonance scattering and absorption of anti-EGFR antibody conjugated gold nanoparticles in cancer diagnostics: applications in oral cancer *Nano Lett.* **5** 829–34

[43] Zou L *et al* 2016 Current approaches of photothermal therapy in treating cancer metastasis with nanotherapeutics *Theranostics* **6** 762–72

[44] Collins C B *et al* 2014 Radiofrequency heating pathways for gold nanoparticles *Nanoscale* **6** 8459–72

[45] Costantini P E *et al* 2021 Spiky gold nanoparticles for the photothermal eradication of colon cancer cells **11** 1608

[46] Park S *et al* 2019 Reversibly pH-responsive gold nanoparticles and their applications for photothermal cancer therapy *Sci. Rep.* **9** 20180

[47] Elbialy N S *et al* 2019 Multifunctional magnetic-gold nanoparticles for efficient combined targeted drug delivery and interstitial photothermal therapy *Int. J. Pharm.* **554** 256–63

[48] Zhang H *et al* 2018 Magnetic nanoparticles based cancer therapy: current status and applications *Sci. China Life Sci.* **61** 400–14

[49] Hervault A and Thanh N T 2014 Magnetic nanoparticle-based therapeutic agents for thermo-chemotherapy treatment of cancer *Nanoscale* **6** 11553–73

[50] Liu X L *et al* 2015 Magnetic vortex nanorings: a new class of hyperthermia agent for highly efficient *in vivo* regression of tumors *Adv. Mater.* **27** 1939–44

[51] Khan A *et al* 2019 Magneto-plasmonic stimulated breast cancer nanomedicine *External Field and Radiation Stimulated Breast Cancer Nanotheranostics* ed N D Thorat (Bristol: IOP Publishing)

[52] Ali A *et al* 2016 Synthesis, characterization, applications, and challenges of iron oxide nanoparticles *Nanotechnol. Sci. Appl.* **9** 49–67

[53] Mukherjee S, Liang L and Veiseh O 2020 Recent advancements of magnetic nanomaterials in cancer therapy *Pharmaceutics* **12** 147

[54] Khan A and Sahu N K 2020 Folate encapsulation in PEG-diamine grafted mesoporous Fe_3O_4 nanoparticles for hyperthermia and *in vitro* assessment *IET Nanobiotechnol.* **14** 881–8
[55] Tran N and Webster T J 2010 Magnetic nanoparticles: biomedical applications and challenges *J. Mater. Chem.* **20** 8760–7
[56] Farzin A *et al* 2020 Magnetic nanoparticles in cancer therapy and diagnosis *Adv. Healthcare Mater.* **9** 1901058
[57] Gupta A K and Gupta M 2005 Synthesis and surface engineering of iron oxide nanoparticles for biomedical applications *Biomaterials* **26** 3995–4021
[58] Dutta B *et al* 2021 Malic acid grafted Fe_3O_4 nanoparticles for controlled drug delivery and efficient heating source for hyperthermia therapy *J. Alloys Compd.* **883** 160950
[59] Adimoolam M G *et al* 2018 A simple approach to design chitosan functionalized Fe_3O_4 nanoparticles for pH responsive delivery of doxorubicin for cancer therapy *J. Magn. Magn. Mater.* **448** 199–207
[60] Afzalipour R *et al* 2021 Thermosensitive magnetic nanoparticles exposed to alternating magnetic field and heat-mediated chemotherapy for an effective dual therapy in rat glioma model *Nanomedicine* **31** 102319
[61] Bouchoucha M *et al* 2016 Size-controlled functionalized mesoporous silica nanoparticles for tunable drug release and enhanced anti-tumoral activity *Chem. Mater.* **28** 4243–58
[62] Farjadian F *et al* 2019 Mesoporous silica nanoparticles: synthesis, pharmaceutical applications, biodistribution, and biosafety assessment *Chem. Eng. J.* **359** 684–705
[63] Gao Y *et al* 2020 A review of mesoporous silica nanoparticle delivery systems in chemo-based combination cancer therapies **8** 1086
[64] Gao Y *et al* 2011 Controlled intracellular release of doxorubicin in multidrug-resistant cancer cells by tuning the shell-pore sizes of mesoporous silica nanoparticles *ACS Nano* **5** 9788–98
[65] Singh N *et al* 2011 Bioresponsive mesoporous silica nanoparticles for triggered drug release *J. Am. Chem. Soc.* **133** 19582–5
[66] Wu X, Wu M and Zhao J X 2014 Recent development of silica nanoparticles as delivery vectors for cancer imaging and therapy *Nanomed. Nanotechnol. Biol. Med.* **10** 297–312
[67] Yang Y and Yu C 2016 Advances in silica based nanoparticles for targeted cancer therapy *Nanomedicine* **12** 317–32
[68] Liao T *et al* 2021 A chitosan/mesoporous silica nanoparticle-based anticancer drug delivery system with a 'tumor-triggered targeting' property *Int. J. Biol. Macromol.* **183** 2017–29
[69] Porrang S *et al* 2021 Preparation and in-vitro evaluation of mesoporous biogenic silica nanoparticles obtained from rice and wheat husk as a biocompatible carrier for anti-cancer drug delivery *Eur. J. Pharm. Sci.* **163** 105866
[70] Amin M U *et al* 2021 Enhanced efficacy and drug delivery with lipid coated mesoporous silica nanoparticles in cancer therapy *Eur. J. Pharm. Biopharm.* **165** 31–40
[71] Tripathi P K *et al* 2002 Dendrimer grafts for delivery of 5-fluorouracil *Pharmazie* **57** 261–4
[72] Tripathi P K and Tripathi S 2020 Dendrimers for anticancer drug delivery *Pharmaceutical Applications of Dendrimers* ed A Chauhan and H Kulhari (Amsterdam: Elsevier) ch 6 pp 131–50
[73] Zhu J and Shi X 2013 Dendrimer-based nanodevices for targeted drug delivery applications *J. Mater. Chem.* B **1** 4199–211

[74] Singh J *et al* 2016 Dendrimers in anticancer drug delivery: mechanism of interaction of drug and dendrimers *Artif. Cells Nanomed. Biotechnol.* **44** 1626–34

[75] Karimi S and Namazi H 2021 Fe_3O_4@PEG-coated dendrimer modified graphene oxide nanocomposite as a pH-sensitive drug carrier for targeted delivery of doxorubicin *J. Alloys Compd.* **879** 160426

[76] Pooja D *et al* 2020 N-Acetyl-D-glucosamine-conjugated PAMAM dendrimers as dual receptor-targeting nanocarriers for anticancer drug delivery *Eur. J. Pharm. Biopharm.* **154** 377–86

[77] Du X *et al* 2018 Hyaluronic acid-functionalized half-generation of sectorial dendrimers for anticancer drug delivery and enhanced biocompatibility *Carbohydr. Polym.* **202** 513–22

[78] Pugazhendhi A *et al* 2018 Synthesis and characterization of silver nanoparticles using *Gelidium amansii* and its antimicrobial property against various pathogenic bacteria *Microb. Pathog.* **114** 41–5

[79] Sur S *et al* 2019 Recent developments in functionalized polymer nanoparticles for efficient drug delivery system *Nano-Struct. Nano-Objects* **20** 100397

[80] Conde J *et al* 2014 Gold-nanobeacons for gene therapy: evaluation of genotoxicity, cell toxicity and proteome profiling analysis *Nanotoxicology* **8** 521–32

[81] Oerlemans C *et al* 2010 Polymeric micelles in anticancer therapy: targeting, imaging and triggered release *Pharm. Res.* **27** 2569–89

[82] Alsehli M 2020 Polymeric nanocarriers as stimuli-responsive systems for targeted tumor (cancer) therapy: recent advances in drug delivery *Saudi Pharm. J.* **28** 255–65

[83] Maeda H *et al* 2000 Tumor vascular permeability and the EPR effect in macromolecular therapeutics: a review *J. Control. Release* **65** 271–84

[84] Ting C-W *et al* 2021 Indocyanine green-carrying polymeric nanoparticles with acid-triggered detachable PEG coating and drug release for boosting cancer photothermal therapy *Colloids Surf.*, B **208** 112048

[85] Palanikumar L *et al* 2020 pH-responsive high stability polymeric nanoparticles for targeted delivery of anticancer therapeutics *Commun. Biol.* **3** 95

[86] Sowmya S 2019 Nanohybrid scaffold structures for smart drug delivery applications *Biomimetic Nanoengineered Materials for Advanced Drug Delivery* ed A R Unnithan *et al* (Amsterdam: Elsevier) pp 53–9

[87] Israel L L *et al* 2020 Magnetic iron oxide nanoparticles for imaging, targeting and treatment of primary and metastatic tumors of the brain *J. Control. Release* **320** 45–62

[88] Sindhwani S *et al* 2020 The entry of nanoparticles into solid tumours *Nat. Mater.* **19** 566–75

[89] Ngoune R *et al* 2016 Accumulating nanoparticles by EPR: a route of no return *J. Control. Release* **238** 58–70

[90] Barui A K *et al* 2020 Cancer-targeted nanomedicine: overcoming the barrier of the protein corona . *Adv. Therap.* **3** 1900124

[91] Yu M and Zheng J 2015 Clearance pathways and tumor targeting of imaging nanoparticles *ACS Nano* **9** 6655–74

[92] Liu J *et al* 2016 Rapid degradation and high renal clearance of cu3bis3 nanodots for efficient cancer diagnosis and photothermal therapy *in vivo ACS Nano* **10** 4587–98

[93] Chauhan D S *et al* 2018 Disintegrable NIR light triggered gold nanorods supported liposomal nanohybrids for cancer theranostics *Bioconj. Chem.* **29** 1510–8

[94] Poon W *et al* 2019 Elimination pathways of nanoparticles *ACS Nano* **13** 5785–98

[95] Zhou H *et al* 2020 Biodegradable inorganic nanoparticles for cancer theranostics: insights into the degradation behavior *Bioconj. Chem.* **31** 315–31

[96] Zhao Y, Sultan D and Liu Y 2019 Biodistribution, excretion, and toxicity of nanoparticles *Theranostic Bionanomaterials* ed W Cui and X Zhao (Amsterdam: Elsevier) ch 2 pp 27–53

[97] Liu Y *et al* 2019 Double switch biodegradable porous hollow trinickel monophosphide nanospheres for multimodal imaging guided photothermal therapy *Nano Lett.* **19** 5093–101

[98] Nguyen K and Khachemoune A 2019 An update on topical photodynamic therapy for clinical dermatologists *J. Dermatol. Treat.* **30** 732–44

[99] Zhang P *et al* 2016 Recent progress in light-triggered nanotheranostics for cancer treatment *Theranostics* **6** 948–68

[100] Rastinehad A R *et al* 2019 Gold nanoshell-localized photothermal ablation of prostate tumors in a clinical pilot device study *Proc. of the National Academy of Sciences.* 116 18590–6

[101] Szebeni J, Muggia F and Barenholz Y 2013 Case study: complement activation related hypersensitivity reactions to pegylated liposomal doxorubicin—experimental and clinical evidence, mechanisms and approaches to inhibition *Handbook of Immunological Properties of Engineered Nanomaterials* ed M A Dobrovolskaia (Singapore: World Scientific) pp 331–61

[102] Havel H A 2016 Where are the nanodrugs? an industry perspective on development of drug products containing nanomaterials *AAPS* J **18** 1351–3

[103] Xia W and Low P S 2010 Folate-targeted therapies for cancer *J. Med. Chem.* **53** 6811–24

[104] Peng H *et al* 2020 Controlled phage therapy by photothermal ablation of specific bacterial species using gold nanorods targeted by chimeric phages *Proc. Natl. Acad. Sci.* **117** 1951–61

[105] Wong X Y *et al* 2020 Nanomaterials for nanotheranostics: tuning their properties according to disease needs *ACS Nano* **14** 2585–627

Chapter 2

Introduction to imaging modalities

Sandeep B Somvanshi and Nanasaheb D Thorat

In everyday life, a number of people are undergoing imaging examinations to evaluate the different stages of a medical condition. The appropriate expansion of the potential of imaging modalities yields in the important medical condition of the patient. On the other hand, like all medical processes, most of the imaging analysis is connected with the risk to the patient and cost to the patient and society as well. These shortcomings are particularly noteworthy when the research studies fail to get the important information, such as when unsuitable studies are ordered or when an imaging modality is not designated. Thus, information about the various kinds of imaging techniques and their respective costs and benefits is imperative for the accurate supervision of patients. Moreover, these imaging techniques are helpful for the patient's follow-up with respect to the development of diseases, which are pre-diagnosed or/and are undergoing treatment. The present chapter is focused on a brief introduction to the currently available imaging modalities and their imaging mechanism along with the applications. Also, the imaging modalities for cancer treatment are discussed briefly in this chapter.

2.1 Introduction

The invention of x-ray computed tomography (CT) 40 years ago transformed medical imaging [1]. Computed tomography offered the very first cleared cross-section image of the human body with the considerable contrasts in between the different types of soft tissues. The long-term inheritance of CT is, on the other hand, the impetus it provided to the ensuing introduction of tomography imaging modality in the diagnostics nuclear medicines and the particularly rapid development of magnetic resonance imaging (MRI) over this time frame. Recently, the various imaging modalities such as MRI, positron emission tomography (PET), CT, optical imaging (OI), photo-acoustic imaging (PAI), ultrasound (US) imaging, single-photon emission computed tomography (SPECT) etc were focused in order to diagnose the cancer tumor and monitor the drug released for treatment of the tumor [2–5]. It is noteworthy to determine that the inventions and progression of these

doi:10.1088/978-0-7503-3675-8ch2

© IOP Publishing Ltd 2022

imaging techniques were implied on historical advances within the field of physics, chemistry and not to provide the requisition of the oncology field. The basics of different radio-imaging techniques are explained in figure 2.1 [6].

Cancer incidences and mortalities are rising day by day all over the globe. The global cancer burden was projected to have risen to 18.2 million new incidences and 9.7 million deaths in the year of 2018 [7, 8]. As per the estimated predictions, by 2030, around 30+ million deaths will be caused by cancer every year. To cure cancer in a successful manner, early diagnosis and detection are key factors by which cancer mortalities can be substantially decreased. Although the field of diagnosis radiology is very much advanced, the detection and imaging of cancerous diseases remain compromised. The significant impact of cancer monitoring, its stages and therapy is unlikely to arise until the cancer tumor-to-surroundings ratio progresses by three to four orders of magnitude, i.e. 10^3 to 10^4 fold, which subsequently advances the sensitivity and contrasting ability.

Type and Example Image	Description	Technique (Use of Radiation)	Applications	Cost	Current Use
Computed tomography (CT) 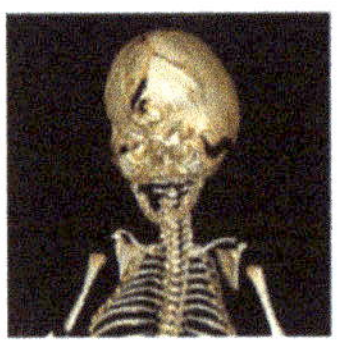	Uses X-rays to generate geometrically accurate 3D information about body structures. 2D cross-sectional (axial) images are first reconstructed using a computer, then reformatted to generate 2D images representing other planes or 3D surfaces or volumes. Also referred to as computed axial tomography (CAT).	Yes (yes)	• Whole body assessment • Trauma (e.g., spinal, thoracoabdominal, head), particularly skeletal trauma • Presence of pathological air or fluid collections • Identification of calcifications, stones • maging foreign objects (e.g., bullet, medical intervention) • Human identification • Skeletal remains, anthropology	$$	Often (less often in the USA)
Magnetic resonance imaging (MRI) 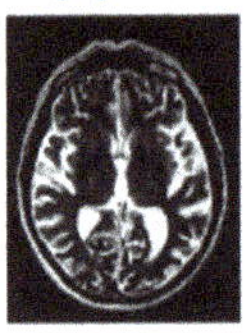	Imaging using a magnetic field, radio waves, and computational methods to produce geometrically accurate, detailed 2D or 3D images of soft tissues such as organs, fat, muscle, connective tissues, and body fluids.	Yes (no)	• Imaging soft tissues/organs in specific body regions • Trauma (e.g., spinal, thoracoabdominal, head), particularly soft tissue trauma • Assessing disease or congenital defects involving complex soft tissue structures (e.g., heart, brain) • Identification of pathological fluid or air collections • Fetal imaging	$$$	Rare
Magnetic resonance spectroscopy (MRS) 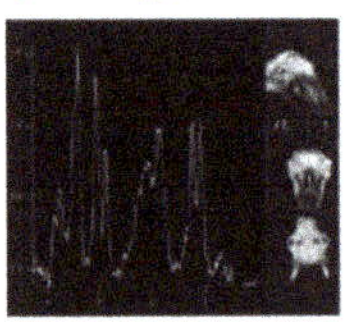	MRS characterizes chemical composition of the tissue.	Yes (no)	• Measuring metabolite levels in normal vs. abnormal tissue (e.g., tumors) • Most frequently applied to the brain • Assessing post-mortem chemical changes	$$$	Very rare
X-ray radiographs 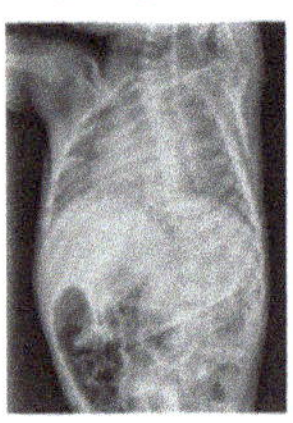	A single image prepared through radiation exposure. Dense objects, such as bone, block the radiation and appear white in an X-ray picture.	No (yes)	• Document fragments, fractures • Human identification	$	Routine, most often

(continued)

Figure 2.1. Basics of different radio-imaging techniques (image reproduced with permission from [6]).

All the individual imaging techniques have their limitations in the case of sensitivity or/and resolutions, which prohibit the capability of the imaging modality to tackle most of the imperative clinical level issues in cancer monitoring, stage determination and therapies. Amongst these imaging modalities, MR, CT and USI can be employed with or without contrasting agent. In the case of contrasting agent employment, pre-scanning is needed to conclude the background levels of MR, CT and USI signals preceding to contrasting agents incorporation. This type of base measurement is required to enumerate the molecular level or functional imaging information. On the other hand, in hot-spot techniques like SPECT, PET or OI, no such type of background signal is detected in the absence of contrasting agent, and thus no pre-scanning is required. However, these hot-spot imaging modalities do not offer any anatomy related information and thus they are required to couple with one of the imaging modalities like MR or CT, which is extremely beneficial for anatomy and morphology related imaging. This gives rise to the hybrid system of imaging in combination as CT–PET, CT–SPECT, MRI–PET etc, in which the anatomy related information acquired through CT or MR imaging is employed for assistance in assigning the molecular level or functional level hot-spot information to the accurate organ or tissues. Most importantly, the above discussed imaging techniques are applicable for different rationales depending upon their specificity, sensitiveness, and abilities. Figure 2.2 [9] shows a schematical representation of the imaging modalities with their benefits and drawbacks. Moreover, the advantages and disadvantages of different imaging techniques employed with targeted or/and non-targeted imaging agents are tabulated in table 2.1 [10].

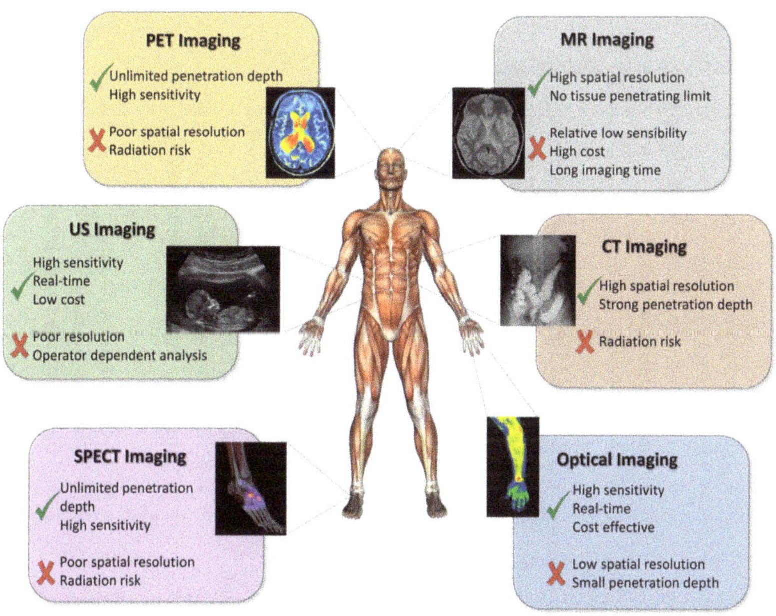

Figure 2.2. Schematical representation of the imaging modalities with their benefits and drawbacks. All the images reproduced with permission from [9], copyright 2021 Elsevier Ltd. All rights reserved.

Table 2.1. Advantages and disadvantages of different imaging techniques employed with targeted or/and non-targeted imaging agents (reproduced with permission from [10], copyright 2014 Sivasubramanian, Hsia and Lo).

Modality	Advantages	Disadvantages	Contrast agents	Radiation
CT	• Unlimited tissue depth penetration • High spatial resolution • Can be used for whole body imaging • Low acquisition time • Anatomical imaging	• Radiation exposure • Poor soft tissue contrast	• Krypton • Xenon • Iodine • Barium	X-rays
Positron emission tomography (PET)	• Unlimited tissue depth penetration • Can be used for whole body imaging • Detailed anatomical information can be obtained when combined with CT or MRI	• Radiation exposure • Low spatial resolution and long acquisition time • Expensive	• ^{11}C • ^{18}F • ^{64}Cu	High energy γ-rays
MRI	• Unlimited tissue depth penetration • Non-ionizing radiation High spatial resolution and excellent soft tissue contrast • Whole body imaging possible	• Expensive • Long acquisition time and limited sensitivity	• Gd^{3+} • SPIO, • USPIO	Radio waves
Ultrasound	• High spatial resolution • Real-time imaging with low acquisition time • Highly sensitive and inexpensive	• Cannot be used for whole body imaging	• Microbubbles	High frequency sound
OI	• High spatial resolution • Real-time imaging with low acquisition time • Highly sensitive and inexpensive	• Cannot be used for whole body imaging limited tissue depth penetration	• Fluorescent dyes and molecules • Light sensitive NPs	Visible or near infrared light

In view of the fact that all these imaging techniques express different types of anatomy, molecular or functional level imaging information and they have some benefits as well as limitations, thus it is essential to have an appropriate understanding of the properties, specificity, and translational ability of each imaging modality, in order to appropriately examine the appropriateness for diagnosis of cancer tumor and for monitoring the therapy. This chapter is intended to give introductory information about the medical imaging techniques. It covers the introductory principle of the currently available imaging modalities, taking cancer related imaging as its main theme. The first section of the chapter covers a brief introduction to the general imaging modalities along with their fundamental information. The subsequent sections of the chapter are focused on cancer related imaging modalities and their role in cancer management.

2.2 Different types of imaging modalities

In the ideal world, health systems need to be capable to diagnose and treat cancer-like diseases without any damaging side effects. To attain this, medical imaging is one of the finest ways which can allow doctors to visualize the ongoing activities in the body without any need for surgery or other invasive protocols. Different imaging modalities can be employed for diagnostic as well as therapy purposes, which makes them potential candidates accessible for the effectual and intensive care of the patient. The different types of medical imaging techniques available today are presented in figure 2.3 [11].

Common imaging types include:

- Computer tomography imaging (CT);
- Magnetic Resonance Imaging (MRI);
- Ultrasound imaging (US);
- X-ray imaging;
- Nuclear medicine imaging (including positron emission tomography (PET)).

All these imaging modalities are somewhat different from each other as they generate images of the inside of the body by different principles, as discussed below.

Computed tomography

CT, also called computed axial tomography (CAT) employs x-rays to generate the cross-sectional image of the inside body [12]. CT scanners have large circular shaped structures (figure 2.4) which make the patient able lie on a computer operated table. The source of x-rays and detectors rotate around the patient which produces a narrower beam of x-ray. These generated x-rays pass through the particular regions of the body which further creates the snapshot of the particular organ. Further, these snapshots can be assembled into single or multiple images of the organ or tissues. CT images provide superior clarity over conventional x-ray images by generating images with more details of the internal organ, bone, soft tissues and blood vessels. The advantages of employing CT imaging go beyond the risks, including increased chances of cancer, harm to the unborn child or a side reaction of the contrasting

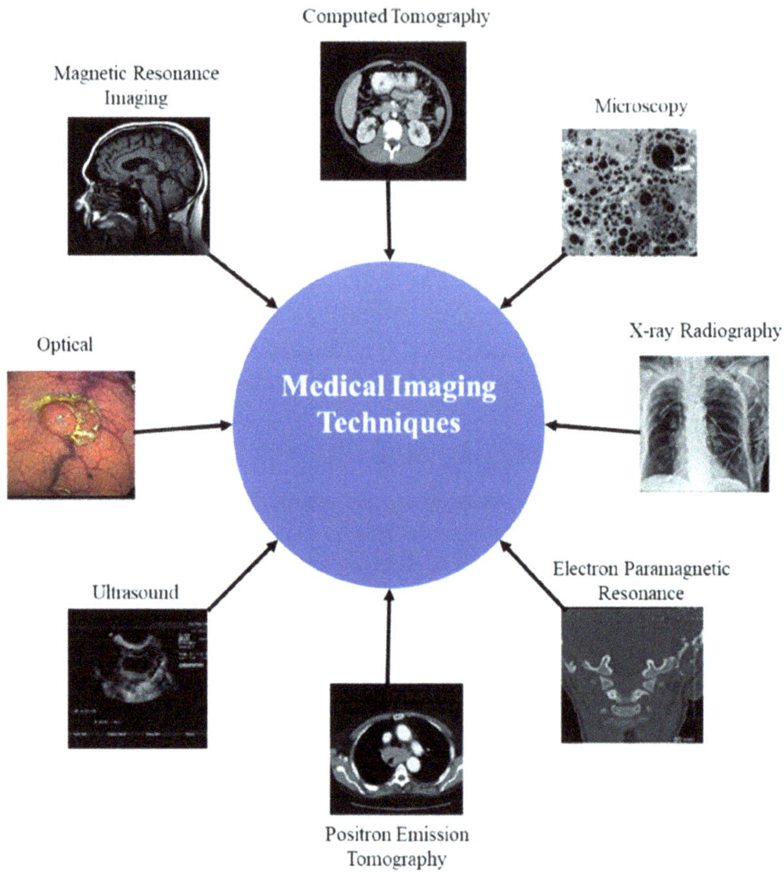

Figure 2.3. Different types of medical imaging techniques available in the present world (image reproduced from [11], copyright 2021 with permission of Springer).

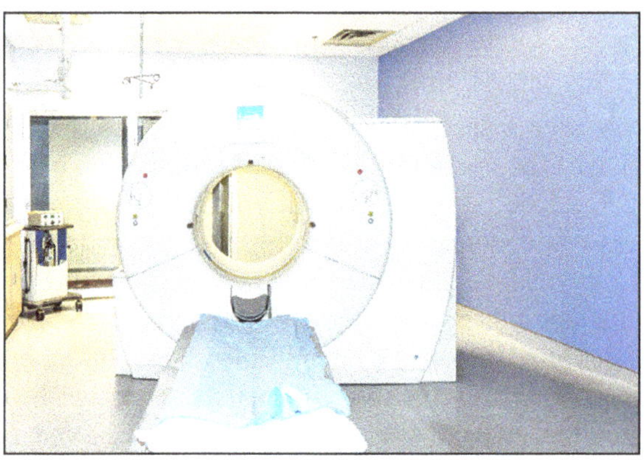

Figure 2.4. Computed tomography (CT) imaging setup.

agents or dyes used for imaging. In a number of cases, the employment of CT imaging prevents the requirement for examining surgeries.

Magnetic resonance imaging (MRI)

Magnetic resonance imaging (MRI) generates the diagnosis images without employing any harmful radiation [13]. It employs a stronger magnetic field and radio signals to produce a detailed image of the organ, soft tissue, bone, ligaments or cartilage. It is most frequently employed to inspect the internal body structure in order to evaluate:

- Abnormal conditions in brain and spinal cord;
- Other abnormalities related to breast, prostate, liver;
- Abnormal conditions in joints or injury;
- Injuries related to the spinal cord;
- Structure and functioning of the heart;
- Activated areas in the brain;
- Flowing of blood through the vessels and arteries;
- Chemical compositions of tissue;
- Internal organs like liver, kidneys, heart, spleen etc.

It is well known that most of the human body contains water, and water molecules contain a hydrogen nucleus (proton). In an MRI scanner, these protons forcefully get aligned after introduction of the stronger magnetic field. Then radio waves are applied to stimulate the protons and spin them out of equilibrium. After tuning of the radio frequency, protons get back to their initial alignments, which results in release of energy which is detected by the MRI scanner. Protons in the various human body parts or tissue return to their initial alignment at different rates, which allows MRI to differentiate between the various kinds of tissues and recognize any kind of abnormality in organs. The way in which the molecules get flipped and returned to the initial spin alignments is recorded and converted into images. The setup of an MRI scanner is shown in figure 2.5. Although, MRI scanners do not

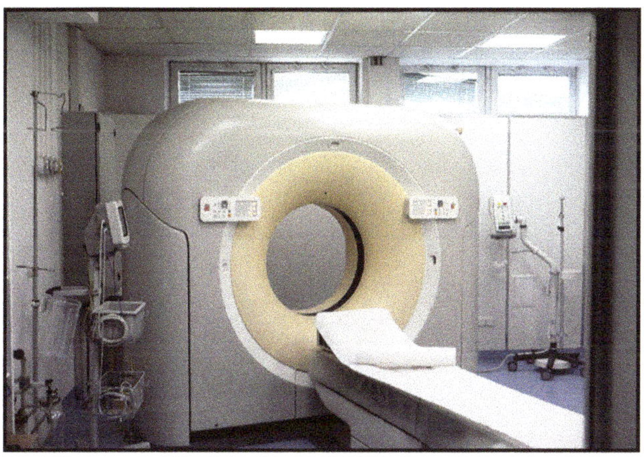

Figure 2.5. Magnetic resonance imaging (MRI) setup.

employ ionizing radiation, there are still some disadvantages with their use in medical imaging. As it contains a stronger magnetic field, a metallic implant such as a pacemaker or implanted metallic organs in the patient's body can create a hazard as the implanted metal can be heated up under the stronger magnetic field. There are several reported cases of patients with pacemakers dying through MRI scanning.

Other drawbacks of MRI imaging include:

- A loud noise generated from the MRI scanner requires appropriate protections for ears;
- Long operating procedures;
- Metallic objects (sensitive to strong magnetic field) can get converted into harmful projectiles and thus, objects entering an MRI scanner need to be screened with intense care;
- Heat generation in the body;
- Adverse reactions to the contrasting agents;
- Patients may feel claustrophia;
- The patient needs to be still for the whole time of the procedure.

Ultrasound imaging (US)

US is a non-invasive and safer imaging modality which possess a wide range of applications [14, 15]. US employs sound waves instead of ionizing radiation. The typical setup of US is shown in figure 2.6. High frequency sound waves get transmitted from an ultrasonic probe to the patient's body by the conduction of gel. These sound waves get bounced back when they interact with different body-structures to create real-time images. The other type of US is Doppler imaging that allows visualization of the blood circulation through the veins and arteries. As it possesses minimal risk of hazard, US is the frequently used technique to visualize the fetus during pregnancy. On the other hand, as it can be applied for a wide range of applications, it tends to be the first choice for many patients.

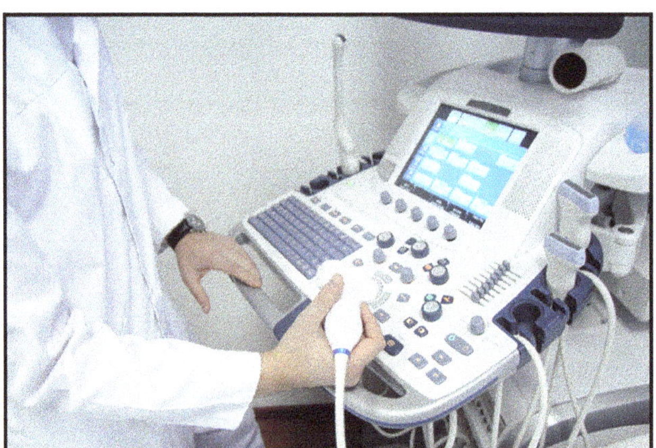

Figure 2.6. US imaging setup.

US is useful in diagnosing different conditions inside the body, which include:

- Joints;
- Kidneys;
- Blood vessels;
- Breast;
- Muscles;
- Pelvis;
- Abdomen;
- Bones.

X-ray imaging

X-ray imaging is the conventional but most used imaging modality in the medical field. X-rays are nothing more than one of the forms of electromagnetic radiation, which were discovered back in 1895 [16, 17]. The typical setup of x-ray imaging is shown in figure 2.7. It works only in the wavelength and frequency range that are non-visible to the naked eye. On the other hand, they can easily penetrate through the skin to generate an image of what is below. Beyond the fact that x-rays are typically used for diagnosing issues affecting the skeleton, they may also be employed to identify other issues like breast cancer (via mammographic images) and investigate related issues. X-ray imaging is broadly employed in medical imaging as it is rapid and comparatively easy for the patient to tolerate. On the other hand, there are some risk factors related to the use of x-ray radiation.

Whenever a patient undergoes x-ray imaging they receive a particular dose of ionizing radiation which can cause issues like:

- Slight chance of getting cancer in later life;
- Cataracts;
- Skin reddening;
- Hair loss;

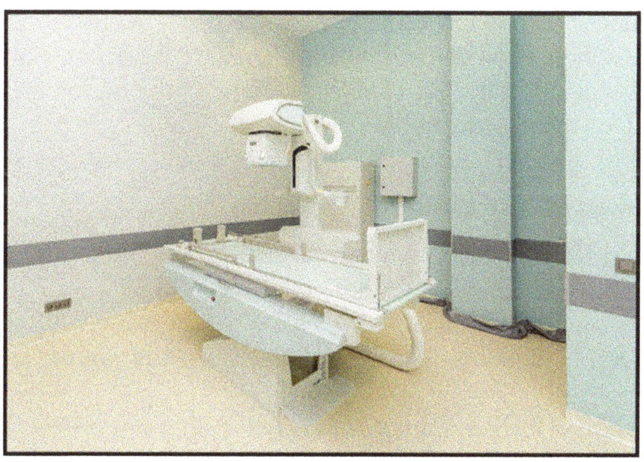

Figure 2.7. X-ray imaging setup.

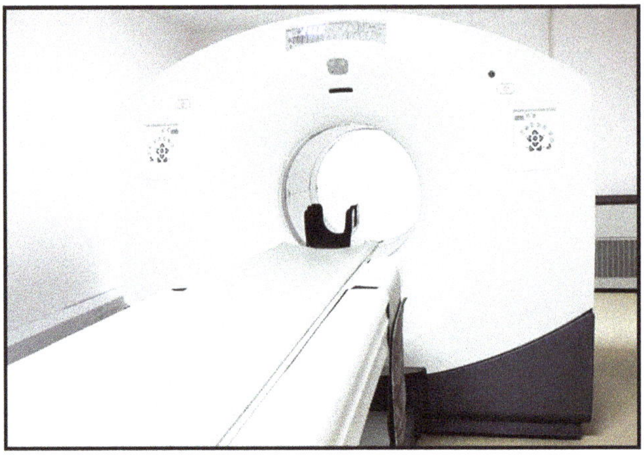

Figure 2.8. Positron emission tomography (PET) setup.

- Growth of fetus or embryo can be disturbed in a pregnant patient;
- Side effects related to the contrasting agent or dye used for better visualization.

Many of these risks can be tackled by employing x-ray imaging with strict and correct shielding of the patient's body.

Positron emission tomography (PET)

PET mainly involves injection and inhalation of radiological agents known as tracers [18]. The patient then lies in a PET scanning machine (figure 2.8), a larger doughnut-like setup that detects gamma rays received from the tracer and converts it into an image. A brighter spot on the image indicates high chemical activities caused by a disease in a potential way. PET scanners are mostly employed for diagnostics of conditions like tumor, heart disease and brain disorder. They can be employed to evaluate the whole body or a specific part of the body. Although PET scanning is normally painless, it does involve exposure to ionizing radiation. Another drawback of PET scanning includes the risk of side reactions to the radiological material and potential feeling of the claustrophobia.

Differences between PET, CT and MRI scanning

- A CT or MRI scan can evaluate the size and shape of body organs and tissues, but it cannot evaluate how they are working.
- A PET scan can visualize how organs are working, but without a CT or MRI image it can be tricky to identify the precise position of movement inside the body.
- Combination of PET scanning with CT scanning can provide a clearer image of the patient's condition.

More comparative details of PET, CT and MRI scanning are provided in figure 2.9 [19].

Parameter	CT	MR imaging	PET
Imaging basis	Ionizing x-radiation	Non-ionizing radiofrequency radiation	Ionizing radiation (positron emitting radiotracer ± x-radiation for concurrent low dose CT scan
Preparation	None needed	None needed	Fasting × 6 h (diabetic patients require close glucose monitoring); no strenuous activity before study to avoid muscular deposition of radiotracer;
Contraindications	Avoid in pregnant women and pursue with caution in women of childbearing age	Avoid in patients with metallic implants (e.g., pacemakers, aneurysm clips)	If concurrent low dose CT scan obtained, avoid in pregnant women and pursue with caution in women of childbearing age
Acquisition time	Short (5 min)	Long (30–90 min)	Long (60 min for radiotracer to reach target tissue + 30 minutes for imaging)
Contrast material	Iodinated contrast material; may cause contrast-induced nephropathy	Gadolinium contrast material; may cause nephrogenic systemic fibrosis	None

CT, computed tomography; MR, magnetic resonance; PET, positron emission tomography.

Figure 2.9. Comparison between CT, MRI and PET (figure reproduced with permission from [19], copyright 2019 Faraji and Gaba).

2.2.1 Basics and fundamentals of imaging techniques

Various non-invasive techniques of medical imaging exist viz. MRI, US, PET, CT, SPECT and OI. Each of them have their individual benefits and drawbacks related to the differentiation in terms of the image resolutions, sensitiveness, and depth of signaling penetration, and preference for the suitable imaging modality relies upon the type of requisite information. OI is most often useful for *in vivo* imaging of the small animal as this imaging is safe, timely and economical. On the other hand, imaging of deep tissue or big animals is not practically convenient by OI. To tackle this issue, radionuclide based imaging modalities like PET or SPECT have emerged offering deeper tissue imaging with higher sensitiveness. However, PET or SPECT provide comparatively low resolution and lack anatomy information. To gain anatomical detail, PET or SPECT are thus frequently coupled with CT and MRI, which facilitate selectivity and tissue visualization with higher resolution.

Current advancements in molecular level imaging have modified the approach we utilize for diagnosis and monitoring of the different diseases such as cancer. Molecular level imaging modalities need specific instruments for the diagnostic and therapy monitoring of diseases comprising PET, MRI, SPECT, PAI and OI, as shown in figure 2.10 [20].

Currently, clinically used imaging techniques can be classified in two groups, i.e. primary anatomical imaging modalities and higher spatial resolutions imaging modalities such as CT, MRI and US, and the others are primary molecular level imaging modalities such as OI, PET or SPECT. For possible clinical diagnosis and therapy, all these techniques are inimitable for doctors as they all have different kinds of features and applicability for different tissue in view of the different properties such as sensitivity and in-depth or spatial resolutions.

Magnetic resonance imaging (MRI)

Although MRI, a non-destructive imaging modality, is time consuming and costly, it offers higher resolution bio-images and penetrates deeply into tissues to visualize

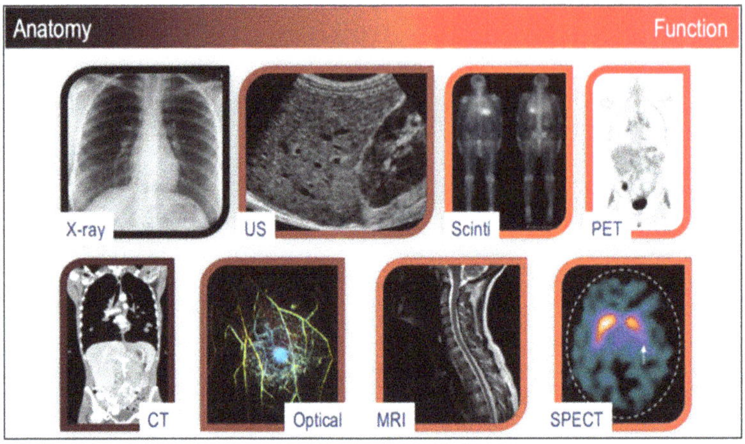

Figure 2.10. Different molecular level imaging techniques utilized for cancer imaging and therapy monitoring (all the images are reproduced with permission from [20], copyright 2020 The Authors).

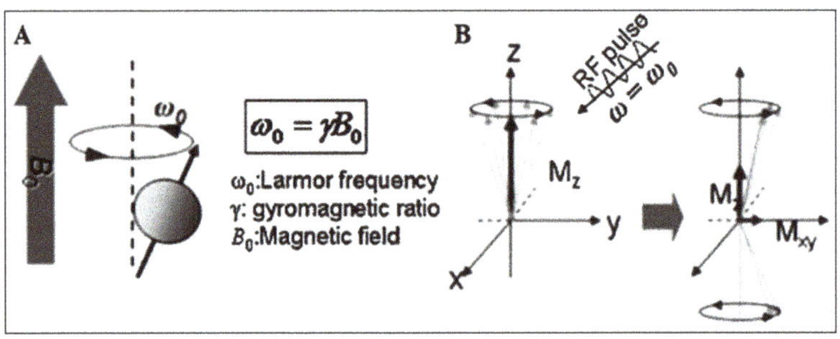

Figure 2.11. Principle of MRI. (a) Spins align parallel or anti-parallel to the field and process under Larmor frequency. (b) After induction of radio frequency (RF) pulse, magnetization of spins changes. Reproduced with permission from [21], copyright 2009 John Wiley & Sons.

the anatomy of soft tissues. The fundamental basis of MRI is primarily on the nuclear magnetic resonance (NMR) technique and relaxations of the nuclei of the protons spin in the presence of stronger magnetic field. After exposure to the stronger magnetic field, the nuclei of protons are spin aligned parallel or anti-parallel towards the applied fields and precess under the Larmor frequencies, as shown in figure 2.11(a) [21]. The proton absorbs energies and excites to a higher energy state after applying radio frequency (RF) to the systems. With removal of RF field, the activated nuclei relax instantaneously to their initial energy state. The relaxation process can be of two types and both can be employed for recording an MR image to differentiate the two different types of tissues. One of them is the T_1 relaxations involving decreasing net magnetizations recuperating towards the initial energy states and offers a bright image. On the other hand, the transverse or T_2 relaxations refer to the induced magnetizations onto the horizontal planes vanishing and offer a dark image (figure 2.11(b)).

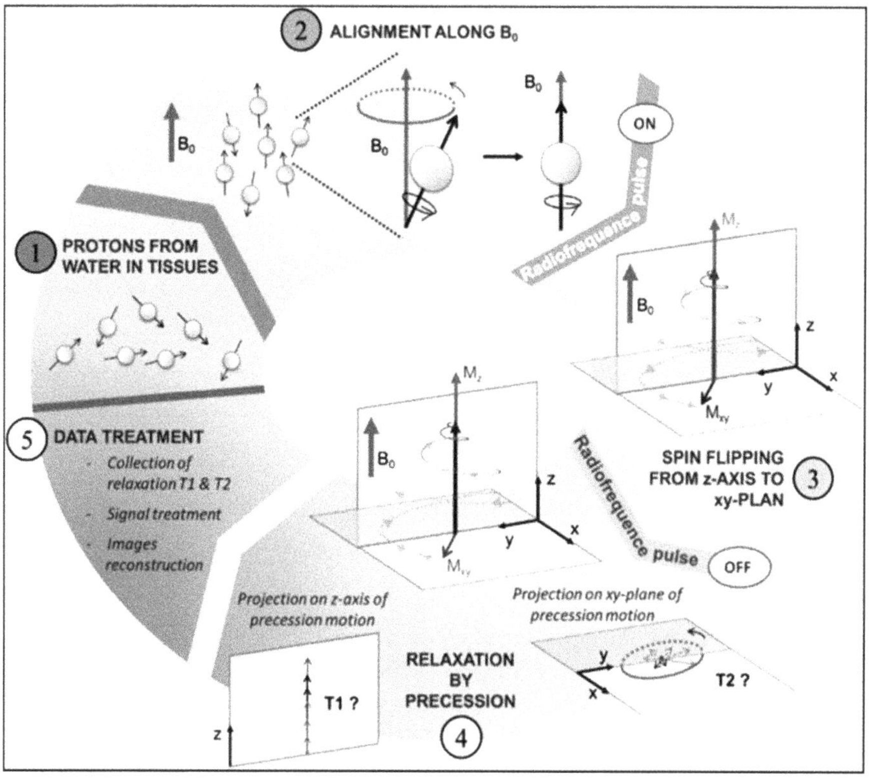

Figure 2.12. Schematic representation of the MRI effect on the magnetic moment of hydrogen nuclei from water molecules contained in tissues to yield reconstructed images (images reproduced with permission from [22], copyright 2019, Springer Science Business Media, LLC, part of Springer Nature).

Depending on these two relaxation processes, the contrast enhancing agent can also be grouped into T_1 and T_2 contrasting agents to distinguish the signals and parameters in MR images of diverse tissue. The previously used transition metal ions and rare earth metals with unpaired electron are Fe^{3+}, Cu^{2+}, Mn^{2+} and Gd^{3+}. Thus, nanoparticles with the combination of transition or rare earth metallic ions such as MnO, Gd_2O_3, $GdPO_4$ and GdF_3 can be of great interest for T_1 MRI contrasting agents as they have higher magnetic moment. Another type of contrast materials are magnetic NPs based on iron oxide which possess stronger magnetic moment when exposed to exterior magnetic fields. Fascinatingly, iron oxide nanoparticles offer both the T_1 and T_2 contrasting ability in MRI by tuning the NPs size. Ultra-small nanoparticles of iron oxide with size less than 6 nm show great ability for T_1 weighted MR imaging. There are several commercially available MR imaging agents related to iron oxide, viz. Combidex, Feridex, Resovist etc. In addition to this, the spinel type ferrite materials such as $NiFe_2O_4$, $CoFe_2O_4$ and $MnFe_2O_4$ were found to be good candidates for T_2 contrasting agents. The schematical representation of the MRI effect on the magnetic moment of hydrogen nuclei from water molecules contained in tissues to yield reconstructed images is shown in figure 2.12 [22].

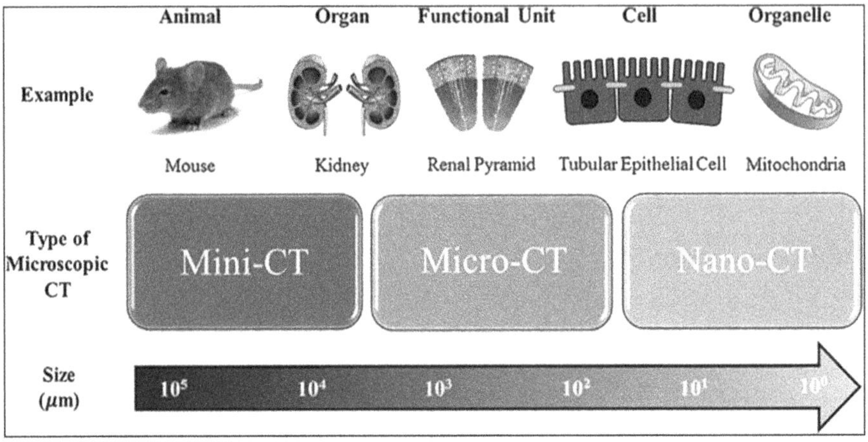

Figure 2.13. Types of CT with their representative *in vivo* scale at which investigations can be carried out (image is reproduced with permission from [23], copyright 2014 John Wiley & Sons).

Computed tomography (CT)

CT, being one of the important radiological modalities, is the most convenient imaging technique in current clinical practice as it is very cost-friendly, easily available, and efficient. CT is able to visualize bone structure in a clear manner due to automatic contrasting among the soft tissue and electronically denser bone. On the other hand, CT is constrained in differentiating soft tissue with the same density, as the mechanism of CT differentiates tissue depending on the dissimilar degree of x-rays attenuation of different tissue. For improved contrast in the CT image and advanced illustration of the soft tissues with the same contrast, promising contrasting enhancer agents are required in CT modality. The chief component in choosing the CT contrasting agent is material with higher atomic number. The original and presently used clinical CT contrasting agents are primarily dependent on iodine (I) based material with higher atomic number, which are effectual in x-ray absorption but are rapidly excreted out of the body by the kidneys. Iodine based materials with larger size may tackle this problem. In addition to this, the metallic nanoparticles such as gold (Au), tantalum (Ta) and bismuth (Bi) are found to be promising for the production of high contrasting images as compared to the iodine based materials. Figure 2.13 [23] shows the types of CT with their representative *in vivo* scale at which investigations can be carried out.

Optical imaging (OI)

OI is mainly based on the behavioral properties of UV–vis and infrared rays. OI is one of the non-invasive and cost effective imaging methods which offers moderate imaging as compared to the other imaging modalities. It includes bio-luminescent, chemiluminescent, fluorescent, optical coherence tomography, after glow imaging and Raman scattering imaging techniques. Among them, fluorescent imaging is the one most extensively employed in clinical practice and it is based on the absorptions and emissions of energies gained from exterior light via fluorophores. As compared to visible light, near infrared light with wavelength in the range of 700–1100 nm gets absorbed minimally and deeply penetrates inside biological tissue. To tackle the photonic attenuation and lower penetrating power occurring due to visible light, fluorescence materials with longer emission at near infrared are being hastily developed. The quantity of near infrared probes is increasing day by day due to advancement in nanomaterials like quantum dots comprising semiconducting nanoparticles possessing optical properties, different rare earth ions driven by photonics, carbon nanotubes with NIR emission tuning and Au based nanoscale materials with plasmonic resonances. Significantly, fluorescent imaging modality in the NIR-II region having wavelength range 900–1400 nm is more advantageous than that of the NIR-I region having wavelength range 700–900 nm due to the deep tissue penetration, reduction in photonic scattering, and auto-fluorescence. The promising NIR-II region fluorescent imaging agent comprises carbon nanotubes, quantum dots, and different small molecular dyes.

Positron emission tomography (PET) and single-photon emission computed tomography (SPECT)

PET and SPECT are the imaging modalities primarily dependent on the phenomenon of NMR. Although, both PET and SPECT are capable of imaging the *in vivo* bio-distribution of positrons emitting radionuclides inside the body, both still have some dissimilarities. First of all, PET has higher resolution and higher precision in imaging than SPECT and is currently broadly applied in clinical practice of the evaluation of tumors. PET scan images provide resolution of the order of 5–7 mm in cardio tissue, whereas SPECT scan images provide resolution of the order of 12–15 mm. Thus, the PET modality can easily recognize anatomical as well as biological structures which may be not possible with the SPECT modality. Moreover, the SPECT modality needs a compound with two or more radionuclides for labeling of the biological structures. On the other hand, as per the clinical application concern, SPECT is inexpensive as compared to the PET modality. Commonly used PET radioisotopes include carbon (^{11}C), copper (^{64}Cu), yttrium (^{86}Y), fluorine (^{18}F), gallium (^{68}Ga) and zirconium (^{89}Zr), and commonly used radioisotopes in SPECT include indium (^{111}In), iodine (^{123}I), technetium (^{99m}Tc), iodine (^{125}I), iodine (^{131}I) and gallium (^{67}Ga). The half-life of the radionuclide is the main distinction for radioisotopes used in PET and SPECT. The PET radionuclides have comparatively shorter half-life than those used in SPECT. In recent reports, researchers used nanoscale materials for the handling of nuclear radionuclides in the biological atmosphere. A schematic of the principle behind PET and SPECT along with their comparison is shown in figure 2.14 [24].

Photo-acoustic imaging (PAI)

PAI is nothing but a hybrid imaging technique, which comprises the higher contrasts of OI and the higher spatial resolutions of US together. PAI primarily depends on the phenomenon of photo-acoustical effect, in which biological tissues can be

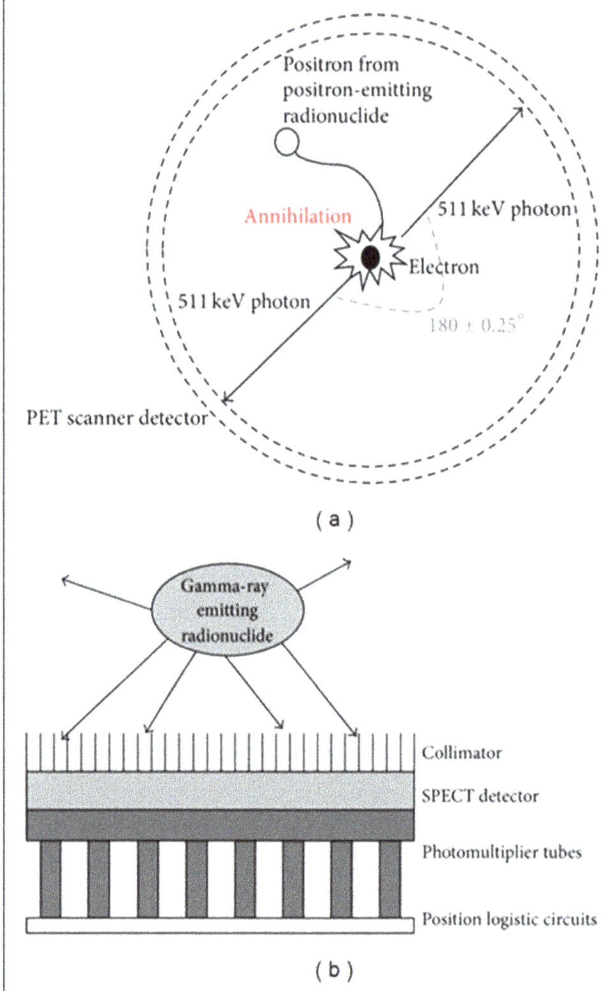

PET	SPECT
Detect positron-emitting radionuclides	Detect gamma ray-emitting radionuclides
Higher resolution	Lower resolution
Costly	Relatively inexpensive

(c)

Figure 2.14. Comparison of PET and SPECT. Schematics of the principle behind PET (a) and SPECT (b) along with its comparison (c) (all the images reproduced with permission from [24], copyright 2013 Fan-Lin Kong *et al*).

inductively heated by the absorptions of non-ionizing laser pulse or absorption by contrasting agent and following this process it generates a wider acoustical wave of the order of MHz frequency due to the momentary thermo-elastic expansions. These photo-acoustical waves can be sensed and perceived by the US transducer at the

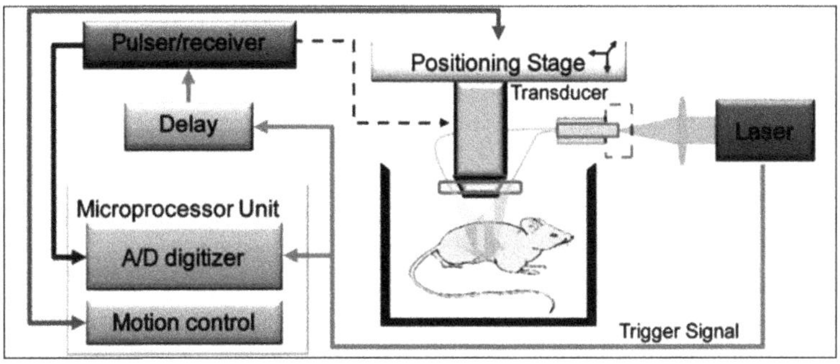

Figure 2.15. Block diagram of a typical PAI system. Reproduced with permission from [25], copyright (2009) American Chemical Society.

tissues surfaces and can be reconstructed to generate the US image (figure 2.15) [25]. PAI modality is being demonstrated as an excellent platform for the visualization of the biological structure with contrast, penetrating depths and spatial resolutions which overcomes the boundaries of OI or US. To improve PAI an exogenous contrasting agent might be employed. The main feature of the contrasting agent should be the capacity to transform the absorbed light into the US wave. Metallic NPs such as Ag, Au, C and quantum dots possess this functionality. These nanostructures have a particular role in PAI for differentiating between infected and normal tissues by reconstruction of the compositions, sizes and shapes.

2.3 Imaging modalities for cancer management

It is a challenging task to detect cancer, but in particular forms of cancer early detection is beneficial to treat the cancer in an effective way. Different imaging modalities to produce images of bodies are an important factor in earlier detection of various cancers. But the imaging cannot be used for detection in a simple way. Cancer imaging is also beneficial in determination of different stages of the cancer and the exact location of the tumor to assist in surgery and other treatments or to verify whether cancer has returned or not. Different kinds of clinical trial, research studies involving human beings, play an important role in determination of effectiveness and safe nature of the imaging modalities. Cancer imaging may not be considered as a treatment itself but it can be used as an aid to make the best decision for therapies. Similar imaging modalities can aid doctors and surgeons in locating the cancer, to visualize the spread of the cancer, monitor image-guided drug delivery and to determine whether the treatment is working or not. Different stages in cancer imaging are discussed below:

- **Cancer screening:** Imaging is used in determination of suspicious spots or abnormal areas in a person who may be affected with cancer cells. Mammogram is a good example of the imaging modality employed in screening of breast cancer. Cancer screening is mainly recommended for people who have a high risk of cancer development due to family history, lifestyle or age.

- **Cancer diagnostics and different stages:** Imaging is useful in locating the cancer in the body, its spread through the body and the level of spreading. Used in this way, image modality can assist in determining the stages of the cancer and locate whether it is near a vital organ or blood vessel. If a biopsis (a small amount of the tumor taken out for laboratory examinations) is required, the image modality can be employed to assist doctors in guiding towards the tumor and to extract a small piece of it.
- **Image-guided cancer treatment:** Image-guided drugs delivery can be employed for cancer treatment in multiple approaches. Image modalities can be useful for non-invasive treatment of cancer by targeting the tumor region only. For example, US, MRI or CT can be employed for the determination of the precise tumor area so that treatment procedure can be focused particularly on the tumor, which minimizes the harm to the normal tissues residing in the cancer tumor.
- **Determination of treatment efficacy:** Image modalities can be employed to observe whether a tumor is shrinking or whether the shape of the tumor is changed or not. For instance, in currently employed treatments, x-rays, CT and MRI scan are executed at intervals to observe whether treatments are working and whether the tumor is reducing or not. PET and nuclear medicines are employed in monitoring the way the tumor uses the body resources. MRI is often used in studying the chemical change in the tumor site.
- **Monitoring of cancer spread and reappearance:** After some timespan of treating the cancer tumor, it disappears from the body and thus, post-treatment monitoring is important for effective cancer management. Imaging modalities can be employed to monitor the recurrence of the cancer tumor or the spread of the cancer tumor into other regions of the body.

In the last two decades, many conventional biomedical imaging modalities have been demonstrated for regular pre-clinical and clinical practices. These imaging techniques like OI, CT, US, MRI, PET, SPECT etc are being broadly employed for superior performance in early diagnosis and therapies of cancer-like diseases. The molecular level imaging modalities differ from the conventional techniques in which biomarkers are employed to offer the imaging of the targeted sites. It is requisite that these biomarkers should interface in a specific manner in the biological environment and provide the imaging with respect to the molecular level change that has occurred at the desired site. Molecular level imaging candidates are endogenously activated molecules or exogenously activated probes employed for the visualization, characterization, and quantification of the biological process within the living system. Amongst all the molecular imaging techniques, none of the single imaging techniques is ideal to concentrate all the requisites for biomedical applications. Consequently, the current inclination is in the direction of hybrid imaging techniques such as CT–PET, MRI–PET, CT–SPECT, OI–CT etc. Moreover, the combinational approach of MRI and US is appealing as it predominantly holds accuracy for the real-time supervision of high range US treatments. Therefore, the development of multimodal imaging techniques for both MRI and US and combination of these two offers synergistically activated benefits to present significant diagnosis information and therapeutic approaches. Though it is exigent to combine dual-mode or multi-mode imaging techniques into a unique probe, this perception is certainly the most capable and suitable to tackle the present shortcomings of the individual imaging technique.

2.3.1 Diagnostics

The detection of cancer at an early stage is connected with the patient's prognosis as it enables timely intervention, at this early stage, to avert cancer cell growth. However, it is not the regular scenario, as cancer is ordinarily diagnosed after its growth and when it reaches a detection level at which it can be visualized. For such situations, the imaging can be utilized to verify the diagnostics, and it may require biopsies to be acquired from the suspected cancer tumor to be verified in histology or cytology technique to authenticate whether cells are cancer affected or not. The other issue in complication of cancer diagnosis is the heterogeneous nature inside the cancer lesion. Cancerous cells are normally present with pre-cancer cells and also even with healthy cells like immuno-cells. This heterogeneous nature may obstruct estimation of samples at the cell or molecule level. In the case of molecule level estimations, the gathered samples need to be homogenous, and therefore the attendance of healthy tissues inside the sample can lead to the false decrement or increment at the level of the tested molecule.

The aims of cancer detection is: (i) detection of the pre-cancer change or detection of cancer at earlier stages when very few cells are starting to transform into cancer cells, in the conditions of non-visible cancer also, i.e. the aim is to achieve greater sensitivity in detection; (ii) monitoring progress of cancers and their response to therapy. The diagnostics of cancer mainly involves screening of the biomarker, utilization of imaging to observe the cancer or its early development, or detection of the biomarker inside the biopsy of the patient (figure 2.16) [26]. Nanoscale

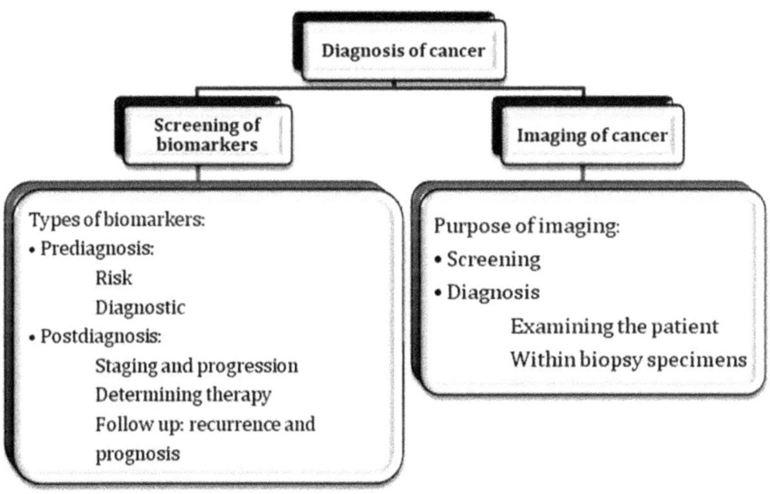

Figure 2.16. Steps involved in diagnosis of cancer (image reproduced with permission from [26], copyright (2020), with permission from Elsevier).

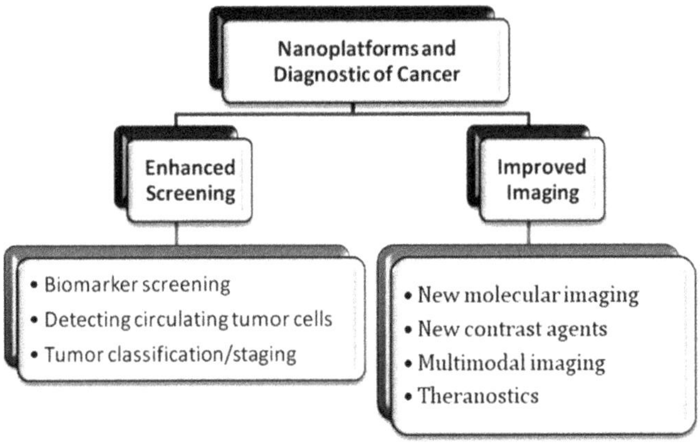

Figure 2.17. Contribution of nanoplatforms for advancement of cancer diagnostics (image reproduced with permission from [26], copyright (2020), with permission from Elsevier).

technologies have the potential to enhance the cancer diagnostics by improving both the screening and imaging modalities (figure 2.17) [26] via utilization of nanoscale materials and nanoscale fabrications that may generate a newer diagnosis platform with superior features for earlier detection of cancer. Moreover, the miniaturizing of nanomaterials eliminates the distress of destructiveness for the patient, especially the distress that is connected to the endoscopic level technique. A range of nanoscale materials are being employed in the area of diagnostics of cancer which include quantum dot, carbon nanotube, fullerene, metal organic framework, gold nanomaterials, silver nanomaterials, zinc oxides, liposomes, polymeric nanomaterials, dendrimer etc. These nanoscale materials have desired features which can promote their use for screening and imaging of the cancer growth. The special feature includes size and shape tuning along with superior surface-to-volume ratio. The high surface-to-volume ratio enables the functionalization of these nanomaterials with different targeting and imaging agents, i.e. it becomes multifunctional. For instance, the surface functionalizing with specifically opted moiety which can be recognized binds to the explicit biomarkers which enables their utilization for specific targeting. In parallel, these nanoscale materials can be functionalized with multiple imaging candidates alongside the therapeutics. An additional benefit of the nanoscale materials is that they can produce signals of their own which can be used in biosensing. Such features lead to improved imaging modalities that were not achievable in the absence of nanoscale materials. For instance, metal nanoscale materials enable surface plasmonic resonance microscopes as they enhance light scatterings for *in vitro* imaging.

The area of non-destructive diagnosis is progressing day by day as the imaging techniques are advancing very fast. Due to growth in computational power, currently available imaging modalities aim to provide comprehensive visualization starting from molecular level to the cell level, organs, tissues and the entire biological scale [27]. The armory of the techniques devoted to imaging has been emerging in recent

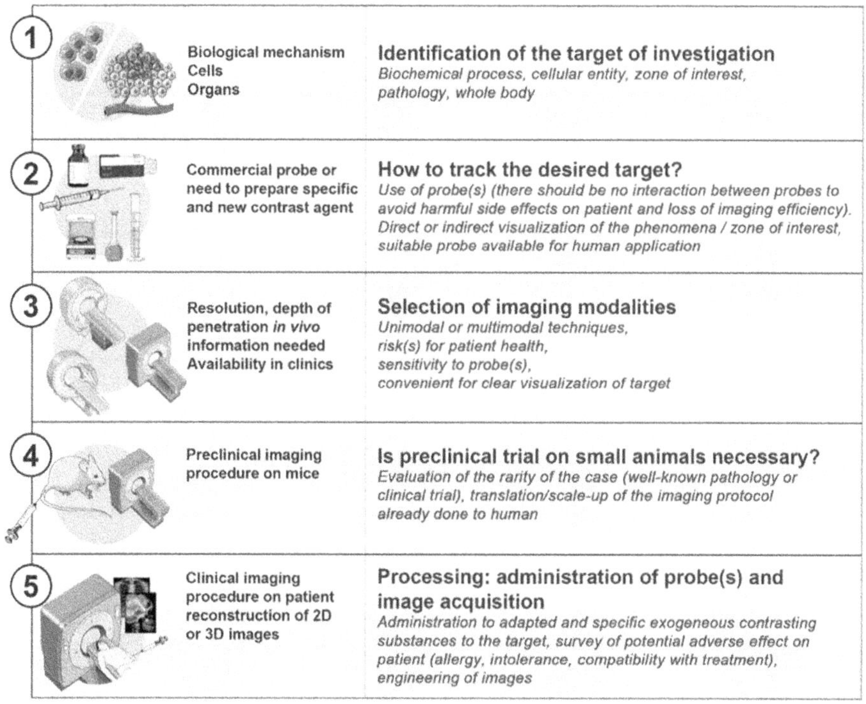

Figure 2.18. Schematics for the stepwise guide to execute radiological diagnosis process (the image is reproduced from [22], copyright 2019 with permission of Springer).

decades and allows us to recognize and inspect the biomedical profiles of patients by constructing the two-dimensional and three-dimensional images without destructive supervision of the patient. Due to the dissimilarity in the region-to-region contrasts, the image displays apparent description of the interior biology (anatomical), morphologies, and physiology related functions at varying scales. Therefore, a bioengineered image provides a base for detecting the earlier stages pathological tests, estimation of the disease progress, stages of cancer, efficiency of the therapy etc and it also assists in clinical level decisions for patient disease administration. Advanced and quick monitoring of cancer-like diseases by imaging modalities is the necessary and proficient non-destructive technique to lessen the mortalities caused by insufficient information on the *in vivo* environment. To attain the perceptible structures of the interior body by varying the contrasts in between the normal and abnormal area, the contrast enhancing material, i.e. contrast agent needing to be incorporated into the human body to increase the sensitivity and specific behaviour of the modalities to a target area. Through this approach, all the imaging modalities offer valuable information at their level and limitations. The preference of the technique is defined by the kind of information one can want to gain from the modalities. Analysis of the imaging modalities by stepwise approaches is a suitable approach to build up competent and pertinent diagnosis procedure. Figure 2.18 [22] shows a schematic for the stepwise guide to execute the diagnosis process.

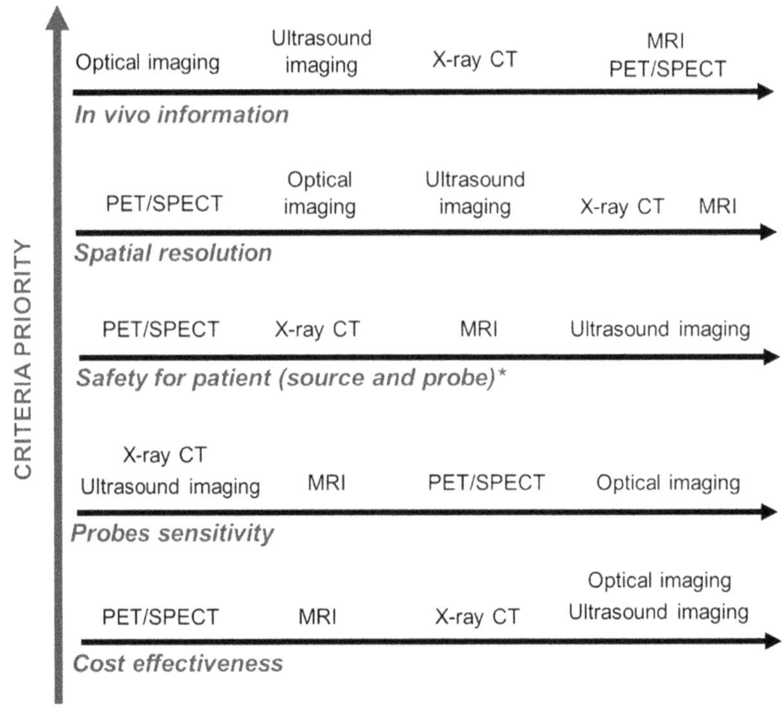

Figure 2.19. Comparative classification of the imaging techniques (the image is reproduced with permission from [22], copyright 2019 with permission of Springer).

Figure 2.19 [22] shows the comparative classification of the imaging techniques. The criteria for the classification was chosen as comparatively less (bottom) to the most important (top) points to be considered in the case of diagnosis. Comparison of the imaging techniques alongside all the criteria apparently shows that in comparison to the clinical level imaging technique, CT and MRI are superior because of the gathering of significant information from their superior resolutions. It can also be observed that they are insensitive as compared to SPECT and PET, even though radiological contrast agents and magnetic formulation are safe. Moreover, none of them has in-depth penetrating limits, which means that biological entities might be absolutely visualized.

According to this classification, x-ray scanner and MRI are the broadly employed modalities and the more proficient imaging instruments. Advancements in preclinical research have made these techniques extremely attainable and therefore increased their use in clinical level research. However, alone they cannot ensure which imaging modality will be more useful for the particular disease. Therefore, in multiple approaches, x-ray and MRI scanners are applied as an instrument or complementing devices with greater efficacy to achieve diagnostics free from unclear information.

2.3.2 Therapy monitoring

Image-guided therapy monitoring is the employment of imaging modality during the therapy to improve the accuracy and precision of treatments. Image-guided therapy monitoring is used for the treatment of tumor in a particular area of the body that is moving such as the lungs. The therapy machine should be well equipped with the imaging modality in order to assist doctors in visualizing the tumor before, during and after treatment. Design configurations for image-guided therapy monitoring are shown in figure 2.20 [28]. By comparison of the generated images with the reference images acquired during the simulation, the patient's position or the radiative beam may be regulated with more precision to target the radiative doses to the tumors. Schematical representation of radio-imaging guided therapy monitoring is shown in figure 2.21. To help in alignment and targeting of the radiation equipment, some image-guided therapy monitoring may employ biomarkers, US, MRI, x-ray image of the bone structure, CT scans, 3D body surface mappings or coloring ink tattoo. While undergoing image-guided therapy, doctors will most likely employ CT scanning to perform the treatment for simulation sessions and to generate the reference image. Other image-guided therapy processes like PET scan on MRI imaging can be employed to determine the exact shape and position of the tumor and special devices may be designed to assist in sustaining the exact position for each treatment.

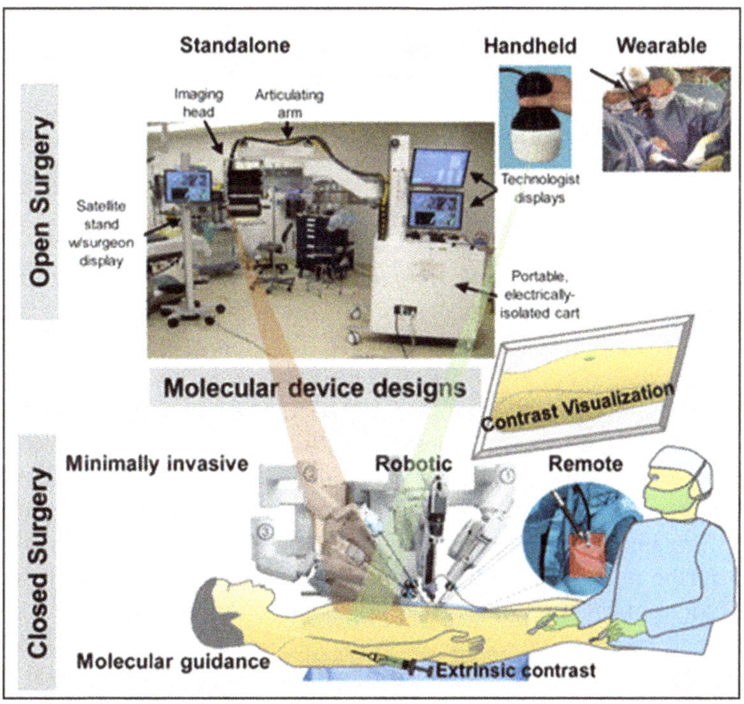

Figure 2.20. Design configurations for image-guided therapy monitoring (all the images are reproduced with permission from [28], copyright Society of Nuclear Medicine and Molecular Imaging (SNMMI)).

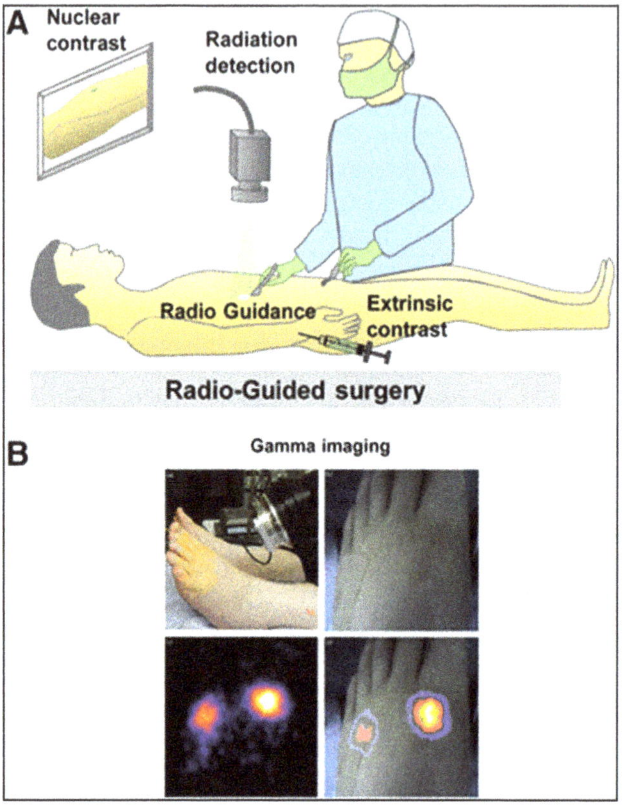

Figure 2.21. Schematical representation of radio-imaging guided therapy monitoring (all the images are reproduced with permission from [28], copyright Society of Nuclear Medicine and Molecular Imaging (SNMMI))).

In image-guided therapy monitoring, the machine that delivers the radiation, like linear accelerators or synchrotron/cyclotron, are well equipped with the imaging modality that enables physicians to visualize the tumor in real time before/after exposure to the radiation, while the patient remains in the same position of the treatment. By opting special computer software, these captured images are compared with the reference image generated during simulations. Any kind of adjustment can be made with the patient position to visualize the tumor with more precision and to circumvent the radiation damage to the normal tissues located near the tumor. Imaging techniques such as CT, MRI, US and x-ray imaging can be employed during image-guided therapy monitoring by visualization of the bone or soft tissues anatomical surgeries. Other imaging modalities for therapy monitoring use a marker to be delivered inside the patient's body or the surface. Image-guided therapy monitoring is mainly employed to treat the tumor in particular regions of the body that are prone to movement like lungs, prostate gland, liver, pancreas, as well as tumors located close to critical organs and tissue. It is frequently used to conjugate with intensity modulated radiological therapies, proton beam therapies, stereotactic radio surgeries, or stereotactic body radio therapies which advance the mode of highly precise radio therapy that utilizes computer operated x-ray accelerator to deliver precise radiation dose to a tumor or specific regions inside the tumor. Schematic representations for optical image-guided and multimodal image-guided therapy monitoring are shown in figures 2.22 and 2.23.

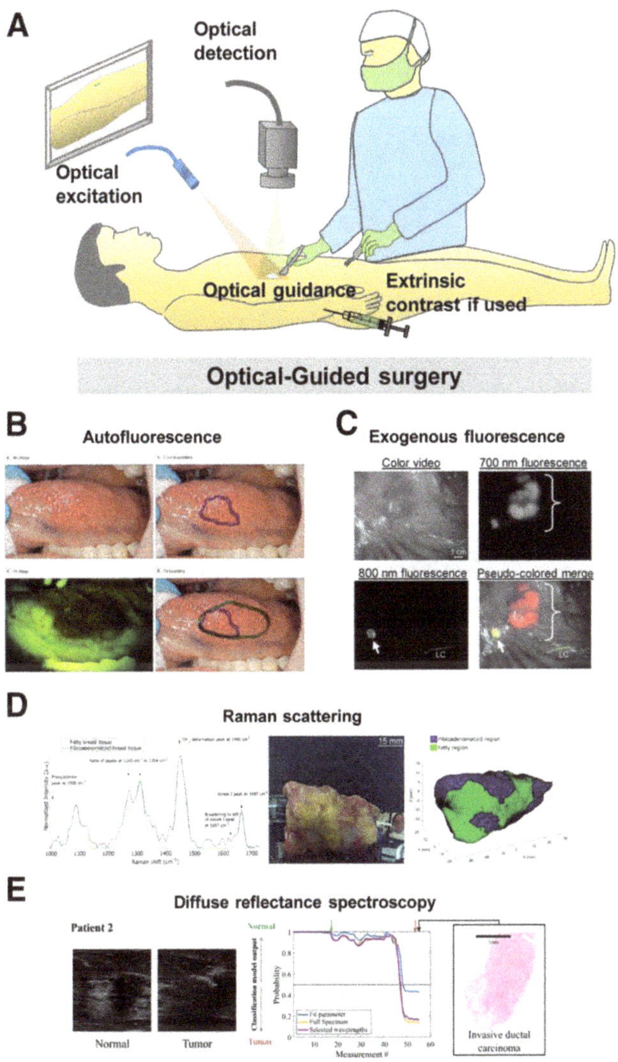

Figure 2.22. Schematic representation of optical image-guided therapy monitoring. (a) Reproduced with permission from [28], (a) copyright Society of Nuclear Medicine and Molecular Imaging (SNMMI)). (b) Reprinted from [27], copyright (2019), with permission from Elsevier. (c) Reprinted from [29], copyright 2009, Society of Surgical Oncology, with permission of Springer. (d) Reprinted from [30], copyright 2017, The Authors. With permission of Springer. (e) Reprinted from [31], copyright 2018, The Authors, with permission of Springer.

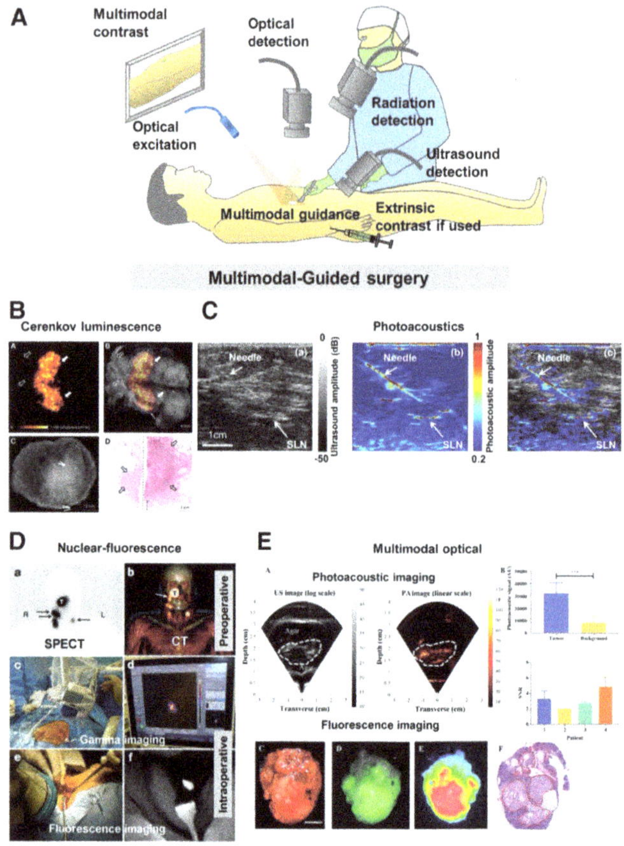

Figure 2.23. Schematic representation of multimodal imaging guided therapy monitoring (all the images are reproduced with permission from [28], (a) copyright Society of Nuclear Medicine and Molecular Imaging (SNMMI)). (b) Reprinted with permission from [32], copyright Society of Nuclear Medicine and Molecular Imaging (SNMMI). (c) Reprinted with permission from [33], copyright 2015, The Authors, with permission of Springer. (d) Reprinted with permission from [34], copyright 2011, The Authors, with permission of Springer. (e) Reprinted from [35], copyright 2018, with permission of Springer.

Delivery of radiological therapies requires a treatment team, which includes an oncologist, therapist, radiological officers, and dosimetry experts. The oncologist is a physician who assesses the patients and determines suitable therapies or combinational therapy and the type of image-guided therapy monitoring. The physician determines the area of interest to treat and how much dosage needs to be delivered. Together with the therapist and the dosimetry experts, the radiation oncologist determines what technique to employ for the delivery of the predefined dose. Further, physicians and dosimetry experts make the calculation required for the therapy. Radiological therapists are especially trained technology experts who acquire images and deliver the daily treatment. The radiation oncologist may also assess patients and provide them with additional information about the treatments and possible side reactions. The radiation oncologist also helps to manage side effects caused by the treatment that may occurr, in collaboration with the physician.

Radiation therapies can cause earlier and late side effects. Earlier side effects occur during or immediately after the treatments and are typically gone within a few weeks. Ordinary earlier side effects of radiation therapies include tiredness or skin problems. Skin in the treatment areas may become more sensitive, swollen or irritated.

Depending on the area being treated, other early side effects may include:

- Loss of hair in the treatment region;
- Oral problems and complexity swallowing;
- Digestive and eating issues;
- Diarrhea;
- Vomiting and nausea;
- Headache;
- Swelling and soreness in the treatment region;
- Urinal problems.

Late side effects, which are unusual, take place months or years following treatment and are often permanent.

They include:

- Brain issues;
- Spinal cord issues;
- Lung issues;
- Kidney issues;
- Colon and rectal issues;
- Infertility issues;
- Joint issues;
- Lymphedema;
- Oral issues;
- Secondary cancers.

There might be an insignificant risk of developing cancer from radiological therapies. Following radiation treatment for cancer, the patient will be evaluated frequently by the radiological oncologist for complications as well as recurrent or new cancer. Using techniques such as image-guided therapy monitoring, imaging specialists are exploiting its effects on healthy tissue and organs and the side effects of the treatment itself.

2.4 Conclusion

In this chapter, we have exemplified the different types of imaging techniques and their application in medical imaging techniques such as CT, PET, MRI, SPECT, OI and florescence etc. Current investigations of the imaging technologies for cancer

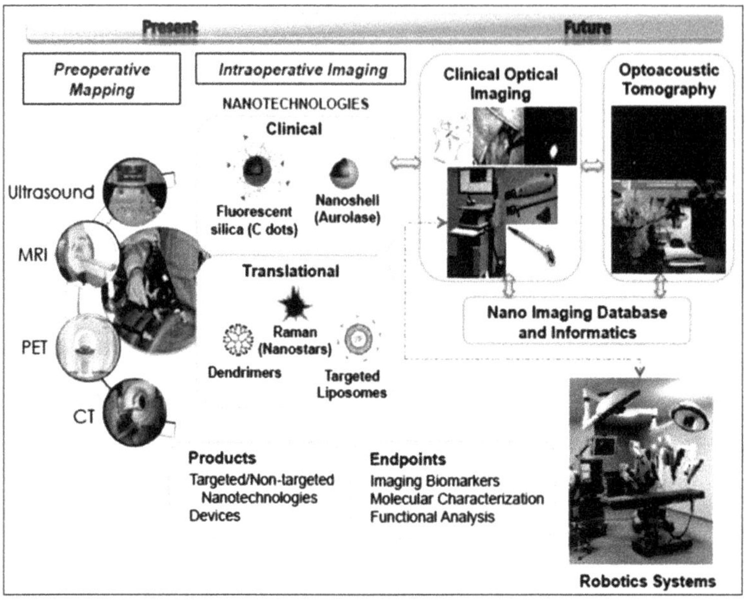

Figure 2.24. Current and upcoming nano-imaging guided surgical suites (image reproduced with permission from [36], copyright (2018) American Chemical Society).

therapeutics and diagnostics display their benefits for cancer management. The current basic as well as translational efforts of imaging modalities show their extent with multiple emerging fields. From a technology perspective, this area has undergone incredible growth and success. On the other hand, the deficient understanding of human cancer biology persists comparative to the applications of advanced imaging techniques. Although the technical improvement in large-scale imaging modalities like CT–PET or MRI have led to an enhancement in pre-operative cancer diagnosis and stages, their utilization is restricted by attainable spatial resolution, sensitivity and practical issues of intra-operative implementation. Moreover, image-guided imaging strategies have conventionally been hindered in surgical practice by the small number of presented targeting near infrared agents, superficial tissues penetration, constrained contrast resolutions, quick photo-bleaching and inability to detect multiple cancers or healthy tissues. Noteworthy progress, on the other hand, is being made to tackle the drawbacks, with notable efforts promoted toward development of optically activated and targeting imaging agents, inclusive of particles based probes for clinical level practice. Aimed at promoting improved sensitivity, specific nature and depth penetration, these probes promise noticeable improvements in real-time early stage molecular level detection and treatment of diseases in combination with a multi-channel fluorescent camera system with clinical grade precision (figure 2.24) [36].

References

[1] Kalender W A 2006 X-ray computed tomography *Phys. Med. Biol.* **51** R29
[2] Kunjachan S, Ehling J, Storm G, Kiessling F and Lammers T 2015 Noninvasive imaging of nanomedicines and nanotheranostics: principles, progress, and prospects *Chem. Rev.* **115** 10907–37
[3] Louie A 2010 Multimodality imaging probes: design and challenges *Chem. Rev.* **110** 3146–95
[4] Janib S M, Moses A S and MacKay J A 2010 Imaging and drug delivery using theranostic nanoparticles *Adv. Drug Deliv. Rev.* **62** 1052–63
[5] Fan Z, Fu P P, Yu H and Ray P C 2014 Theranostic nanomedicine for cancer detection and treatment *J. Food Drug Anal.* **22** 3–17
[6] Jones N, Ropero-Miller J, Waltke H, McLeod-Henning D, Weiss D and Barcus H (eds) 2017 *Proceedings of the International Forensic Radiology Research Summit May 10–11, 2016, Amsterdam, The Netherlands* (Research Triangle Park, NC: RTI International)
[7] Wild C P 2019 The global cancer burden: necessity is the mother of prevention *Nat. Rev. Cancer* **19** 123–4
[8] Bray F, Ferlay J, Soerjomataram I, Siegel R L, Torre L A and Jemal A 2018 Global cancer statistics 2018: GLOBOCAN estimates of incidence and mortality worldwide for 36 cancers in 185 countries *CA: Cancer J Clin* **68** 394–424
[9] Luengo Morato Y, Ovejero Paredes K, Lozano Chamizo L, Marciello M and Filice M 2021 Recent advances in multimodal molecular imaging of cancer mediated by hybrid magnetic nanoparticles *Polymers* **13** 2989
[10] Sivasubramanian M, Hsia Y and Lo L-W 2014 Nanoparticle-facilitated functional and molecular imaging for the early detection of cancer *Front. Mol. Biosci.* **1** 15
[11] Dang N, Tiwari S, Khurana M and Arya K V 2021 Recent advancements in medical imaging: a machine learning approach *Machine Learning for Intelligent Multimedia Analytics: Techniques and Applications* ed P Kumar and A K Singh (Singapore: Springer) pp 189–212
[12] Cierniak R 2011 *X-ray Computed Tomography in Biomedical Engineering* (Berlin: Springer Science & Business Media)
[13] Lundervold A S and Lundervold A 2019 An overview of deep learning in medical imaging focusing on MRI *Z. Med. Phys.* **29** 102–27
[14] Wells P N 2006 Ultrasound imaging *Phys. Med. Biol.* **51** R83
[15] Chan V and Perlas A 2011 Basics of ultrasound imaging *Atlas of Ultrasound-Guided Procedures in Interventional Pain Management* (Berlin: Springer) pp 13–19
[16] Chapman H N 2009 X-ray imaging beyond the limits *Nat. Mater.* **8** 299–301
[17] Russo P 2017 *Handbook of X-ray Imaging: Physics and Technology* (Boca Raton, FL: CRC Press)
[18] Jerusalem G, Hustinx R, Beguin Y and Fillet G 2003 PET scan imaging in oncology *Eur. J. Cancer* **39** 1525–34
[19] Faraji F and Gaba R C 2019 Radiologic modalities and response assessment schemes for clinical and preclinical oncology imaging *Front. Oncol* **9** 471
[20] Beyer T, Bidaut L, Dickson J, Kachelriess M, Kiessling F, Leitgeb R, Ma J, Shiyam Sundar L K, Theek B and Mawlawi O 2020 What scans we will read: imaging instrumentation trends in clinical oncology *Cancer Imaging* **20** 38
[21] Na H B, Song I C and Hyeon T 2009 Inorganic nanoparticles for MRI contrast agents *Adv. Mater.* **21** 2133–48

[22] Wallyn J, Anton N, Akram S and Vandamme T F 2019 Biomedical imaging: principles, technologies, clinical aspects, contrast agents, limitations and future trends in nanomedicines *Pharm. Res.* **36** 78

[23] De La Vega J C and Häfeli U O 2015 Utilization of nanoparticles as x-ray contrast agents for diagnostic imaging applications *Contrast Media Mol. Imaging* **10** 81–95

[24] Kong F-L, Ford R J and Yang D J 2013 Managing lymphoma with non-FDG radiotracers: current clinical and preclinical applications *BioMed Res. Int.* **2013** 626910

[25] Mallidi S, Larson T, Tam J, Joshi P P, Karpiouk A, Sokolov K and Emelianov S 2009 Multiwavelength photoacoustic imaging and plasmon resonance coupling of gold nanoparticles for selective detection of cancer *Nano Lett.* **9** 2825–31

[26] Zeineldin R 2013 Nanotechnology for cancer screening and diagnosis: from innovations to clinical applications *Biomaterials for Cancer Therapeutics* (Cambridge: Woodhead Publishing) pp 137–64

[27] Kozakai A, Ono K, Nomura T, Takano N and Shibahara T 2020 Usefulness of objective evaluations by fluorescence visualization device for differentiating between superficial oral squamous cell carcinoma and oral lichen planus *J. Oral Maxillofac. Surg. Med. Pathol.* **32** 26–32

[28] Mondal S B, O'Brien C M, Bishop K, Fields R C, Margenthaler J A and Achilefu S 2020 Repurposing molecular imaging and sensing for cancer image–guided surgery *J. Nucl. Med.* **61** 1113–22

[29] Troyan S L, Kianzad V, Gibbs-Strauss S L, Gioux S, Matsui A, Oketokoun R, Ngo L, Khamene A, Azar F and Frangioni J V 2009 The FLARE™ intraoperative near-infrared fluorescence imaging system: A first-in-human clinical trial in breast cancer sentinel lymph node mapping *Ann. Surg. Oncol.* **16** 2943–52

[30] Thomas G *et al* 2017 Evaluating feasibility of an automated 3-dimensional scanner using Raman spectroscopy for intraoperative breast margin assessment *Sci. Rep.* **7** 13548

[31] de Boer L L, Bydlon T M, van Duijnhoven F, Vranken Peeters M-J T F D, Loo C E, Winter-Warnars G A O, Sanders J, Sterenborg H J C M, Hendriks B H W and Ruers T J M 2018 Towards the use of diffuse reflectance spectroscopy for real-time in vivo detection of breast cancer during surgery *J. Trans. Med.* **16** 367

[32] Grootendorst M R *et al* 2016 Intraoperative assessment of tumor resection margins in breast-conserving surgery using ^{18}F-FDG Cerenkov luminescence imaging: A first-in-human feasibility study *J. Nucl. Med.* **58** 891–8

[33] Garcia-Uribe A, Erpelding T N, Krumholz A, Ke H, Maslov K, Appleton C, Margenthaler J A and Wang L V 2015 Dual-modality photoacoustic and ultrasound imaging system for noninvasive sentinel lymph node detection in patients with breast cancer *Sci. Rep.* **5** 15748

[34] Brouwer O R, Klop W M C, Buckle T, Vermeeren L, van den Brekel M W M, Balm A J M, Nieweg O E, Valdés Olmos R A and van Leeuwen F W B 2011 Feasibility of sentinel node biopsy in head and neck melanoma using a hybrid radioactive and fluorescent tracer *Annals of Surgical Oncology* **19** 1988–94

[35] Tummers W S 2018 Intraoperative pancreatic cancer detection using tumor-specific multimodality molecular imaging *Ann. Surg. Oncol.* **25** 1880–8

[36] Hartshorn C M, Bradbury M S, Lanza G M, Nel A E, Rao J, Wang A Z, Wiesner U B, Yang L and Grodzinski P 2018 Nanotechnology strategies to advance outcomes in clinical cancer care *ACS Nano* **12** 24–43

Chapter 3

Nanoplatforms for cancer imagining

Sandeep B Somvanshi and Nanasaheb D Thorat

Cancer is perhaps the most destructive global disease and is causing millions of deaths annually. Recently, nanotechnology, as a one of a kind innovation, has been widely applied in the treatment of cancer-like diseases through diagnostics, imaging and therapy. Furthermore, with the rise of cutting-edge biomaterials equipped for being applied in biomedical areas, research in cancer nanotechnology has gained critical ground. In particular, nanomaterials with dimensions under a few hundred nanometers are significantly investigated among these high level biomaterials. In the past years, various organic, inorganic and hybrid nanomaterials have arisen as novel probes for cancer diagnosis and therapy because of their special attributes, similar to their solubilization impact, inactive/dynamic tumor focusing, controlled drug deliverance which bring about improved anti-cancer viability while decreasing the negative results. In this chapter, we initially give a short depiction of the nanomedicines used for cancer imaging. The significant objective of this chapter is to sum up the accomplishments that have been made in the advancement of the use of nanomaterials for cancer imaging, alongside a short portrayal of their overall attributes and future perspectives.

3.1 Introduction

Cancer is one of the leading reasons for global deaths and it is increasing very rapidly. According to the WHO report, it was projected that cancer incidences in 2018 were around 18.2 million and the estimated deaths due to cancer were around 9.7 million [1–3]. Also, predictions suggest that there will be 30+ million deaths every year by the year 2030. Early stage diagnosis and the detection of the cancer can treat it efficiently in timely manner with fewer side effects. Even though the areas of detection and diagnosis have improved during the last decade, the accuracy and the efficiency of the imaging techniques are still underdeveloped.

Recently, the various imaging modalities such as magnetic resonance imaging (MRI), positron emission tomography (PET), computed tomography (CT), optical imaging (OI), photo-acoustic imaging (PAI), ultrasound (US) imaging, single-photon

doi:10.1088/978-0-7503-3675-8ch3

© IOP Publishing Ltd 2022

emission computed tomography (SPECT) etc have been focused on diagnosing the cancer tumor and monitoring the drugs released for treatment of the tumor [4–7]. It is noteworthy to determine that the inventions and progression of these imaging techniques are implied on historical advances within the field of physics, chemistry and not to provide the requisition of the oncology field. All the individual imaging techniques have their limitations in the case of sensitivity or/and resolutions, which prohibit the capability of the imaging modality to tackle most of the imperative clinical level issues in cancer monitoring, stage determination and therapies. Among these imaging modalities, MR, CT and USI can be employed with or without contrasting agent. In the case of contrasting agent employment, pre-scanning is needed to conclude the background levels of MR, CT and US imaging signals preceding to contrasting agents incorporation. This type of base measurement is required to enumerate the molecular level or functional imaging information. On the other hand, in hot-spot techniques like SPECT or PET or OI, no such type of background signal is detected in the absence of contrasting agent, and thus no pre-scanning is required. However, these hot-spot imaging modalities do not offer any anatomy related information and thus they are required to couple with one of the imaging modalities like MR or CT, which is extremely beneficial for anatomy and morphology related imaging. This gives rise to the hybrid system of imaging in combination as CT–PET, CT–SPECT, MRI–PET etc, in which anatomy related information acquired through CT or MR imaging is employed for assistance in assigning the molecular level or functional level hot-spot information to the accurate organ or tissues. Most importantly, the above discussed imaging techniques are applicable for different rationales depending upon their specificity, sensitivity, and abilities. Figure 3.1 shows a schematic of the different imaging modalities along with their in detail applications and limitations. In view of the fact that all these imaging techniques express different types of anatomy, molecular or functional level imaging information and they have some benefits as well as limitations, thus it is essential to have an appropriate understanding of the properties, specificity, and translational

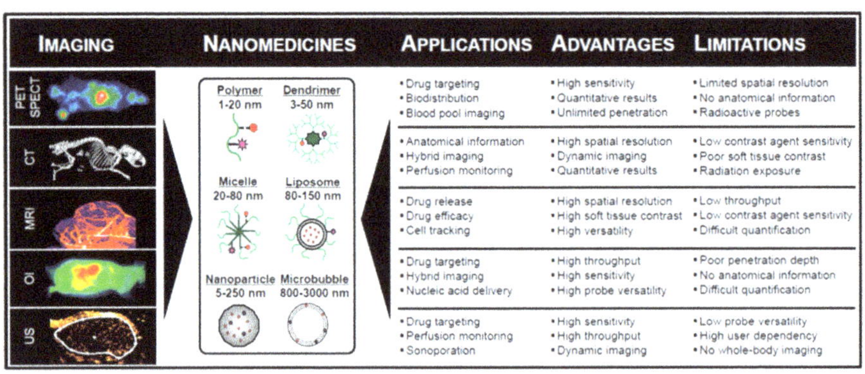

Figure 3.1. Schematic representation of different imaging modalities regularly employed in clinical research and their specific applications, advantages, and limitations (all the images reproduced with permission from [4], copyright (2015) American Chemical Society).

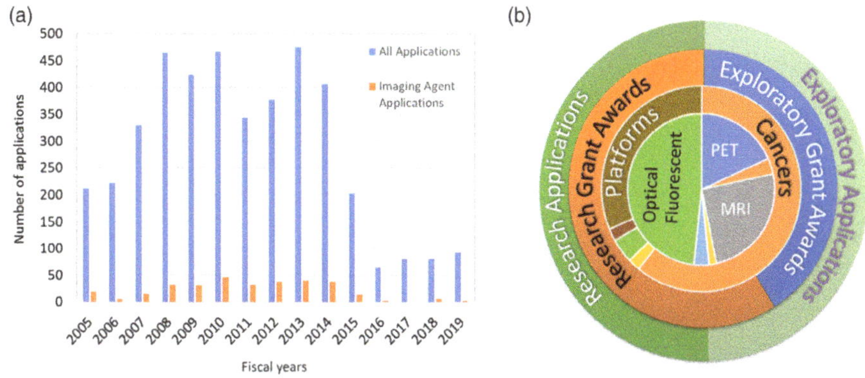

Figure 3.2. NIH-sponsored grant proposals (applications) for nano-enabled imaging applications. (a) Comparisons between the number of imaging agent applications versus all applications submitted to the nanotechnology funding opportunity applications (FOAs) between 2005 and 2019. Data were extracted from the NIH and NCI nanotechnology FOAs referenced in the main text. Imaging agent applications were defined as applications with keywords 'imaging agent' or 'imaging probe' in the titles or abstracts. (b) Additional breakdown of the imaging agent applications and awards. The outermost ring depicts the type of applications received. The series of inner rings highlight the focus of those applications that were awarded, whereby research grants with a cancer focus using optical/fluorescent imaging were predominant (all the images reproduced with permission from [8], copyright 2020 John Wiley & Sons).

ability of each imaging modality, in order to appropriately examine the appropriateness for diagnosis of cancer tumor and monitoring the therapy.

The US National Institute of Health released a lot of funding for nanotechnology after the foundation of National Nanotechnology Initiatives in 2000. This includes announcement of funds related to Nanotechnology in Biology and Medicine for 2003–2011, Nanotechnology in Cancer Program for nanotechnologies in cancer for 2005, 2010 and 2014, Innovative Nanotechnology Platform for 2005, 2010, 2014 and 2017, and most recently the program of translational cancer nanotechnology in 2020. These funding initiatives boosted the nanotechnologies in creating noteworthy progression in developing the therapeutic approach. However, it is observed that less consideration has been given to nanoscale based imaging agents. The probable cause for this non-progression is that most of the translational funding did not incorporate imaging agents in the keywords of the call. This resulted in fewer research proposals focusing on imaging agents submitted to NIH. Depending on the analysis of the collections of applications submitted to NIH for funding during the period of 2005–2019, around 6.3% of the total proposals are related to imaging agents (figure 3.2(a)). Overlapping circular shapes describe supplementary information of the imaging agent application as shown in figure 3.2(b). Only a small number of nanoscale imaging candidates have been endorsed for clinical use. Table 3.1 shows the list of approved nanoparticle imaging agents [8].

3.2 Nanomedicines for cancer imaging

Various non-invasive techniques of medical imaging exist viz. MRI, US imaging, PET, CT, SPECT and OI [9]. Each of them have their individual benefits and

Table 3.1. Approved nanoparticle imaging agents (table reproduced with permission from [8], copyright 2020 John Wiley & Sons).

Nanoparticle type	Trade name	Manufacturer	Approval	Current status
Radionuclides for SPECT		Mallinckrodt	1974 (United States)	Discontinued
^{99m}Tc sulfur colloid	TechneColl	Phamalucence	1978 (United States)	Active
^{99m}Tc sulfur colloid	AN-sulfur colloid	CIS BIO international	1993 (Finland)	Active
^{99m}Tc rhenium sulfide colloid	Nanocis		1995 (Denmark) 2001 (Norway) 2002 (Sweden)	
^{99m}Tc albumin colloid	Nano-albumon	Medi-Radiopharma	1993 (Hungary) 1994 (Czech Republic) 1998 (Romania)	Active
^{99m}Tc albumin colloid	Nanocoll	GE Healthcare S.r.l	1995 (Denmark)	Active
^{99m}Tc albumin colloid	Senti-Scint	Medi-Radiopharma	1999 (Hungary) 2001 (Czech Republic) 2004 (Slovakian Republic) 2004 (Turkey)	Active
^{99m}Tc tin fluoride colloid	Hepatate	Gipharma S.r.l.	2002 (France)	Active
^{99m}Tc albumin colloid	Nanotop ROTOP-NanoHSA (Spain, France, Finland) NanoHSA (Sweden)	ROTOP Pharmaka AG	2011 (Germany) 2014 (EU)	Active
^{99m}Tc albumin colloid	Nanoscan Nano-albumon (Italy) Nanoscint (Belgium)	Medi-Radiopharma	2011 (Denmark)	Active
		Iron oxides for MRI		
Ferristene (polystyrene coating)	Abdoscan (Sweden, Finland, UK, Norway)	Nycomed imaging	1993	Discontinued in 2002
Ferumoxide (dextran coating)	Feridex (United States) Endorem (Britain)	Amag pharmaceuticals	1996	Discontinued in 2008

Ferumoxsil (silicone coating)	Lumirem (EU) Gastromark (United States)	Geurbet, Amag pharmaceuticals	1996	Discontinued in 2012
Ferucarbotran (carboxydextran coating)	Resovist (EU) Cliavist (France)	Bayer Schering pharma	2001	Discontinued in 2009 in EU. Active in Japan.
Ferumoxtran-10 (dextran coating)	Sinerem (EU) Combidex (United States)	Guerbet	(Netherlands)	Withdrawn from FDA in 2005, EMA in 2007
Ferumoxytol (polyglucose sorbitol carboxymethylether coating)	Feraheme (United States)	Amag pharmaceuticals	2009	Active (off-label use for MRI)
(carboxydextran coating)	Magtrace (United States)	Endomagnetics, Ltd.	2018	Active (for use with Sentimag magnetic localization system)

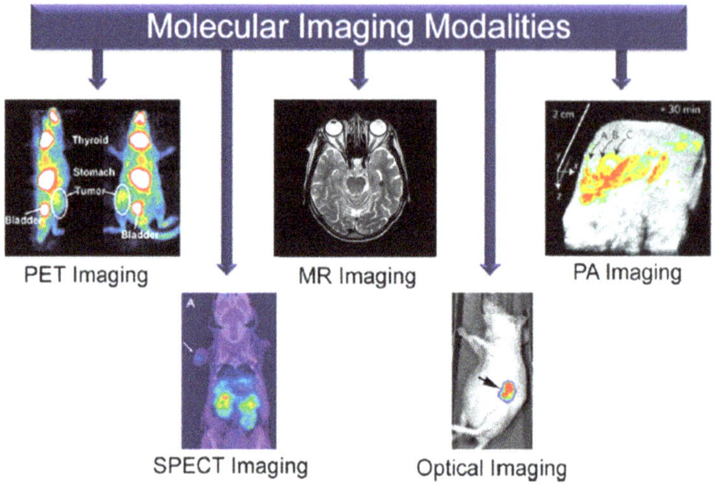

Figure 3.3. Different molecular level imaging techniques utilized for cancer imaging and therapy monitoring comprising PET, MRI, SPECT, PAI and OI. Images reproduced with permission from [13] copyright 2014, Nature Publishing Group, with permission of Springer, [14] copyright (2014) American Chemical Society, [15] copyright 2014, The Authors and [16] copyright (2011), with permission from Elsevier. Top right image has been obtained by the authors from the Pixabay website where it was made available under the Pixabay License (https://pixabay.com/service/terms/#license). It is included within this article on that basis.

drawbacks related to differentiation in terms of the image resolution, sensitivity, and depth of signaling penetration [10, 11], and preference for the suitable imaging modality relies upon the type of requisite information [4]. OI is most often useful for *in vivo* imaging of the small animal as this imaging is safe, timely and economical. On the other hand, the imaging of deep tissue or big animals is not practically convenient by OI. To tackle this issue, radionuclide based imaging modalities like PET or SPECT have emerged as they offer deeper tissue imaging with higher sensitivity. However, PET or SPECT provide comparatively limited resolution and lack anatomical information. To gain information about anatomy, PET or SPECT are thus frequently coupled with CT and MRI, which facilitates selectivity and tissue visualization with higher resolution.

Current advancements in molecular level imaging have modified the approach we utilize for the diagnostics and monitoring of different diseases such as cancer [12]. Molecular level imaging modalities need specific instruments for the diagnostic and therapy monitoring of the diseases, comprising PET, MRI, SPECT, PAI and OI, as shown in figure 3.3.

Currently, clinically used imaging techniques can be classified in two groups, i.e. primary anatomical imaging modalities and higher spatial resolution imaging modalities such as CT, MRI and US imaging, and the others are primary molecular level imaging modalities such as optical imaging, PET or SPECT [17, 18]. For possible clinical diagnosis and therapy, all these techniques are

Table 3.2. Features of various cancer imaging modalities (table reproduced with permission from [17]).

Modality	Benefits	Drawbacks	Ref.
Magnetic resonance imaging	Higher spatial resolutions; provides molecular level as well as physiological info; no limiting tissues penetration.	Lower sensitiveness; requires longer period for imaging; costly.	[20, 21]
Computed tomography	Higher spatial resolutions; No limiting tissues penetration.	Exposable to radiations; harder to distinguish soft tissue.	[22]
Fluorescent imaging	Highly sensitive, higher temporal resolutions; easier to discriminate.	Limiting tissue penetration; lower spatial resolutions.	[23–25]
Positron emission tomography	Highly sensitive; no limiting tissues penetration; appropriate for entire body.	Exposable to radiations; costly.	[26]
Single-photon emission computed tomography	Highly sensitive; no limiting tissues penetration.	Exposable to radiations; limiting spatial resolution.	[26, 27]
Photo-acoustic imaging	Higher spatial resolutions and penetration depth; highly sensitive; provides functional as well as molecular level information.	Limited in imaging agents.	[28, 29]

inimitable for doctors as they all have different kinds of features and appropriate for the different tissue in view of the different properties such as sensitiveness and in-depth or spatial resolutions [19]. The different features of the different imaging modalities are tabulated in table 3.2.

Magnetic resonance imaging (MRI)

Magnetic resonance imaging (MRI) is one of the most widely used imaging techniques which provides high resolution imaging and penetrates deep in the tissues to view the anatomy in a clear manner [20, 21, 30, 31]. The basic mechanism of MRI mainly depends on nuclear magnetic resonance (NMR) and relaxation of the nucleus of the proton spin in the existence of strong magnetic fields. In the presence of the strong magnetic field, the nuclei of the proton spin align in a parallel way or anti-parallel way towards the applied magnetic field and precess under the Larmor frequencies, as shown in figure 3.4(A). After applying external

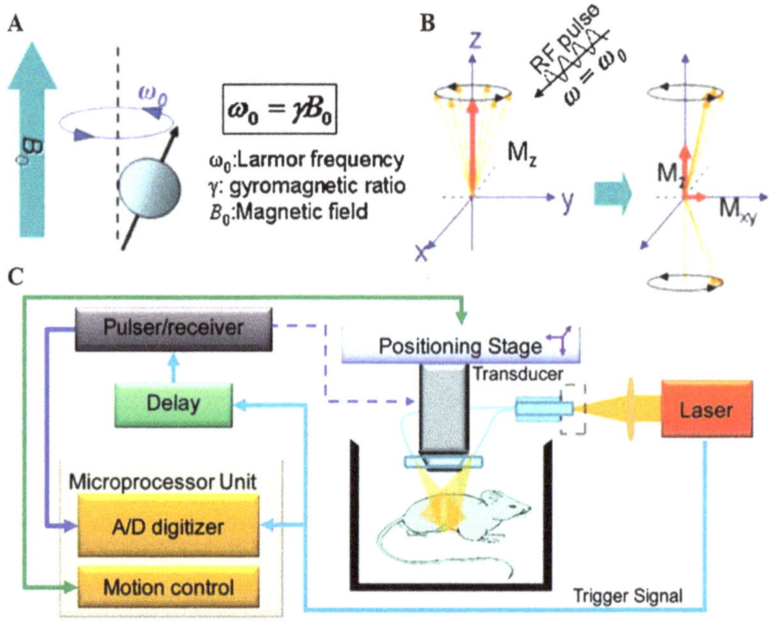

Figure 3.4. Principle of magnetic resonance imaging. (a) Spins align parallel or anti-parallel to the field and precess under Larmor frequency. (b) After induction of RF pulse, magnetization of spins changes. Reproduced with permission from [32], copyright 2009 John Wiley & Sons. (c) Block diagram of a typical PAI system. Reproduced with permission from [31], copyright 2009 American Chemical Society.

radio frequency, the proton gets energized and excited to the higher energy level. After removing the external radio frequency, the energized nuclei relax down instantly to their original energy states. This relaxation process can be further divided into two types, i.e. T_1 and T_2 relaxation and can be used to generate the MRI images to distinguish the tissues (figure 3.4(B)). On the basis of these two relaxation types, the contrast enhancing agents can be divided into the T_1 and T_2 specific contrast agents. The nanoscale materials combining transition metal ions or rare earth metal ions like MnO [32], Gd_2O_3 [33], $GdPO_4$ [34] and GdF_3 [33] are of great interest for T_1 contrast agents as they possess higher magnetic moments [35]. Magnetic nanoparticles based on Fe_3O_4 are also of great interest as they show superior magnetic moment when exposed to the applied magnetic field. Interestingly, Fe_3O_4 nanoparticles show T_1 and T_2 contrast enhancing in MR imaging with the modification the nanoparticles size [36, 37]. A number of contrast agents based on Fe_3O_4 on commercial level are available and some of them are Combidex, Feridex, Resovist etc [38]. Similar to Fe_3O_4, the nanoscale spinel ferrites like $MnFe_2O_4$, $NiFe_2O_4$, $CoFe_2O_4$ etc have shown great T_2 contrast ability [36]. The illustration of the MRI effect on the magnetic moment of hydrogen nuclei from H_2O molecules contained in tissues to yield reconstructed images is shown in figure 3.5.

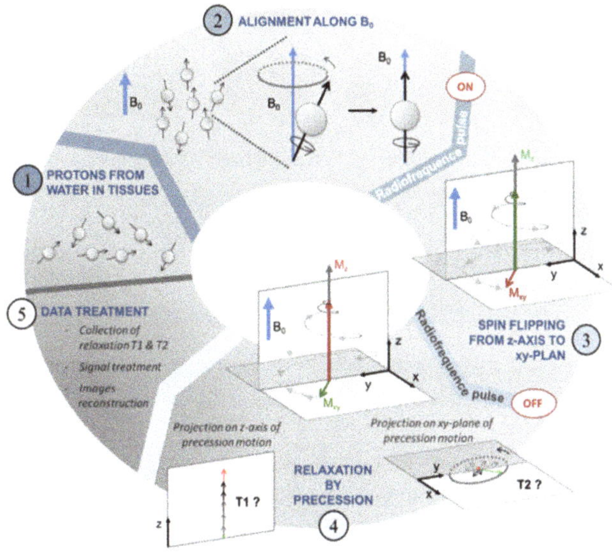

Figure 3.5. Schematic representation of the MRI effect on the magnetic moment of hydrogen nuclei from water molecules contained in tissues to yield reconstructed images (images reproduced from [39], copyright 2019, Springer Science Business Media, LLC, part of Springer Nature, with permission of Springer).

Computed tomography (CT)

Computed tomography (CT) has proved a handy imaging modality among the others and it is cost effective and competent. CT enables the visualization of the bones with better clarity because of its contrast ability in between the dense bone and soft tissues [22]. To get superior contrast in CT imaging for advanced imaging of soft tissue with similar contrast, a contrast agent is necessary in CT imaging. The prime factor in selecting the CT contrast agent is elements with higher atomic number. In the current scenario, clinically used contrast agents are mostly made up of iodine (I) based materials with higher atomic number, and are efficient in x-ray absorption and they get exerted rapidly [40]. Moreover, metal nanoparticles like gold (Au) [40], tantalum (Ta) [41] and bismuth (Bi) [42] are of great interest for the generation of high contrast images. Figure 3.6 shows the types of CT with their representative *in vivo* scale at which investigations can be carried out.

Optical imaging (OI)

Optical imaging (OI) is the imaging technique based on the properties of UV-visible light and infrared rays. It is a nondestructive and cost efficient imaging modality which provides reasonable imaging in comparison with the other imaging techniques. Optical imaging includes photoluminescent, fluorescent,

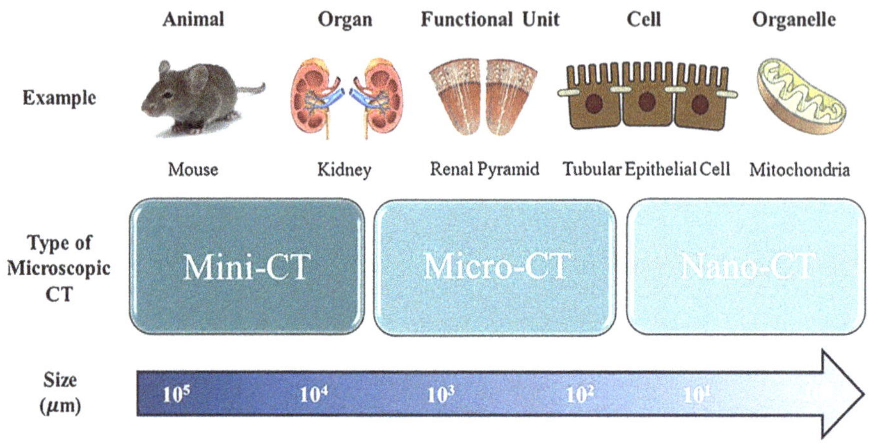

Figure 3.6. Type of computed tomography with their representative *in vivo* scale at which investigations can be carried out (image is reproduced with permission from [43], copyright 2014 John Wiley & Sons).

Raman scattering and other related imaging techniques [44–49]. Fluorescent imaging is broadly used in clinical applications and is based on the absorption and emission of energy gained from external light. In comparison with visible light, near infrared rays with wavelength range of 700–1100 nm get absorbed and penetrate within the tissues. The use of near infrared probes is increasing currently because of the involvement of nanoscale materials like quantum dots [50], rare earth ions [51], carbon nanotubes [52] and gold (Au) [53]. The fluorescence imaging technique in the near infrared region II with wavelength scope of 900 to 1400 nm is more helpful as compared to the near infrared region I with wavelength scope 700 to 900 nm. The potential near infrared region II fluorescence imaging agents consist of carbon nanotubes [23, 24], quantum dots [54], and different small molecular dyes [55].

Positron emission tomography (PET) and single-photon emission computed tomography (SPECT)

PET and SPECT are the imaging techniques which mainly rely on NMR. PET scanning image gives a resolution of the order of 5–7 mm, whereas SPECT scanning image offers resolution of the order of 12–15 mm [56]. So, the PET imaging technique can identify the anatomy easily which cannot be achievable with SPECT. Also, the SPECT imaging technique requires compounds with two or more radionuclides to label the biological entities [26, 27]. But, in clinical application SPECT is cost-effective in comparison with the PET imaging technique. The most frequently employed PET radioisotopes consist of fluorine (^{18}F), gallium (^{68}Ga), carbon (^{11}C), copper (^{64}Cu), zirconium (^{89}Zr) and yttrium (^{86}Y) [57], and most frequently employed radioisotopes in SPECT consist of iodine (^{123}I), iodine (^{125}I), iodine (^{131}I), indium (^{111}In), technetium (^{99}mTc), and gallium (^{67}Ga) [6]. In recent reports, researchers used nanoscale materials for the handling of nuclear radionuclides in the biological environment [58].

Photo-acoustic imaging (PAI)
PAI is a hybrid type of imaging modality which consists of the combination of optical imaging and ultrasound imaging. PAI is mainly based on the photoacoustic effect in which tissues are heated in an inductive way by absorbing non-destructive laser energy and following this procedure it produces a wide acoustical wave of the order of MHz frequency due to momentary thermoelastic expansion [28]. These photoacoustic waves can be detected and distinguished by ultrasound transducers at the surface of the tissues and can be reconstructed to produce the ultrasound images (figure 3.4(C)). PAI imaging provides an outstanding platform for visualizing biological entities with good contrast, penetration depth and spatial resolution and has conquered the limitations of OI and US imaging [29]. Metallic nanoparticles like silver (Ag), gold (Au), carbon (C) and quantum dots show better contrasting ability in PAI imaging [59, 60].

3.2.1 Types of nanoplatforms as imaging agents

Although progress in the biomedical field sustain cancer diagnostics and therapy with better survival propects, these techniques still have some constraints. In recent years, the applicability of the non-destructive imaging of cancer diagnostics and treatment has turned out to be a crucial part of clinical level practice. On the other hand, currently available contrasting agents and tracers that are broadly employed in clinical practices, have their own inherent constraints and drawbacks. Nanoscale technologies with advanced *in vivo* diagnosis and improved targeted efficacy of cancer have the ability to conquer these constraints of cancer diagnostics and therapies. Theranostics nanomaterial has superior ability to act as a therapeutics representation, which possesses the capability to load the targeting molecules for both imaging and therapy function. The obtained nano-systems will be expected to be crucial with the advancement of customized medicines due to their diagnosis potentiality, efficacy in drug transportation and capability to supervise patient response to the therapeutics. Nanoscale structures are found to be able to deliver different types of probe for imaging purposes, which in turn advance early stages of cancer diagnosis by multi-modal imaging techniques. The employment of multifunctional nanoscale materials for imaging techniques with different modalities has the prospect of overcoming the constraints of individual imaging modality by advancing the resolution, tissue penetration depth, probe sensitivity, temporal resolution period, gathering data, economical factor and clinical significance. Surface functionalized nanostructures have been disclosed to perform as a drug or as gene transporters and they can also be enclosed within the agent that targets the molecules like antibodies and aptamers, which may be utilized for diagnostic and therapeutic puropses. The different type of nanostructures viz. organic nanostructures, inorganic nanostructures and hybrid nanostructures are discussed below.

3.2.1.1 Organic nanostructures

Scientific investigations in nanoscale platform based molecular level imaging and drug transportation have promoted significant progression in cancer diagnosis and therapy, the synchronized applications of cancer therapeutics and diagnostics. Theranostics nanoscale materials have expanded their applicability by utilizing the various materials, and organic nanomaterials are of foremost attention in synthesis and preparation. A range of organic nanomaterials have individual benefits depending on different physical, chemical and biological features of the base material.

Effectual imaging modalities assist in timely diagnosis of cancer tumors and offer a non-destructing surveillance of theranostics responses. Timely diagnosis and therapy monitoring are necessary to improve the survival of patients. Therefore, novel image contrast enhancing agents are much needed for successful clinical trials. Scientists and technologists have demonstrated diverse approaches for the advancement of novel imaging techniques by effectual use of proteins, viruses, antibodies and peptides as targeting agents [61]. In 1993, the FDA approved the very first radio-labeled antibodies which were employed for cancer imaging [62]. Extremely precise imaging contrasting agents are requisite for non-destructive monitoring of the molecular level process via molecular level imaging. Although scientists have developed a number of imaging candidates for cancer diagnosis and therapy monitoring, many of them are constrained by sub-optimal tumor growth [63]. To address this issue, antibodies are being developed as promising candidates for molecular level imaging. The different features of the antibody such as highly specific nature, comparatively lower immunogenicity, clinical relevance etc makes them appropriate for molecular level imaging. Consequently, many antibodies are available in the market which are approved and validated by the FDA and some of them are in process of the FDA approval [64]. Moreover, the chances of off-site toxicity of antibodies with chemotherapy is low as they are highly specific for proteins. Figure 3.7 shows the assembly of antibodies-based molecular level imaging which necessitates a contrast enhancing material specifically for the imaging techniques.

Recently, some nanobodies have been integrated for cancer imaging at molecular level [65]. They are of particular interest due to their stability, specificity, rapid distribution, and binding ability, and can be easily evacuated from the body [66, 67]. These properties makes nanobodies perfect for beneficial molecular level cancer imaging. Various molecular level imaging techniques are being developed clinically such as PET, oi technique, SPECT etc [68, 69].

Nuclear level imaging in a targeted manner uses the various types of radionuclide such as zirconium-89, technetium-99m, gallium-68 with half-lives of 78, 6 h and 68 min respectively. Huang *et al* investigated anti-epidermal growth factor receptor

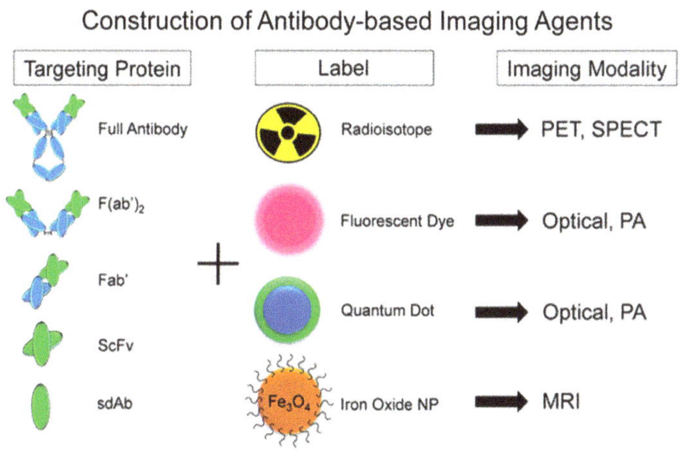

Figure 3.7. Assembly of antibodies-based molecular level imaging necessitates a contrast enhancing material specifically for the imaging techniques. Full as well as fragmented antibody can be utilized as a targeting agent. Radioisotope is utilized for PET and SPECT imaging. Fluorescence dye and quantum dot are employed for OI and PAI. Magnetic (e.g., Fe_3O_4) NPs are frequently employed in MRI (reprinted with permission from [12], copyright (2016) American Chemical Society).

(EGFR) nanobodies as a targeting agent in SPECT [70]. These nanobodies were labeled with technetium-99m as a radionuclide. The *in vivo* studies carried out by them displayed that a clear differentiation between tumors is probable. They also have investigated anti-EGFR nanobodies labeled with technetium-99m-7C12 as a radionuclide to supervise the responses of tumor to the tyrosine kinase inhibitor. The uptakes of technetium-99m-7C12 in tumor were concluded by employing SPECT in the mouse model having A431 human tumor cells. From these studies, the authors have demonstrated that technetium-99m-7C12 is a potential candidate to monitor the treatment responses [71].

Nanobodies are also applied in the area of US imaging techniques. In the US imaging technique, the sound waves are employed to record the images reflected by the different tissues and organs. The nanobodies targeted with the vascular cell adhering protein 1, i.e. VCAM1, were demonstrated for micro-bubble targets [72]. The signaling received from nanobodies attached micro-bubbles are seen to be improved in comparison with the control micro-bubbles. When probed with this method, the applicability of nanobodies targeting is helpful as it provides safer, faster and cost-effective imaging together with comparatively superior image quality [73].

Very recently, molecular level OI technique employed with a targeting contrast enhancing agent have been of great interest to biomedical researchers. This was made achievable due to advancements in near infrared fluorescence. Currently, OI is undertaken as it is safer, more sensitive, faster and economically beneficial in comparison with the existing imaging methods [69, 74, 75]. Recently, Oliveira *et al* [67] have demonstrated a potential material for OI with the use of nanobody as a targeted agent. In their investigations, the near infrared fluorophores are coupled to the EGFR targeted nanobodies 7D12 and towards the negative controlled nanobodies R2. Also, mAb cetuximab was incorporated for the sake of comparative study. After infrared coupling, the specific nature and affinity of this nanoprobe was firstly verified *in vitro*. It was clear that the coupling of infrared does not have any detrimental effects on the affinities of 7D12 for EGFR. A similar kind of study was done in which nanobodies as anti-HER2 were demonstrated for OI technique towards human breast cancer [76]. Moreover, 11A4-IR showed its applicability in imaging assisted therapies [76]. In comparison with SPECT and PET in which roughly 60 min are required for a single scanning, nanobodies intermediated OI with near infrared requires significantly less time, i.e. less than 60 sec/ image with pre-clinical systems. Moreover, because of the easily obtainable coupling techniques, the applicability of nanobodies in OI assisted cancer therapies is greatly desirable [76].

Chet and co-workers have demonstrated dimeric BODIPY (BDP) incorporated a liposome conjugated with anti-hypoxia antibody for imaging applications [77]. They utilized the liposome as a carrier by encapsulating dimeric BODIPY into the shells of the liposome, which features BODIPY structures customized with a nitro-group as shown in figure 3.8(a). The surface of the liposome was decorated with Cy

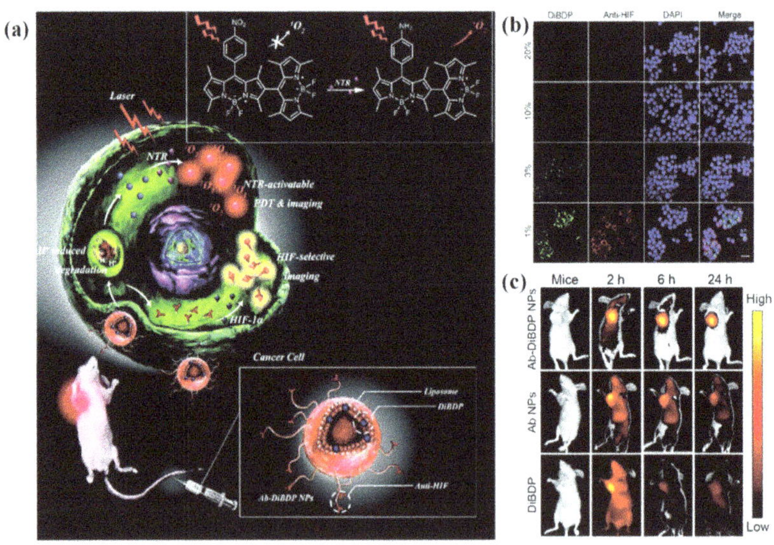

Figure 3.8. (a) Schematic illustration of dimeric BDP-loaded liposome for dual hypoxia marker imaging and activatable photodynamic therapy against tumors. (b) Confocal fluorescence microscopy imaging of cells incubated with nanoprobe under hypoxic conditions. (c) Time-based *in vivo* fluorescence imaging of mice model after injection with nanoprobes (all the images reproduced with permission from [78] with permission of The Royal Society of Chemisty).

7-marked anti-hypoxia antibodies. The fluorescent nanoprobes were receptive to HIF-1a and NTR, and they are extremely up regulating inside the hypoxia cell (figure 3.8(b)). *In vivo* studies showed that, nanoprobes can be utilized for imaging two kinds of hypoxia related biomarker and produce proficient $^1O_2$ under hypoxia condition to attain photodynamic therapy (figure 3.8(c)). Remarkably, concurrent imaging of the manifold hypoxias biomarker may possibly improve the accuracy of tumors hypoxias in contrast with singular markers receptive, as hypoxias are mainly linked with several markers which can be also articulated into the healthy cell.

Previous reports signify that near infrared fluorescence dye in combination with self-assembled smaller bio-molecule and peptides may offer greater imaging modality [79, 80]. Laxman *et al* [79] developed L, Ldiphenylalanine-coupled BF2-oxasmaragdyrin self-assembly as a potential theranostic candidate with better imaging ability. In light of this, non-destructive live animal fluorescent image studies were demonstrated following intravenously injected nanoformulations in mice. After 24 h of injection, considerably stronger fluorescent was observed all though the body of mice which is 100-fold greater than that of the surrounding body signals. It evidently advocates that these nanoplatforms possess potentiality for advanced level tumor imaging (figure 3.9(a–c)). The prepared NPs possess

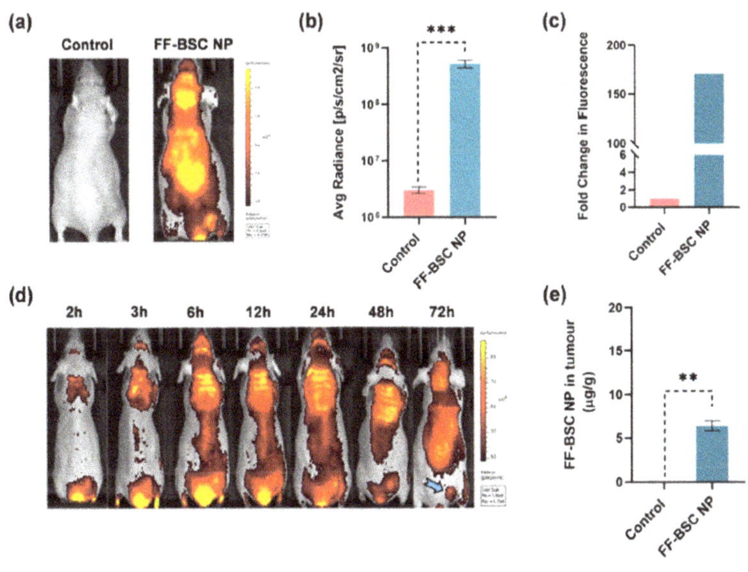

Figure 3.9. Whole-body fluorescence imaging and tumor homing. (a) Whole-body fluorescence imaging of control and FF-BSC NP-injected mice 24 h post material administration. (b) Quantification of total fluorescence from the whole-body of control and FF-BSC NP-injected mice. (c) Fold change in fluorescence output in FF-BSC NP-injected mice compared to control mice. (d) Fluorescence images indicating tumor homing of nanoparticles in FF-BSC NP-injected mice. (e) absolute quantification of the amount of FF-BSC NPs in the tumor tissue of control and FF-BSC NP-injected mice (all the images reproduced with permission from [79], copyright 2020, The Authors, with permission of Springer).

fluorescence all through the body during the starting period as observed in fluorescent imaging. After time periods of 24, 48 and 72 h, the specified homing of a part of the NPs was noted in the tumor (figure 3.9(d)). In addition to this, the tumor tissues were harvested, frozen and homogenized to extract the compounds for the investigation of quantity of materials accreted. The fluorescent images of the compound extracts were noted and the quantity was measured. The measured quantity indicated that a very low quantity, i.e. 6–7 $\mu g\ g^{-1}$ out of 300 μg, was accumulated inside the tumor tissues (figure 3.9(e)).

3.2.1.2 Inorganic nanostructures

The remarkable progression in the preparation, functionalization and characterization of the various inorganic nanostructures with pre-defined sizes, shapes, structures, compositions and surface features has notably elevated their potential in the biomedical area. Inorganic nanostructures have gained enhanced consideration in recent decades as a prospective diagnosis and therapeutics system in the area of oncology. Inorganic nanostructures have displayed considerable outcomes in the area of imaging and therapy of the cancer cell, both *in vivo* and *in vitro*, with promising features for clinical practice. Table 3.3 summarizes the different types of inorganic nanomaterials employed for cancer imaging.

Nanoscale copper sulphides have been of great interest for the diverse imaging techniques due to their significant optoelectronic properties. Copper sulphides have been applied widely in many of the imaging techniques and some of them are discussed further. CuS nanoparticles (CuS-NPs) with an average size below 5 nm possess exceptional physicochemical and pharmacokinetic properties and are promising for many biomedical areas. CuS-NPs are permissible for PAI as they can effortlessly transform the photon energy when exposed to near infrared light. On the other hand, with their lower toxic nature and low cost, the MRI and PET potentiality makes CuS-NPs more desirable multifunctional theranostics agents that show significant advancements in molecular level imaging and cancer therapies [85]. Nanoscale theranostics material based on CuS-NPs was also developed for tri-modal imaging and multi-modal therapies of brain cancer cells. Also, they possess ability in treatment of deep cancer tumors, because of this the near infrared lasers penetrate deep into cancer cells causing little or no harm [86]. As mentioned, CuS-NPs may be applicable for pre-clinical and clinical application in PAI in particular for apparently observed tumors such as breast lesion, limbs, head, neck and lymph nodes.

The applicability of metal NPs as a contrast enhancing agent for MRI is considerably advancing the sensitivity of medical imaging. Amongst the parameters affecting the signaling intensities and contrast in MRI, the relaxation of protons is the main factor which considerably influences the contrasting of tissue. In addition to magnetic NPs, CuS-NPs were also investigated for MRI application. Copper ions have extraordinary photo-thermal properties which can be employed for theranostic applications. Also, they can be combined with other

Table 3.3. Inorganic nanomaterials for cancer imaging (table reproduced with permission from [17], copyright 2020 Wiley Periodicals LLC).

Technique	Material	Reference
Magnetic resonance imaging	Transition metal ions and rare earth metal ions (Cu^{2+}, Mn^{2+}, Fe^{3+} and Gd^{3+})	[36]
	Metal oxides (MnO, GdF_3, Gd_2O_3 and $GdPO_4$)	[34, 35, 81, 82]
	Spinel ferrite NPs ($NiFe_2O_4$, Fe_3O_4, $CoFe_2O_4$, $MnFe_2O_4$)	[32]
Computed tomography	Iodine (I)	[83]
	Gold (Au)	[40]
	Bismuth (Bi)	[42]
	Tantalum (Ta)	[41]
Optical imaging	Quantum dot (QDs)	[50]
	Lanthanide atoms	[51]
	Carbon nanotubes	[52]
	Gold-based nanostructure	[53]
Positron emission tomography	^{11}C, ^{68}Ga, ^{18}F, ^{89}Zr, ^{64}Cu, ^{86}Y	[84]
Single-photon emission computed tomography	^{123}I, ^{99m}Tc, ^{67}Ga, ^{125}I, ^{111}In, ^{131}I	[6]
Photo-acoustic imaging	Metallic and semiconducting NPs (Ag, Au, C, QDs)	[59, 60]

metallic groups having MRI contrasting ability to achieve effective imaging. These things make copper based material more appropriate, particularly in cancer imaging and image guiding therapy [87, 88]. Gadolinium (Gd) is one of the most applied metallic materials in MRI applications. Thus, CuS-NPs coupled with Gd ions have been investigated by many researchers [89]. It was found that, the coupling of CuS-NPs with Gd significantly enhanced the imaging ability in comparison with Gd alone. Alongside Gd ions, other metal ions were also coupled with CuS-NPs for their probable applications in MRI imaging. Liu *et al* investigated surface functionalized CuS-NPs with Mn^{2+} chelate as functional material [90]. They showed that, prepared multifunctional materials possess lower cytotoxic nature and stronger near infrared absorption. The loading of Mn^{2+} in CuS-NPs matrix switched the higher relaxivity and the Cu ions enable image assisted photothermal therapy.

Metallic NPs are being broadly investigated for imaging modalities like PET, MRI and in fluorescence imaging. They possess extraordinary optoelectronic properties which advance the imaging ability of NPs. Copper NPs irrespective of their excellent optical properties, they also possess excellent solubility in water and

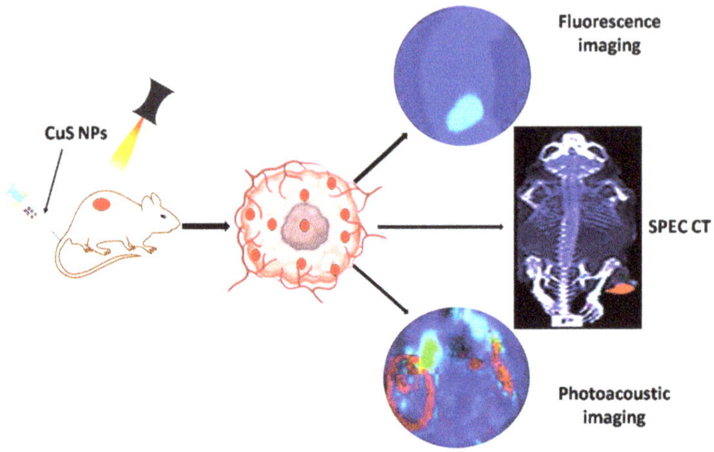

Figure 3.10. Different imaging applications of CuS-NPs (image reproduced with permission from [85], copyright (2020), with permission from Elsevier)).

are economically cheaper. CuS-NPs also exhibits excellent optoelectronic properties depending upon their size. Chen *et al* [91] investigated the CuS-NPs combined with the luminescence NPs for the fluorescence imaging application. The luminescence NPs were offered sustainable luminescence, while CuS has offered the optically enabled activation and the photo-thermal effect. Fluorescent CuS-NPs with surface functionalization of RGD for targeting proves them as a non-invasive multi-modal tumor targeted imaging candidate. Thus, CuS-NPs combined with imaging candidates and targeted agents would be of great interest for the multi-modal diagnosis and therapies specially for cancer-like diseases to reduce the unwanted negative effects of the treatments. Figure 3.10 displays the different imaging applications of CuS-NPs.

Recently, gadolinium based oxide NPs have emerged for several bio-applications owing to their comparatively less toxic nature and potential imaging gesture for MRI [92, 93], cells labeling [94], and as drug carriers [95, 96]. Distinct from gadolinium chelate, the properties of gadolinium oxide NPs could be tailored by altering the size, shape and surface modifications (figure 3.11) [99]. Nanoscale gadolinium oxide NPs are being reported to possess higher T_1 relaxivity due to their higher specific surface area. Recently, Shen and co-workers reported smaller gadolinium oxide NPs with size less than 2 nm and significantly higher r_1 value of the order of 70 $mM^{-1}\ s^{-1}$ [97]. In the meantime, Gd_2O_3 NPs with small particles size facilitated penetration of the blood–brain barrier [100]. Thus, gadolinium oxide NPs are specifically developed with size less than 15 nm. Cho and his research group fabricated nanoplates of gadolinium oxide with average diameters in the range of 2–20 nm. Their outcomes indicate the significant enhancement in r_1 values with the decrement of nanoplates size, and for nanoplates with size 2 nm the r_1 value was found to be 10 times greater as compared to

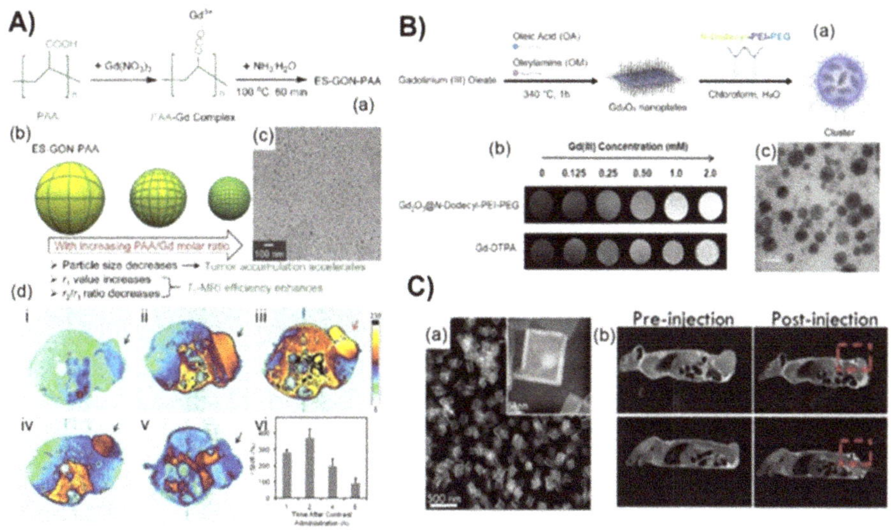

Figure 3.11. Preparation of gadolinium oxide based nanomaterials with different sizes, shapes and surface coatings, and their applications in MR imaging. (A) (a), (b) synthetic schematic of PAA-stabilized exceedingly small gadolinium oxide nanoparticles (ES-GON-PAA); (c) TEM image of ES-GON1–5-PAA; (d) *in vivo* MRI scan of U-87 MG tumor-bearing nude mice with ES-GON5-PAA@RGD2 nanoparticles as a contrast agent and its SNR at different time points. Reprinted with permission from [97], copyright 2019 John Wiley & Sons. (B) (a) Synthetic schematic of Gd_2O_3@N-Dodecyl-PEI-PEG clusters; (b) T_1-weighted MR intensity of the cluster compared with clinical Gd-DTPA; (c) TEM image of the cluster. Reprinted from [98], copyright (2020), with permission from Elsevier. (C) (a) TEM image of Gd_2O_3 nanoscrolls; (b) *in vivo* MRI scans of A-375 tumor-bearing mice before and after the injection of Gd2O3 nanoscrolls. Reprinted with permission from [95], copyright 2019 John Wiley & Sons.

the commercially available Gd-DTPA [101]. In accordance with these outcomes, nanoscale gadolinium oxide as MRI contrast enhancing agent can significantly sharpen the contrast in the images produced from gadolinium and it can also uphold a more biocompatible environment.

Although, gadolinium is one of the most used materials for MRI, the combination of gadolinium with another biomaterial or the imaging probe may offer enhanced imaging quality or may provide multi-modal imaging. In this line, biomaterials such as carbon nanomaterials, luminescence materials, persistent luminescence NPs, gold NPs etc can be coupled with gadolinium ions for enhanced bio-imaging [102–105].

Carbon nanomaterials in the form of quantum dots, nanotubes, fullerene and graphene [106] are promising in the area of cancer diagnosis and therapies. Due to their superior specific surface area, they can offer deliverance of a greater number of imaging agents at the cancer tumor site for possible imaging. In addition, carbon nanomaterials can perform as defensive layers to ensure mono-dispersibility and biocompatibility of the NPs. Carbon nanomaterials enhance the r_1 value of gadolinium NPs via two approaches: offering geometric confinements of the

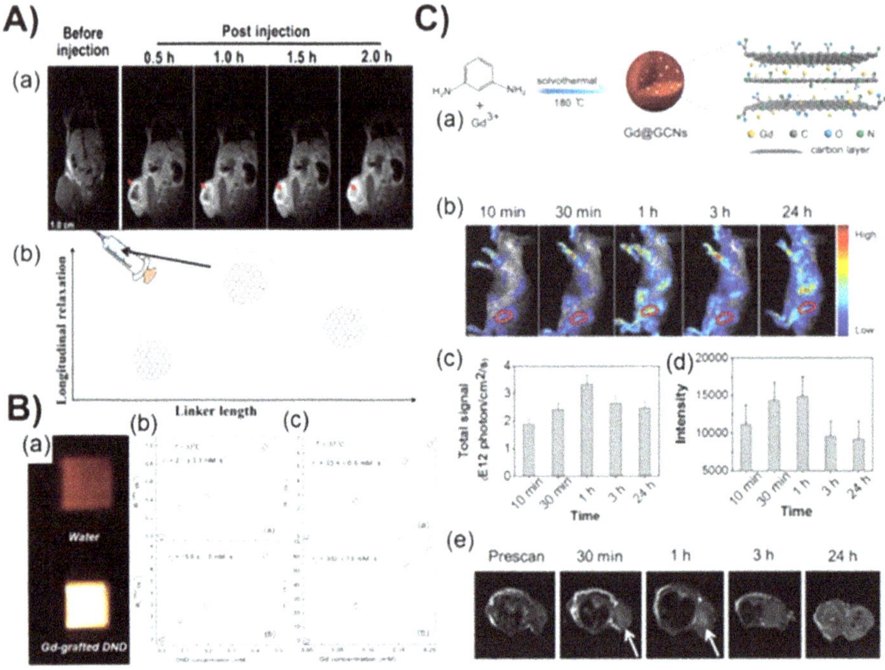

Figure 3.12. Applications of Gd-carbon hybrid-based nanomaterials in MR imaging. (A) (a) T_1-weighted MR images of A549 tumor-bearing mice with paramagnetic graphene quantum dots (PGQD) as a contrast agent; (b) the relationship between longitudinal relaxation of PGOD and the length of PEG in PGOD. Reprinted with permission from [107]. Copyright 2018 American Chemical Society. (B) (a) T_1-weighted MR images of water and Gd-grafted detonation nanodiamond (DND) containing square spectrophotometer cells; R_1 and R_2 relaxation rates of water protons affected by DND (b) and Gd-grafted DND (c). Reprinted with permission from [108]. Copyright 2018 American Chemical Society. (C) (a) Synthetic schematic of Gd-encapsulated Graphene carbon nanoparticles (Gd@GCNs); (b–e) *in vivo* fluorescence images (b) and T1-weighted MR images (e) of tumor-bearing nude mice with Gd@GCNs as a contrast agent and their corresponding signal intensity for fluorescence images (c) and T1-weighted MR images (d). Reprinted with permission from [109], copyright 2018, John Wiley & Sons.

gadolinium ion and/or increments τ_r of gadolinium chelate (figure 3.12). In light of this, carbon coated very small Gd_2O_3 NPs have been fabricated and showed enhanced r_1 relaxivity of the order of 16.26 $mM^{-1}\ s^{-1}$ in *in vitro* studies and 1.5 folded signals improvement in major organs of mice. Moreover, Manus *et al* reported that the agglomeration of nanodiamond particles combined with the Gd chelate directs to an expanded rotational correlation time which results in a considerable increase in the r_1 relaxivity [110].

In recent years, incorporation of metallic ions like Gd and Au in the matrix of organic materials to develop hybrid nanoscale materials has been launched in the areas of cancer diagnostics, detection and surveillance. Generally, metallic ions such

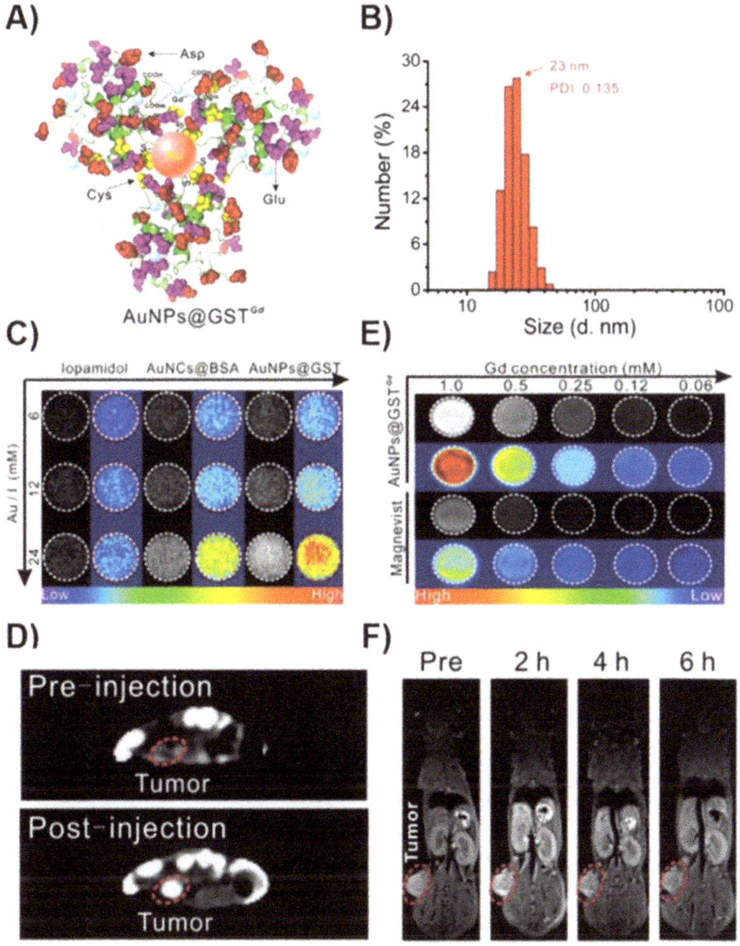

Figure 3.13. Protein-mediated bio-mimetic synthesis of a Gd-Au hybrid nanostructure for tumor bimodal imaging. (a) Model characterization and (b) hydrodynamic diameter of AuNPs@GSTGd; (c) *In vitro* CT images of clinically used iopamidaol, AuNCs@BSA and AuNPs@GST at varying Au/I concentrations, and (d) *in vivo* CT imaging of tumor-bearing mice before and after intratumoral injections of AuNPs@GSTGd. (e) *In vitro* MR images of clinically approved Magnevist and AuNPs@GSTGd at varying Gd concentrations. (f) *In vivo* MR imaging of tumor-bearing mice at different time points before and after intravenous injection of AuNPs@GSTGd (all the images reproduced with permission from [111], copyright (2018), with permission from Elsevier).

as Gd and Au contribute towards cancer imaging and the organic materials assist in improvement of the biocompatibility and stability of the metallic ions. In this line, Yang *et al* [111] developed nanoscale Gd/Au hybrid materials with the help of human proteins, i.e. glutathione S-transferase (figure 3.13). Gadolinium ions were decorated in the Au nano matrix in attendance of glutathione S-transferase. In

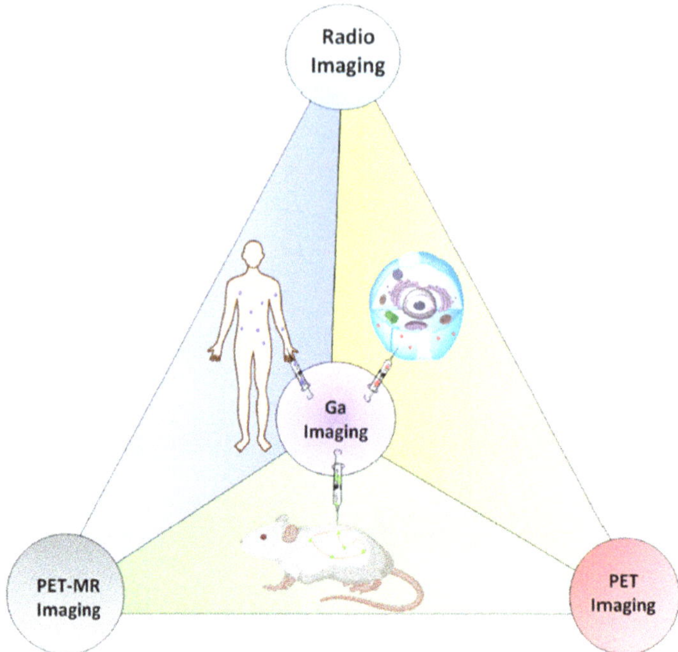

Figure 3.14. Gallium based imaging nanoscale platforms (image reproduced from [112], copyright (2020), with permission from Elsevier).

addition to its outstanding biocompatible nature and reduced immunogenicity, the magnetic resonance signals intensities formed by Au@GSTGd were found to be twice those of the commercially available Magnevist (Gd-DTPA). Furthermore, it displayed excellent contrast in CT images in comparison to the currently used Iopamidaol and accreted in the tumor region, partly assigned to its extending circulation period [111], which may be used as an effectual contrasting enhancer for cancer tumors imaging.

With regards to inorganic NPs, Fe-based NPs have governed the area of bio-imaging alongside gadolinium (Gd) ions [112]. Many Fe-based NPs in pristine form and surface functionalized form were approved by FDA for clinical imaging applications. The major imaging utilities of Fe-based colloid are linked with MRI, whereas only a few of them are being exposed for other imaging applications. Conversely, for imaging engaging Ga-based colloid, the majority of imaging categorizes into radio-imaging. This gap was reduced by engaging Ga and other metallic NPs to develop coupled systems through which Ga-based colloid may be applied for imaging techniques other than radio-imaging like PET or MR. Figure 3.14 shows the Ga-based nanoscale platforms for imaging of cancer tumors.

The most recent tracers utilized for molecular level imaging were formed by the combination of radionuclide and nanoscale materials which influences the sensitivity of the imaging modalities. This potential approach expands its scope for application

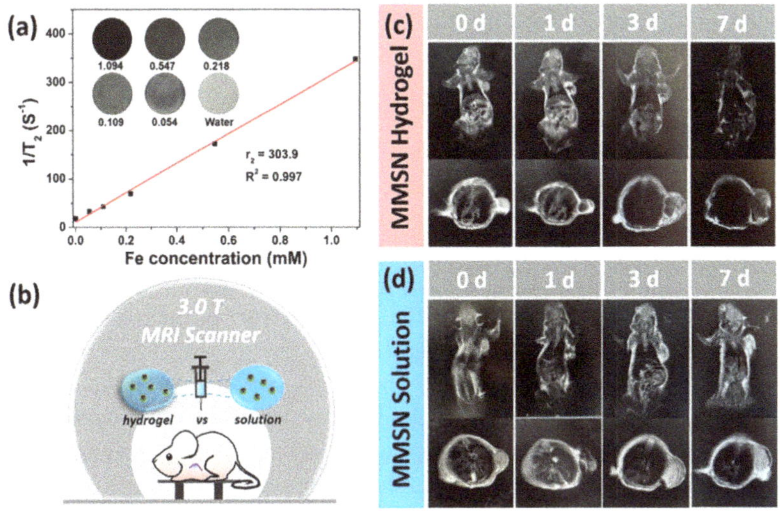

Figure 3.15. (a) T_2-weighted MRI of MMSN-RBITC aqueous dispersion with different Fe concentrations, and T_2 transverse relaxation rate as a function of Fe concentration. (b) A schematic illustration showing the procedure of MRI on the difference of the intratumoral injection. *In vivo* MRI of a tumor-bearing mouse with intratumoral injection of (c) MMSN-RBITC hydrogel and (d) MMSN-RBITC dispersion (all the images reproduced with permission from [115], copyright (2020), with permission from Elsevier).

which may also comprise theranostics applications. The use of Ga-based NPs as a radionuclide was clearly applicable in the area of radio nanoscale materials. Ga-68 was considered as one of the user-friendly isotopes as it can simply produce because of its dual physicochemical properties. This is replicated in previous pre-clinical as well as clinical studies [113, 114].

Wang *et al* [115] reported the design and development of self-healing hydrogels (PULL-CS hydrogels) containing anti-cancer drugs and rhodamine B isothiocyanate (RBITC) labeled Mn–Zn ferrite/silica core–shell (MMSN-RBITC) nanostructure in spherical form for MRI and therapy. Magnetic resonance (MR) bio-imaging was favored in clinics with greater spatial resolutions and no side effects. The T_2 weighted MR contrast evaluation of MMSN-RBITC dispersions were estimated under Fe concentration ranging from 0–1.1 mM (figure 3.15 (a)). MMSN-RBITC displayed the Fe-content based T_2 weighted MR intensity. The transversal relaxations rate ($1/T_2$) was incremented with increase in Fe ion concentration, which yields a relaxivity, i.e. r_2 of the order of 303.9 mM^{-1} s^{-1}. The higher relaxivity showed that the nanospheres possess the ability to significantly enhance the MR contrasting for *in vitro* and *in vivo*. Thus, the *in vivo* MRI of the MMSN-RBITC dispersions and hydrogels were executed with the help of a 3T MRI scanner, as shown in figure 3.15(b). In comparison with the zero-dimensional image without injection, the T_2 weighted tumors image in MMSN dispersions and hydrogels noticeably becomes darker subsequent to the intratumoral injections of nanospheres, whereas the contrasts in hydrogels remained after the seventh day unlike the solutions group due to the hydrogels extending the preservation of the loaded nanospheres (figure 3.15(c) and (d)). All these outcomes showed the coupling effects of MRI and retentive effects of the self-healing hydrogels.

Recently, palladium (Pd)-based nanoscale material is of great interest for bio-applications owing to its excellent optical properties, enhanced stability and better biocompatible nature in a biological environment [116]. In comparison with the broadly investigated nanoscale materials like gold and silver NPs, the studies related to Pd based NPs was undertaken more recently, but due to their extraordinary properties they gained a lot of attention in the area of nanoscale medicines. Pd in different nanoscale forms such as NPs, nanosheets, nanocomposites exhibited stronger absorbing power in the NIR region, stability in photo-thermal conversions and extraordinary biocompatibility. In consideration of these characteristics properties, Pd based nanoscale materials can be promising for imaging cancer tumors.

With extensive advancement in imaging modalities, design and development of superior contrasting agent have been gaining attention of researchers. In view of the imaging mechanism, PAI and CT may be comprehended by Pd based nanoscale materials due to their inbuilt properties, whereas MRI and SPECT mostly depend on combined contrasting agents like Gd or I, which can be decorated on Pd based nanoscale materials and can be transported to the tumor region. All these imaging techniques display exceptional benefits and may accompany each other to attain proper diagnostics in a sensitive and specific manner.

Pd based nanosheet possesses stronger absorbing power in the near infrared range and therefore holds significant potentiality for PAI contrasting agent. For the very first time, Nie *et al* investigated Pd based nanosheet for PAI of cancer tumor [117]. Pd based nanosheets with average diameters of 16 nm have shown stronger near infrared absorption and allowed superior PAI of cancer tumor following intravenously injected nanosheet in tumor containing mice. Unlike Au nanorods, Pd based nanosheet exhibited higher stability and the morphologies can be maintained with absorption after long-term laser irradiations. Pd based nanosheet with size in the range of 5–80 nm possesses superior PAI *in vitro*, whereas significant contrasting effects can be noted in mice after the injection of very small Pd nanosheets (5, 13 and 30 nm) because of the size dependent accumulating nature *in vivo* (figure 3.16(A–B)) [118]. Chen *et al* investigated the preparation of Pd@Au nanoplates using seeded re-growth technique. These nanoplates displayed stronger absorption in the near infrared region and proficiency in accumulations of ultra-high tumors [119]. Therefore, these Pd@Au nanoplates were fruitfully employed for real-time monitoring of the tumors region and PAI guided therapies (figure 3.16(c)).

From the last decade, nanoscale materials are being employed as nanocarriers to control the performance of the radionuclide *in vivo* and the pharmacokinetic and tumors uptake of nanoscale materials can be represented non-destructively via SPECT imaging. Instigated by the stronger coordinating effects between the halide ion and Pd based materials, which follow the ordering iodine (I)>bromide (Br) >chlorine (Cl), many investigations on the applications of Pd based nanoscale materials in SPECT imaging have been reported in literature [120, 121]. Radio-labeled Pd based nanosheets are being achieved by simpler mixing of the Pd

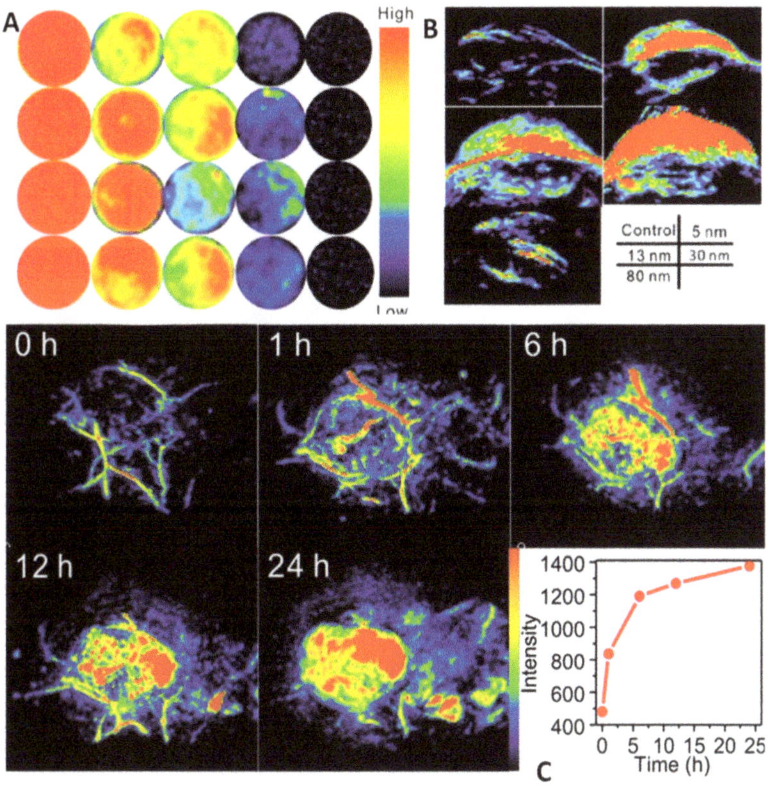

Figure 3.16. PA imaging application of different sized Pd NSs (a) *in vitro* and (b) *in vivo*. Reproduced from [118], copyright 2016, Tsinghua University Press and Springer-Verlag Berlin Heidelberg, with permission of Springer. (c) Application of Pd@Au nanoplates in PA imaging of tumor. Reproduced with permission from [119], copyright 2014 John Wiley & Sons.

nanosheet with ^{131}I, which results in higher labeling efficiency of the order of 98% (figure 3.17(a)). Fascinatingly, the adsorption of radioisotope onto the surfaces of Pd based nanosheet shows pH depending performance and superior stability in acidic solutions, which is a superlative material for tumor imaging. Following intravenous injection, a SPECT image with higher quality was obtained in different tumor models (figure 3.17(b)).

CT imaging is a widely employed non-destructive clinical imaging technique, which provides interior anatomical structure of the tissue depending on absorption of x-rays of various tissues. To improve the image quality and contrasting effects of soft tissue, the contrasting agents are loaded prior to the imaging procedures. On the other hand, the clinically iodinated agent frequently suffers from quick excretion and constrained x-rays absorption ability. To tackle this issue, applications of nanomaterial with higher x-rays attenuating coefficient as CT contrasting agent have achieved attention for achievable *in vivo* behavior by optimizing its compositions, morphologies, sizes and surface functionalization [122, 123]. Amongst all of

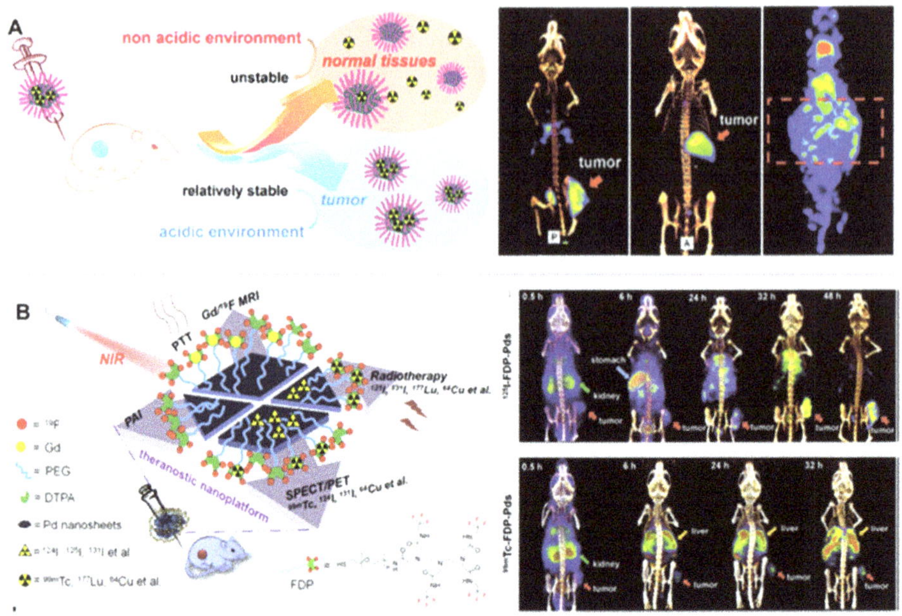

Figure 3.17. pH-sensitive radio-labeled Pd NSs for SPECT imaging in different tumor models, (a) radioactive iodide-labeled Pd NSs ((left) reproduced from [120] with permission of The Royal Society of Chemisty; (right) reproduced from [121], copyright (2018), with permission from Elsevier) and (B) radioactive iodide and ^{99m}Tc-labeled Pd NSs as a multifunctional theranostic platform (reproduced from [121], copyright (2018), with permission from Elsevier).

them, Au based nanoscale materials are gaining interest for CT contrasting agent due to their high atomic number in comparison with iodine, extended blood circulating, improved permeability and are potentially promoted for the development of CT contrasting agent [124, 125]. Even if the atomic number of Pd is much lower than iodine, combination of Pd nanostructure with elements like Au, have made it able to serve as a contrast agents. Recently, Chen *et al* investigated the applications of Pd@Au nanoplates as a CT contrasting agent [119]. Yang *et al* reported the partially coated Pd@Au nanoplate as CT contrasting agent for cancer imaging applications [126].

MRI is one of the promising non-destructive techniques for cellular as well as molecular level imaging with higher spatial resolutions. MRI offers detail information about the soft tissue and organs. For making precise diagnostics of particular diseases, MRI contrasting agents are being frequently employed for the enhancement of the contrasting effects of MRI by upholding relaxations of the surrounded water protons. Similar to the other imaging modalities, coupling with nanoscale materials offers enhanced properties for further advancement of precise diagnostics in pre-clinical as well as clinical level studies. Nanoscale materials with superparamgnetic gesture are promising for MRI imaging by optimizing their size, morphology and surface modifications [127, 128]. Nanoscale materials having no

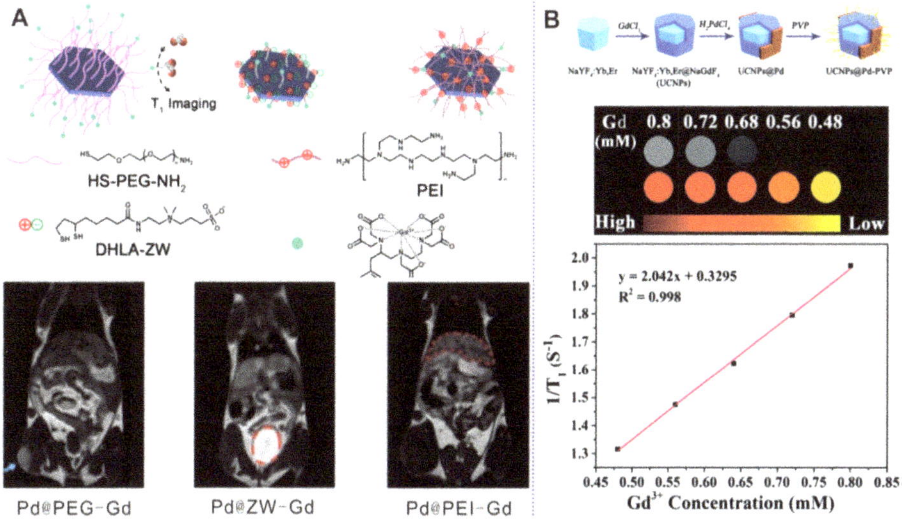

Figure 3.18. (a) Pd nanosheets with different surface modification for MRI imaging. Reprinted with permission from [130], copyright (2015) American Chemical Society. (b) UCNPs@Pd-PVP nanocomposites for T_1-weighted MRI imaging. Reproduced from [131] with permission of The Royal Society of Chemistry.

magnetic features, especially for non-magnetic noble metals like Au nanoparticles, frequently involve chelating with Gd based materials or a combination of MRI contrasting agent by forming heterogeneous structure, core–shell structure, and appropriate surface modifications to obtain the enhancing in contrast of MRI [129]. Via the interactions between polyethylene glycol (PEG), Zwitterionic (ZW) ligand and polyethylenimine (PEI) were modified onto the surface of Pd based nanosheet with Gd at the end of every molecule for real-time MRI for monitoring the effect of surface modification on the biodistribution of Pd nanosheet (figure 3.18(a)) [130]. The outcome of this shows that Pd@PEG-Gd exhibits extended blood circulation period and higher tumor accumulations, whereas Pd@ZW-Gd was quickly cleared via renal. Guo *et al* demonstrated surface functionalized nanoplatforms based on DTPA-PEG-SH decorated Pd nanosheet and employed in MRI imaging application [121]. Additionally, Zhao *et al* demonstrated the fabrication of heterogeneous Pd NPs onto the surface of up-conversion NPs by multiple steps growth technique (figure 3.18(b)) [131]. Due to the incorporation of Gd ions, nanocomposites were effectively employed in MRI contrasting agent by providing a unique way to develop multifunctional nanoscale platforms. Table 3.4 represents the list of Pd based nanoscale materials for cancer imaging applications.

Iron oxide NPs are the most widely studied material for contrast enhancing which is useful for T_2 as well as T_2 weighted MRI. Table 3.5 shows the list of recently developed iron oxide based contrast enhancing agents that are projected for multimodal imaging purposes and drug transportation.

Table 3.4. Palladium based nanomaterials for cancer imaging (table reproduced with permission from [116]).

Imaging modality	Nanomaterials	Ref.
PAI	Pd NSs	[8, 11, 117]
	Pd@Au nanoplates	[6, 12, 119]
	$PdH_{0.2}$ cubes	[132]
	Pd@COS-RGD	[133]
	DOX/Pd@ZIF-8@PDA	[134]
	PdH-MOF	[135]
SPECT imaging	$[^{131}I]$PHPdNPs-DOX	[136]
	^{125}I-Pd-PEG	[137]
	^{99m}Tc-FDP-Pds, ^{125}I-FDP-Pds	[138]
CT imaging	Pd@Au-PEG	[139, 140]
MRI	Pd@PEG-Gd, Pd@PEI-Gd, Pd@ZW-Gd	[130]
	UCNPs@Pd-PVP	[131]
	Gd-FDP-Pds	[138]

Table 3.5. List of different iron oxide based nanoparticles used as MRI probes (table reproduced with permission from [141]).

SPIO-based nanoparticles	Application	Particle size (nm)	Relaxivity (mM^{-1} s^{-1})	Reference
Cy5.5-R_4-SS-CLIO	MR/optical *in vivo* imaging	68 ± 13	r^1 = 27.8; r^2 = 91.2	[142]
Cy5.5-CLIO-EPPT-FITC	MR/optical *in vivo* imaging for uMUC-1 tumor	35.8	r^1 = 26.43; r^2 = 53.44	[143]
Cy5.5-Cltx-PEG-USPIO	MR/optical *in vitro* imaging for glioma brain tumor	10.5 ± 1.5	n.a.	[144]
$CoFe_2O_4$@SiO_2(FITC)	MR/optical *in vitro* imaging	60	n.a.	[145]
$DySiO_2$-(F e3O4)n	MR/optical *in vitro* imaging	46	r^2 = 397	[7, 14, 146]
FePt-Au	MR *in vitro* imaging	6(FePt) −10(Au)	r^2 = 58.7	[148]
PVLA-USPIO	MR *in vivo* imaging for hepatocytes	25.8 ± 6.1	n.a.	[149]
SPIO@SiO_2(FITC)	MR *in vivo* imaging and human stem cell labeling	5 0	r^2 = 128	[1, 15, 150]
USPIO@SiO_2	MR *in vitro* imaging and cell labeling	9.9 ± 1.6	r^1 = 0.55; r^2 = 339.80	[152]
APTMS-USPIO-cRGD	MR *in vitro* imaging for $\alpha_v\beta_3$ integrin	10 ± 3	r^1 = 1.0; r^2= 134.0	[153]

USPIO-4-MC-cRGD	MR *in vivo* imaging for $\alpha_v\beta_3$ integrin	8.4 ± 1.0	$r^2 = 165.0$	[154]
VSOP-Cys-PEG-LCP	MR *in vitro* imaging for lung tumors	6.2 ± 0.9	$r^1 = 11.5$; $r^2 = 142.0$	[155]
SPIO-Doxo@LCP-MFM	MR *in vitro* imaging and drug delivery	48 ~ 60	$r^2 = 400$	[156]

*Abbreviations: CLIO: Cross-linked iron oxide; FITC: fluorescein isothiocyanate; Cltx: Chlorotoxin; PVLA: Polyvinylbenzyl-O-β-D-galactopyranosyl-D-gluconamide; APTMS: Aminopropyl trimethoxysilane; MC: Methylcatechol; Doxo: Doxorubicin; LCP: Lung cancer-targeting peptide; MFM: Multifunctional micelle.

Plasmonically activated gold nanoplatforms provide great applicability in molecular level imaging modalities and cancer therapeutics [157]. In the range of different gold nanoplatforms, star shaped gold nanoplatforms possess flexible behaviour as image contrasting multimodalities for MRI, CT, PET, PAT as well as surface-enhanced Raman imaging. The surface of the gold nanostars are free from surfactants and thus they allow adaptable functionalization to improve cancer cell targeting, and onsite drug delivery. They are also useful for photodynamic as well as photo-thermal therapies. Nanostars of gold having different shapes (figure 3.19(a)), possess enhanced plasmonic gestures in the near infrared tissues optical window and are appropriate for *in vivo* bio-applications. Nanostars of gold offer a significant tool for three-dimensional *in vivo* imaging and diagnosis by complete body scanning. In the case of CT, AuNPs are better than traditionally used contrasting agents as the atomic number of Au is greater ($Z = 79$) and high K-absorption edge (K-edge) value (~80.7 keV). Moreover, water molecules do not affect the x-ray attenuating properties of AuNPs. AuNPs easily absorb x-rays, which consequently produces the photo-electric and Compton effect. This leads to the creation of secondary electrons and reactive oxygen species (ROS). Yielding of this associates with the surface-to-volume ratio of NPs, as Au nanostars display enhanced surface area as compared to spherically shaped AuNPs, and thus nanostars are suitable sensitizers for radio therapies. For MRI, the Gd ion has been attached to Au nanostars surface via DOTA chelators. Figure 3.19(b) displays that a cancer cell encumbered with surface functionalized Au nanostars shows MRI and CT images with higher intensities [158]. PET scans provide very sensible 3D imaging. The sensitivity may reach pico-molar for PET in comparison with micro-molar for MRI. Figure 3.19(c) shows TPL images, where TAT functionalized Au nanostars show high strength signaling within the cell as compared to non-functionalized Au nanostars. Figure 3.19(d) shows PET images for Cu decorated Au nanostars for dynamic images for the period of 24 h. All these outcomes shows the potentiality of the Au nanostars for complete body imaging. Surface functionalized Au nanostars can be employed in the future for cancer therapeutics and diagnosis with different types of imaging. Plasmonic Au nanostars have potential for therapy and diagnosis as they possess combinational abilities with different image modality. Also, Au nanostars show superior applicability for clinical and translational research as a combinational platform for cancer theranostics. Table 3.6 shows a comparative table of the merits and demerits of the various inorganic nanostructures for cancer imaging and therapeutics.

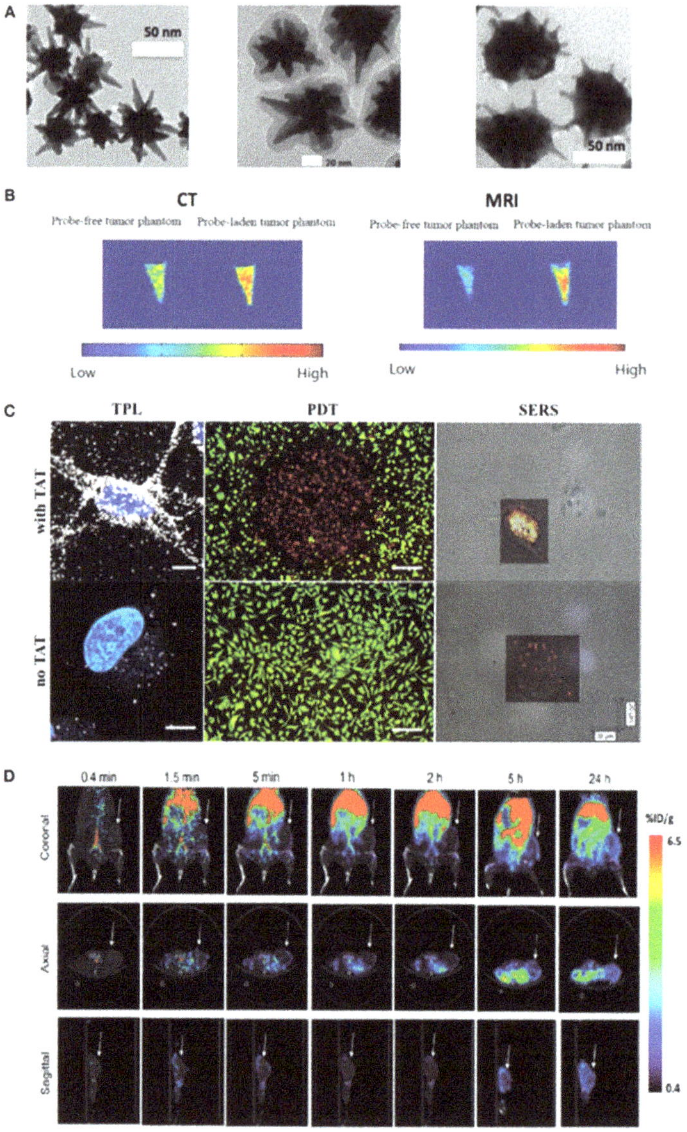

Figure 3.19. (a) TEM images of synthesized AuNS (left), silica-coated AuNS (middle), and silver coated AuNS (right). Adapted with permission from [158], copyright (2015) American Chemical Society and [202], copyright (2011) American Chemical Society. (b) CT (left) and MRI (right) imaging with developed multifunctional AuNS nanoprobe. Reprinted with permission from [205]. (c) Demonstration of TAT-peptide enhanced TPL imaging, photodynamic therapy (PDT), and surface-enhanced Raman scattering (SERS) imaging after 1-h incubation with the AuNS probe. Scale bars for TPL, PDT and SERS image are 10, 250, and 20 μm, respectively. Reprinted with permission from [203], copyright (2013) American Chemical Society (d) PET/CT imaging with ^{64}Cu labeled AuNS probe, which was injected intravenously through tail vein. Dynamic imaging at various time points were acquired. Reproduced with permission from [204], copyright 2013 John Wiley & Sons.

Table 3.6. Comparative table of the merits and demerits of the various inorganic nanostructures for cancer imaging and therapeutics (table reproduced with permission from [159]).

	Cancer imaging/therapeutics		
	Merits	Demerits	Clinical trials for cancer disease
Gold nanoparticles	Biocompatibility [160] Ease of surface functionalization High photo-thermal conversion rate and photostability Intense absorption and scattering greater than organic dyes [162] Micrometer range imaging resolution [163] Single molecule detection limit [164]	Limited penetration depth for imaging and photo-thermal therapy	CYT-6091 (TNF-bound colloidal gold) Phase II [161] AuroShell (gold nanoshells) Phase I (Nanospectra Biosciences, Inc.)
Quantum dots	Higher brightness and photostability than organic dyes [165]	Toxicity Limited imaging resolution and penetration depth	N/A
Carbon nanotubes	Conversion of absorbed light energy into heat [166]	Toxicity [167, 16, 8]	N/A
Magnetic nanoparticles	Biodegradability and biocompatibility [169] Conversion of electromagnetic energy into heat Longer tissue penetration depths for imaging	Opsonization and fast clearance by phagocytes (SPIO) [170]	Feridex I.V. (ferumoxide), Approved Combidex (ferumoxtran-10), Phase I, Phase II [171]
Ceramic nanoparticles	Lower costs materials and relative ease of preparation Biocompatibility [173] High stability [174]	Small pore size (0.5–1 nm) can limit the release of encapsulated drug molecules [172]	N/A

Although inorganic nanostructures have marvelous benefits, advanced translational research related to inorganic nanostructures towards clinical research will need various issues to be tackled in an inclusive way as a component of pre-clinical and clinical practice. The stability of inorganic nanostructures is beneficial as compared to the conventional techniques, however, the extended effects of organic nanostructures still not be studied broadly. Issues connected with long-term tissue damages, toxicity, carcinogenicity, immunogenics and inflammation need to be explicated. It is essential to design and develop inorganic structures with tailored stability, circulation time and localizing ability without compromising their efficiency in order to optimize the need for short period therapy and side effects appearing due to longer exposure time. Altogether, inorganic nanostructures have shown incredible applicability as a theranostic for diagnosis and treatment of cancer. Future studies will establish the translational approach of these inorganic nanostructures toward clinical studies.

3.2.1.3 Hybrid nanostructures

Recently, significant efforts have been made to integrate both the diagnosis and therapeutics functionality within a single nanosized system for effectual treatment of cancer. Nanostructured materials have greater potentiality to attain multi-modal functionality, in particular if more than one type of nanostructured material may be integrated into a nano-assembly referred to as hybrid nanostructures. Several hybrid nanostructures for cancer imaging have emerged and some of them are discussed below.

Jin *et al* developed surface functionalized terpolymeric nanoplatforms for combined imaging and drug transport application [180]. They have coupled diethylenetriamine pentaacetic acid with terapolymers for chelating Gd ions (Gd^{3+}) and studied their applicability for drug transport due to the significant features of surface functionalized terapolymers and the superior contrast enrichment of hydrogel polymers. The features of terapolymers as contrasting enhancer in MRI like T_1 relaxivity and cytocompatibility were investigated *in vitro*. Also, *in vivo* studies with the help of normal and tumor containing mice were investigated for Gd incorporated terapolymers. Figure 3.20(a) shows the T_1 weighted images preceding and for several timings up to 1 h followed by injecting the Omniscan®, Gd incorporated terapolymers (Poly-Gd) and Dox-Gd incorporated terapolymers injected in a single animal. Main organs such as liver, heart, intestine, bladder, and spleen are represented in Slice-A and the other slide, Slice-B, shows kidney, brain and vena cava images. Compared to the Omniscan® dosage, i.e. 0.025 mmol kg^{-1}, both the Gd incorporated terapolymers (Poly-Gd) and Dox-Gd incorporated terapolymers showed significant contrast enhancing in all of the investigated organs. The sequential performance of the whole-body distributions of the contrast enhancing agents were measured by plotting R_1 map at several time periods followed by injecting them into the animal, as shown figure 3.20(b). Figure 3.20(c) displays T_1 weighted magnetic resonance images and the analogous R_1 maps of mice containing tumor cells for before and different time periods followed by the injecting of Poly-Gd and Poly-Gd-Dox with a dosage of 0.025 mmol kg^{-1}. Qualitative investigations of the MR angiographs, shown in

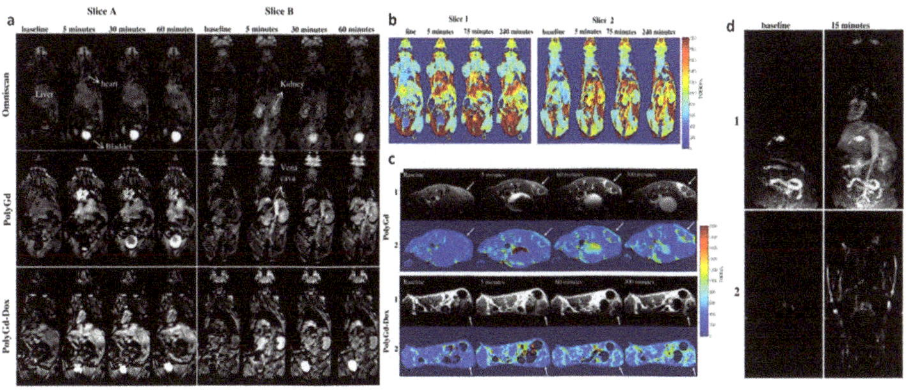

Figure 3.20. (a) T_1-weighted images of mice injected with Omniscan® (0.1 mmol kg^{-1} Gd^{3+}), Poly-Gd (0.025 mmol kg^{-1} Gd^{3+}), and Poly-Gd-Dox (0.025 mmol kg^{-1} Gd^{3+}). The heart, liver, and bladder are represented in Slice A. Slice B shows the kidneys, and vena cava. At one fourth the dose of Omniscan®, the Poly-Gd, and Poly-Gd-Dox produce a much higher contrast over an extended period of time. (b) Quantitative MRI of whole-body distribution: sample R_1 maps of mice injected with Poly-Gd (0.025 mmol kg^{-1} Gd^{3+}). Slice 1 presents the heart, liver and bladder. Slice 2 shows the inferior vena cava and kidneys. (c) Tumor distribution of Poly-Gd and Poly-Gd-Dox (0.025 mmol kg^{-1} Gd^{3+}): T_1-weighted images and the corresponding R_1 maps. (d) MR angiography: MIP angiogram displaying contrast enhancement of the whole body, neck and head regions (all the images reproduced with permission from [174], copyright (2013), with permission from Elsevier).

figure 3.20(d), suggest extended and steady visualizations of the veins and arteries subsequent to the incorporation of contrast enhancing agents. All the outcomes showed that Poly-Gd and Poly-Gd-Dox possess superior properties to advance clinical level imaging modalities.

Abbasi *et al* [175] investigated polymer based theranostics NPs (PT-NPs) enclosing the anti-cancer drug as docetaxel, fluorescence dye, and MnO NPs for dual-mode imaging and therapy. The PT-NPs showed proficient loading of drugs, sustainable drug releasing properties, MRI contrast enhancing and superior cytotoxic nature against human breast cancer cells. The PT-NPs improved the T_1 relaxivity 2.7 fold as compared to individual MnO NPs. Figure 3.21(a) shows the R_1 maps of aMDA-MB-231 tumor-bearing mouse in prone position, at baseline and after 4 and 24 h following IV injection of 0.024 mmol Mn/kg of bodyweight Mn equivalent of PT-NPs. Figure 3.21(b) shows the measured relaxation rates in the liver, kidneys and tumor tissue, at baseline and after 4 and 24 h. The PT-NPs revealed the superior blood circulating, proficient tumor accretion and the improvement in MRI and optical signaling in human breast cancer tumor modeling. The obtained result implies the effectiveness of the PT-NPs for nano theranostics for combined imaging of cancer and drug delivery.

Mao *et al* developed novel NPs with chemically excited near infrared and far infrared emissions and singular oxygen ($^1O_2$) generation for specific imaging and therapy of the tumor [176]. The *in vivo* model containing the breast tumor was developed by incorporating the 4T1 breast cancer cell inside a healthy mouse.

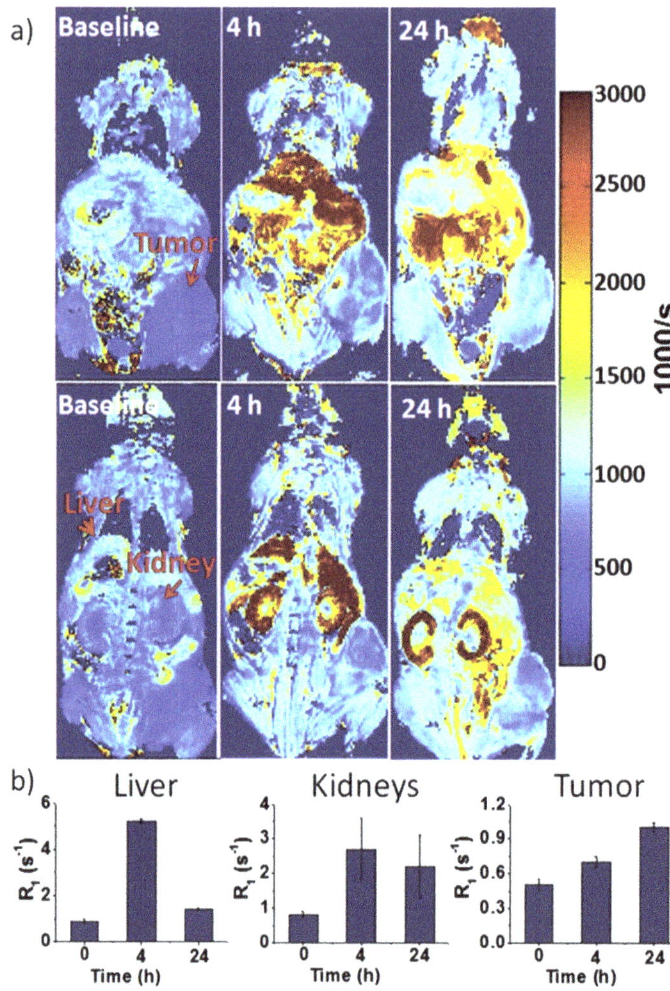

Figure 3.21. (a) R_1 maps of aMDA-MB-231 tumor-bearing mouse in prone position, at baseline and after 4 and 24 h following IV injection of 0.024 mmol Mn/kg of bodyweight Mn equivalent of PT-NPs. The upper region demonstrates a slice at the level of the tumor, while the lower region demonstrates a slice at the level of the liver and kidneys. (b) Measured relaxation rates in the liver, kidneys and tumor tissue, at baseline and after 4 and 24 h (both the images reproduced with permission from [175], copyright (2015), with permission from Elsevier).

Further, the *in vivo* chemiluminescence imaging capability of the prepared NPs was investigated using this tumor model. The prepared NPs were intravenously incorporated into the tumor region and they favorably accumulated in the tumor (figure 3.22(a)). It is observed from the upper region of figure 3.22(b) that, the chemiluminescence signals are only seen inside the tumor region which lasts up to 4 h and is highly intense at around 1.5 h after the incorporation of NPs. In the lower region of figure 3.22(b), the fluorescence signal of the tumor slowly increased with time period and the highest signal was observed at 5 h after the incorporation of

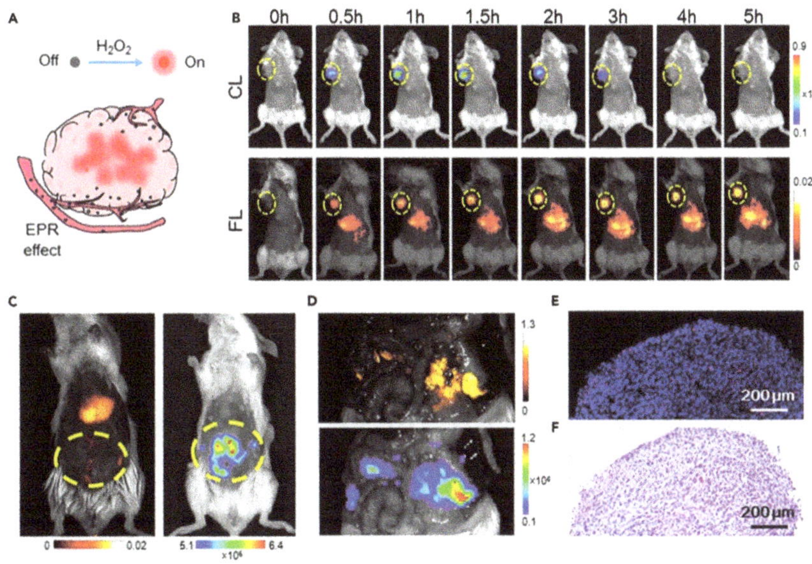

Figure 3.22. Precise and specific abdominal tumor imaging. (a) Schematic illustration of activated C-TBD NPs to image tumor within the H_2O_2-enriched tumor microenvironment. (b) Time-dependent *in vivo* chemiluminescence (top) and fluorescence (bottom) images of mice receiving C-TBD NPs (1 mg ml^{-1} based on C-TBD, 100 ml per mouse) over 5 h periods. Tumor regions are marked with yellow circles. (c) *In vivo* abdominal metastatic breast tumor imaging of a mouse at 1.5 h post intravenous injection with C-TBD NPs (1 mg ml^{-1}, 100 ml per mouse) by fluorescence (left) and chemiluminescence (right) imaging. The tumor region is marked with a yellow circle. (d) *In vivo* abdominal metastatic breast tumor imaging of a mouse with skin and peritoneum removed after intravenous injection with C-TBD NPs (1 mg ml^{-1} based on TBD, 100 ml per mouse) by fluorescence (top) and chemiluminescence (bottom) imaging. (e) Fluorescence imaging of a slice of abdominal metastatic breast tumor in a mouse. The red fluorescence indicates the C-TBD NPs, and the cell nuclei were stained by DAPI (blue). (f) H&E staining of a slice of abdominal metastatic breast tumor (all the images reproduced with permission from [176], copyright (2017), with permission from Elsevier).

NPs. It is observed from the left side of figure 3.22(c) that, after 1.5 h of incorporation of NPs, no evident fluorescence signal was observed from the entire body of the mouse except for the liver area. On the other hand, the right side of figure 3.22(c) shows a chemiluminescence signal noted around the intra-peritoneal region. figure 3.22(d) shows clear fluorescent images of a small intra-peritoneal tumor which are recorded after the surgical elimination of skin and peritoneal. In the meantime, the tumors slice exhibited wider distributions of NPs, showing the specific co-localizing of the chemiluminescence signals and the NPs in all tumor tissue (figure 3.22(e) and (f)). All these outcomes imply that chemiluminescent imaging of C-TBD NPs is appealing for the diagnostics of deeper tumor.

In the past decade, advancement in dendritic polymer materials was noted for the particular field of biomedicines especially for cancer imaging applications [178]. Dendritic polymers, that mainly comprise Dendron, dendrimers, hyperbranched polymer, dendigrafted polymer, and other hybrid polymers [179] are of great interest for the imaging probe in cancer diagnosis and therapy [180, 181]. Their inherent physical and chemical features make dendritic polymers beneficial for cancer imaging and the

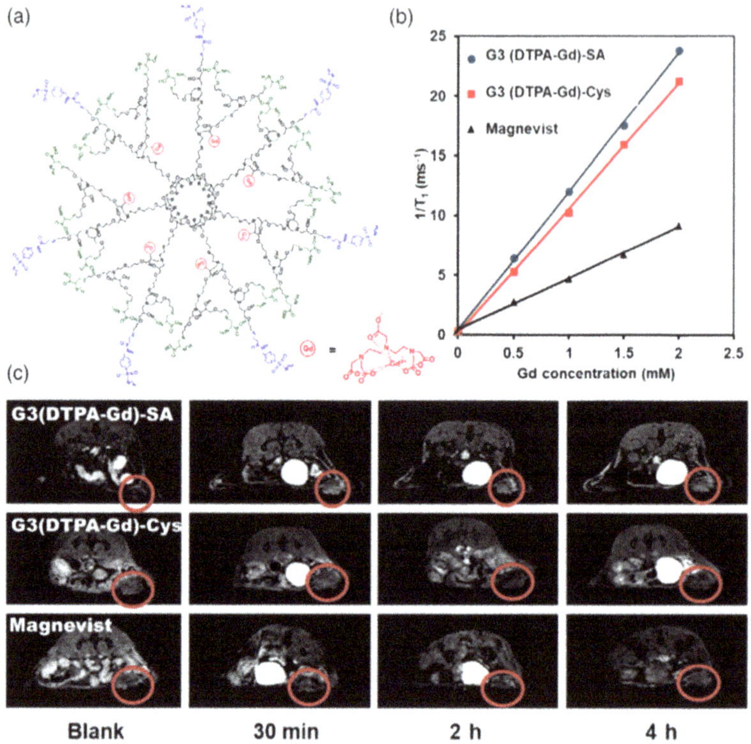

Figure 3.23. Dendritic nanoscale systems for MR imaging of cancer. (a) Scheme representation of a hypoxia-targeting dendritic MR contrast agent with internal hydroxyl groups. (b) *In vitro* longitudinal relaxivity of G3 (DTPA-Gd)-SA, G3(DTPA-Gd)-Cys, and Magnevist. (c) T_1-weighted MR images of orthotopic breast tumor-bearing mice before and after intravenous injection of different MR agents (all the images reproduced with permission from [184], copyright (2019), with permission from Elsevier).

utilization of dendritic polymer based nanoscale medicines are of great interest for effectual diagnosis of cancer tumor at earlier stages as well as monitoring information of tumor metastasis, invasive nature, characterizations and prognosis [182, 183].

Recently, Dendron coated iron oxide NPs were surface functionalized with metronidazole-based ligand to attain hypoxia activated MRI of hypoxia tissue. *In vitro* T_2 weighted MRI imaging of cell pellet demonstrates efficient probes for recognition of tissues derived stem cell and MCF-7 tumors cell under hypoxia conditions. The modification in the R_2 relaxation of hypoxias MCF-7 tumors cell treated with metronidazole functionalised Dendron coated iron oxide NPs was near about 170%, whereas the relaxation modification of ASC treated with the Dendron coated iron oxide NPs was near about 100%. This type of dissimilarity in the relaxation varying percentages may be utilized to differentiate normal cells from the tumor cells [184]. In other investigations, Han *et al* demonstrated sensibly designed and developed hypoxia targeting nanoscale probes with higher molecular weights, G3(DTPA-GD)-SA (figure 3.23) [184]. In these nanoscale probes, β-cyclodextrin

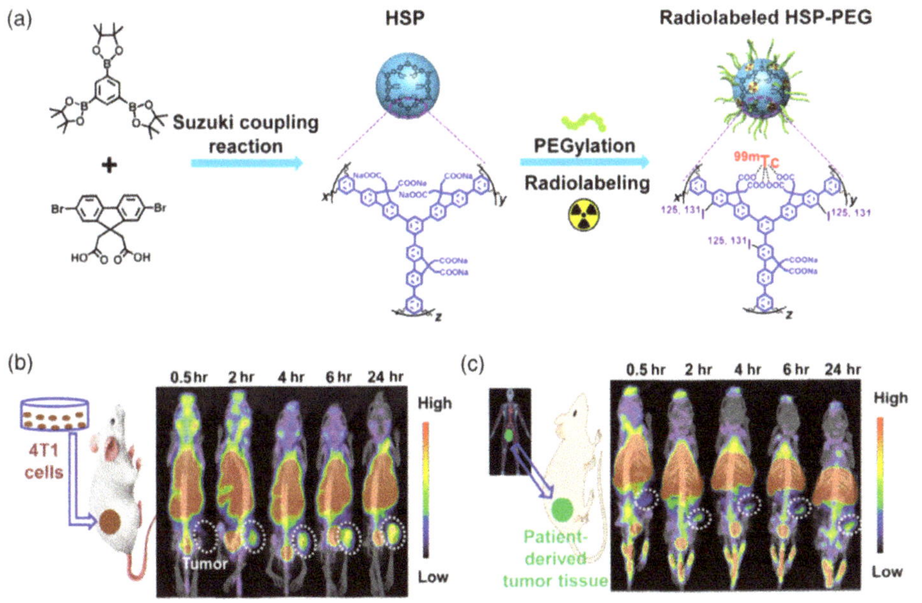

Figure 3.24. Dendritic nanoscale systems for nuclear medical imaging of cancer. (a) Preparation of radiolabeled and PEGylated hyperbranched semiconducting polymeric (HSP-PEG) NPs. SPECT images of mice bearing $4T_1$ tumor (b) and patient-derived prostate tumor tissue (c) after intravenous injection of ^{99m}Tc-labeled HSP-PEG NPs were obtained at different time points (all the images reproduced with permission from [185], copyright (2018) American Chemical Society).

was utilized as a core, Gd was coupled with interior branching cell and the targeting moieties sulfonamide and Zwitterionic moieties were decorated on the peripheral groups of third generation hydroxyl dendrimers.

In other investigations, hyperbranched polymers were utilized for loading the radionuclide for SPECT imaging of cancer tumor (figure 3.24). The hyperbranched semiconducting polymers having sizes around 5 nm were prepared by palladium catalyzed Suzuki coupling reactions and non-covalently functionalized with PEG decorated polymer to form HSP-PEG. PEGylated HSPs labeled with ^{99m}Tc by carboxylic group onto side chains were employed for SPECT imaging of two dissimilar mice tumors models: a 4T1 tumor model and a patient-derived prostate tumor tissue Xeno-grafted tumors model. The fabricated 99mTc labeled HSP-PEG demonstrates a higher tumor cellular uptake and protracted tumor imaging time period in both tumor models. Otherwise, they are excreted from the body via urine as confirmed by SPECT image at different time periods, chromatography based on filer paper chromatography and TEM morphology of the urine [185].

Fluorescence phosphor dendrimers are promising for optical imaging and were reviewed very recently by Qiu *et al* [186]. The series of perylenediimides as a core for polylysine (PDI-PLL) fluorescence dendrimer of the various generations (PDI-PLL G1 to G8) was fabricated in different growths (figure 3.25). Four-amine modified perylenediimides were utilized as core and repeated units commenced in turns.

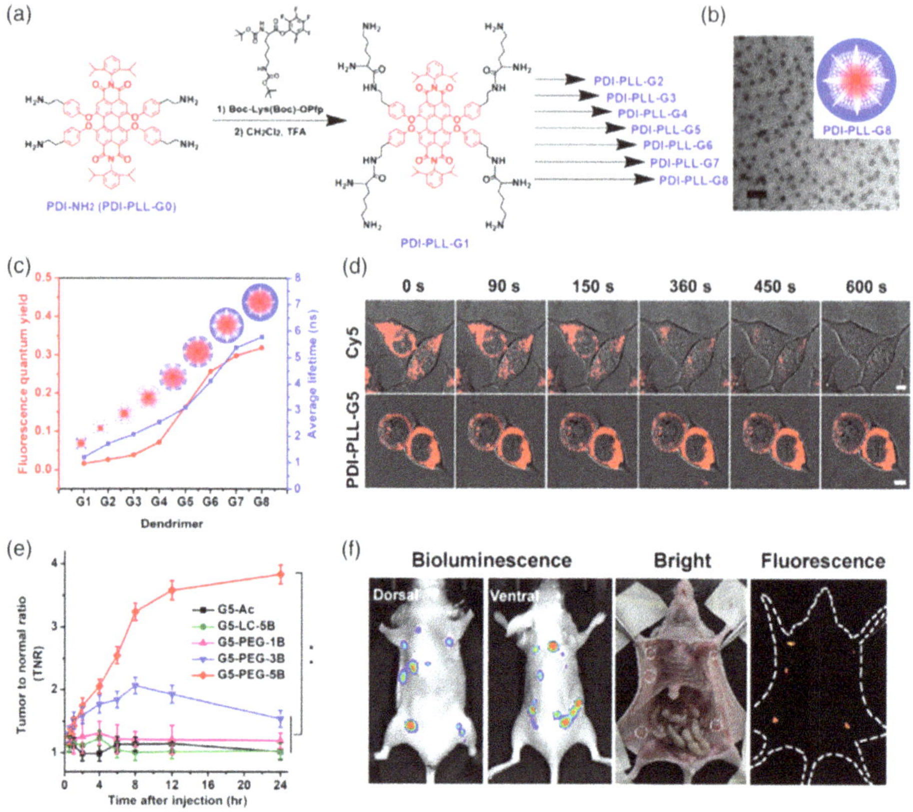

Figure 3.25. Dendritic nanoscale systems for optical imaging of cancer. (a) Preparation route for PDI-PLL dendrimers from generation 0 to generation 8. (b) TEM image of PDI-PLL-G8. (c) Fluorescence quantum yield and average lifetime of PDI-PLL of different generations at 645 nm. (d) Fluorescence images of 4T1 cells preincubated with Cy5 (images above) and PDI-PLL-G5 (images below) at different time points. (e) Tumor-to-normal-tissue ratio of several mice groups at different time points after i.v. injection of various biotin-targeted fluorescent PDI-PLL-G5. (f) Representative bioluminescence/bright/fluorescence pictures of mice bearing systemic metastasis. From left to the right, bioluminescence images of mice 12 days after intracardiac injection of 4T1-Luc cells, bright image and corresponding fluorescence image of lymph node metastasis at 8 h post-injection of fluorescent G5-PEG-5B dendrimers (all the images reproduced with permission from [187], copyright (2020) American Chemical Society).

The fluorescence quantum yields, photostability, anti-photo-bleaching, and average lifetime parameters of the fluorescence dendrimer gradually increases as the generations of the dendrimer increase. This fascinating occurrence was attributed to the shieldings and decreased agglomeration of the internal dye by various sized polylysine shells.

The dendrimer polymer is an ideal nanoscale system for lodging the various contrasting agents because of the easier surface modifications process and adequate interior cavity [189]. Recently, AuNPs were incorporated into G2-NH_2-PAMAM dendrimers by template method, and manganese ions were chelated by NOTA

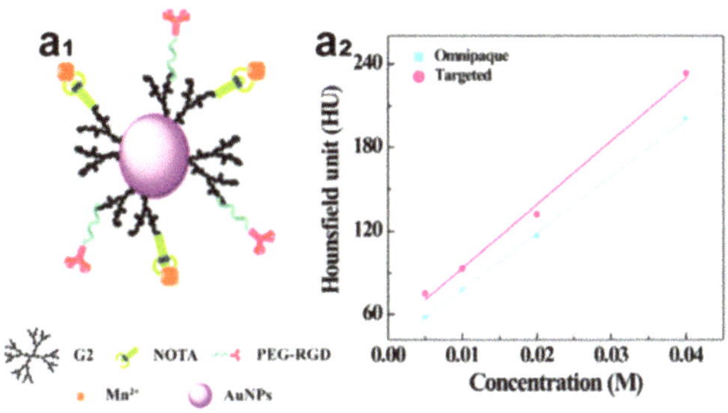

Figure 3.26. Dendritic nanoscale systems for multi-modality imaging of cancer. A low generation dendrimer-based system for dual MR/CT imaging of orthotopic brain gliomas. (a1) Schematic illustration of RGD-Au-Mn DENPs. (a2) X-ray attenuation of RGD-Au-Mn DENPs compared to Omnipaque at various Au or I concentrations. Reproduced with permission from [191] with permission of The Royal Society of Chemisty).

ligand modified onto the periphery group of the dendrimers (figure 3.26). This nanoscale platform possesses a higher r_1 value of 9.88 mM s^{-1} and *in vitro* CT study indicates that it possesses superior x-rays attenuation than that of Omnipaque.

The diagnosis precision in describing tiny pepatocellular carcinoma (HCC) at a size less than 1.0 cm was 29.43% and 10%–33% for MRI and CT with the assistance of usable contrasting agent [191]. To advance the diagnosis sensitivity for tiny HCC, Han *et al* designed and developed endoglin targeted bio-imaging probes that were constructed by G5 dendrimers, onto which aptamers having higher resemblance to endoglin and two imaging candidates, i.e. Gd-DTPA and rhodamine was coupled [184]. This bi-modality probe effectively visualized the orthotopic HCC having sizes in the ranges of 1–4 mm and evidently outlined the tumors margin with higher tumors to the healthy tissues ratios in the NIR fluorescent region and T_1 weighted MRI. The coupling of the MRI and fluorescent imaging may permit for improved diagnostics of cancer and be helpful for precise cancer tumor surgeries [185].

Arami *et al* [190] studied the tumor targeting aptitude of surface modified magnetic particles imaging (MPI) agent in a mouse model with brain cancer Xeno-grafts and assessed the imaging abilities for targeting and tomography imaging of cancerous tumor cells. For the enhancement of specificity in tumor targeting, they have coupled Lactoferrin with the nanoparticles and localized it to the Xeno-grafts via applying exterior magnetic field. The major benefit of this particle imaging is that we are can view only NPs that are attached with the tissue depending upon the inherent magnetic response. Thus, unlike MRI, we do not observe any surrounding interference from the diamagnetic tissue. Figure 3.27 shows near infrared fluorescence images of the tumor Xeno-grafts and figure 3.28 magnetic particle imaging of the mice with tumor Xeno-grafts. Figures 3.27 and 3.28 show lower uptakes in the tumor because of the enhanced permeability and retention (EPR) effects, whereas Lactoferrin coupled with nano-particles is easily internalized and retained in Xeno-grafts and the uptake was improved after exposing magnetic field near to the tumor.

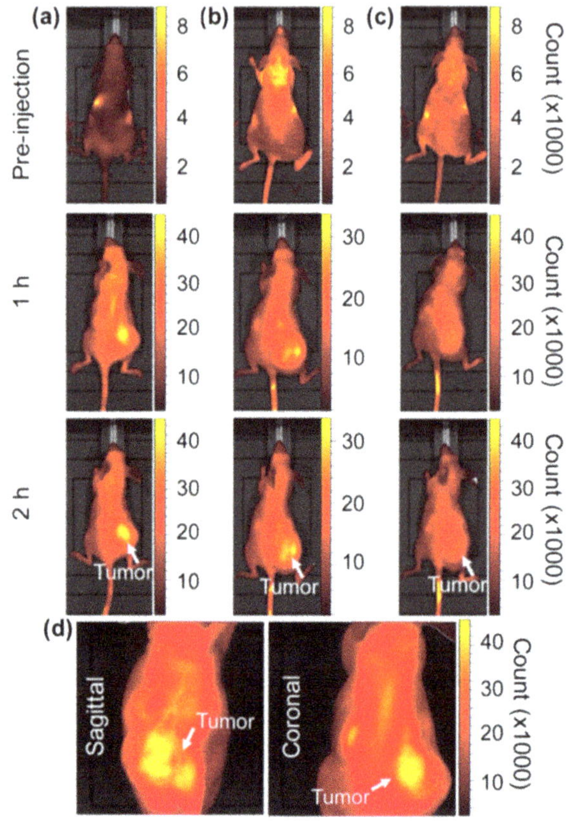

Figure 3.27. Near infrared fluorescent (NIRF) images of the tumor xeno-grafts. Images of the mice injected with Cy5.5-Lactoferrin conjugated NPs, with (a) and without (b) a permanent magnet placed adjacent to the tumor xenograft on the right side flank, compared with mice injected with Cy5.5-labeled NPs, without using lactoferrin and magnetic targeting (c). (d) Higher magnification sagittal and coronal images of the tumors, 2 h after magnetic targeting (all the images reproduced with permission from [190] with permission of The Royal Society of Chemistry).

Tomography studies of the magnetic particle imaging offered the 3D biodistribution of the nanoparticles injected into the tumor and liver. MPI and NIRF imaging of the eliminated tumor shows that the tumor uptake is cumulative and the conjugation of the magnetic and Lactoferrin enabled targeting shows higher uptake. All these outcomes were verified by MPI analysis of the tumor tissue from the eliminated Xeno-grafts as shown in figure 3.29.

Noteworthy advancements in the synthesis and surface functionalization of hybrid nanostructures have been noted in the last decade which offered greater promise for fruitful clinical translations. The chief feature of the hybrid nanostructures is the demonstration of the capability to execute multifunctional behaviour in biological surroundings and some of them are summarized above. If the complex features of the hybrid nanostructures are tailored, the combinations of these functionalities into a hybrid systems shows promis toward superior

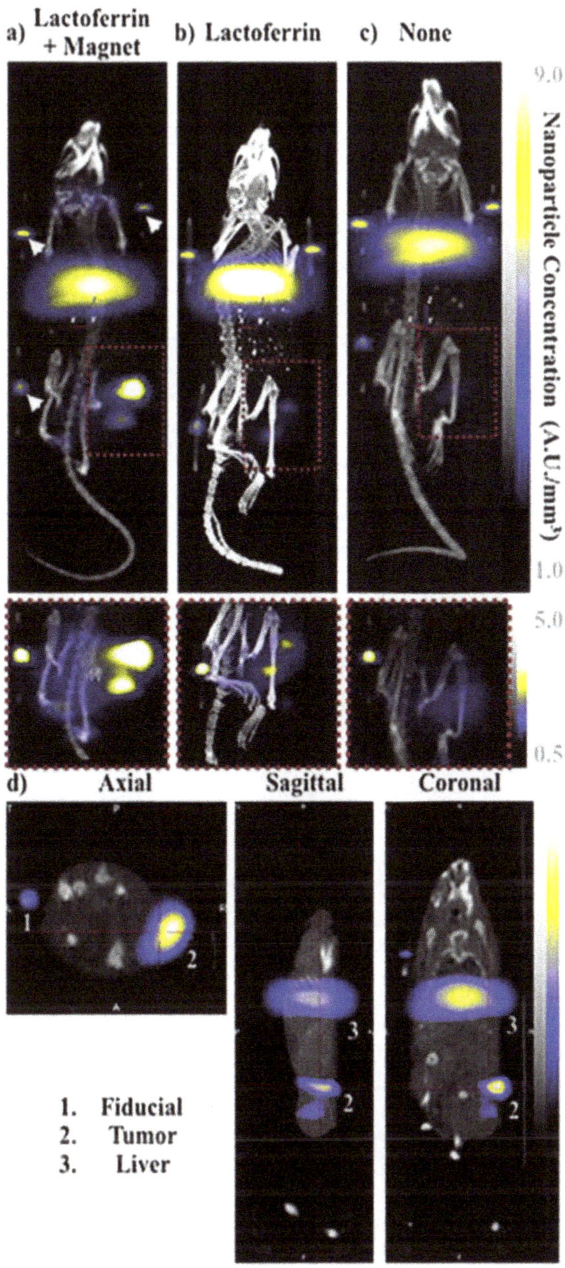

Figure 3.28. MPI images of the mice with tumor xeno-grafts. Two-dimensional (2D) MPI/CT images (2 h post-injection) of mice injected with Cy5.5-Lactoferrin conjugated NPs, with (a) and without (b) a permanent magnet placed adjacent to the tumor xenograft on the right side flank, compared with mice injected with Cy5.5-labeled NPs, without using lactoferrin and magnetic targeting (c). The tumors are marked with the red squares. Rescaled images are shown below each mouse to highlight the tumors. Three fiducial (white arrowheads in (a)) were used for registration of the MPI and CT images. Axial, sagittal and coronal images through the tumor for mouse (a) are shown in (d) (all the images reproduced with permission from [190]).

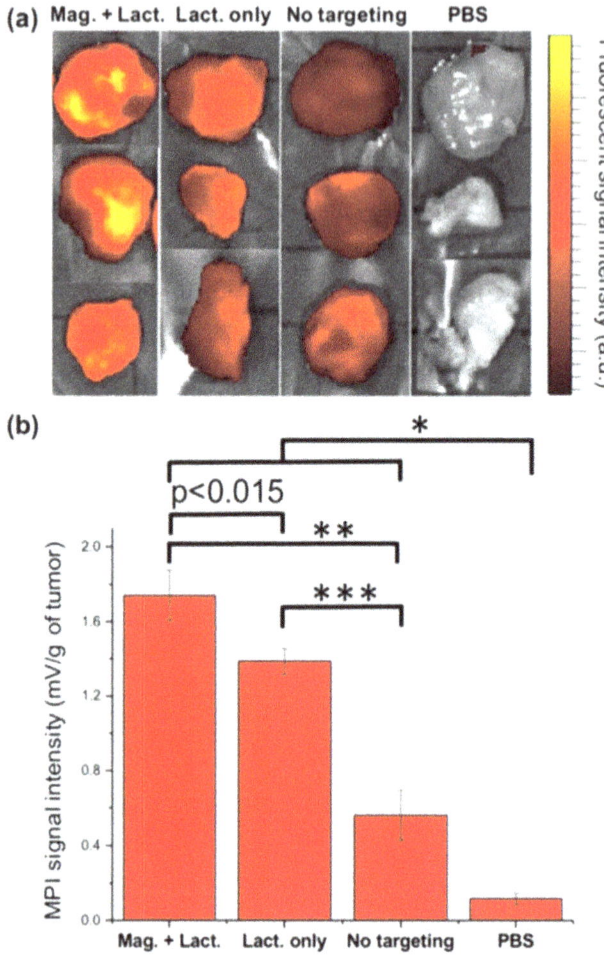

Figure 3.29. *Ex vivo* evaluation of the uptake of MPI contrast agents by tumor xeno-grafts. (a) NIRF images and (b) representative MPI signal intensities (per tumor mass) of the tumor xeno-grafts excised from mice (mean ± standard deviation; $n = 3$) injected with Cy5.5-lactoferrin conjugated NPs, with (Mag. + Lact.) and without (Lact. only) using magnetic targeting, compared with Cy5.5-labeled NPs (without any lactoferrin and magnetic targeting) and PBS as controls (all the images reproduced with permission from [190] with permission of The Royal Society of Chemistry).

advancement in patient outcomes. Moreover, consistent and reproductive synthesis approaches need to be performed and their scalability should be validated. The field of hybrid nanostructures necessitates active participation and collaboration among physicists, chemists, biologists, engineers, materials scientists and clinicians.

3.3 Nanomedicines and radio-imaging techniques

Recently, nanoscience and nanotechnology have been employed in novel modalities of medical imaging. The advance of imaging at the nano level has the capability to improve the area of medicine by supplying in-depth images of the biological process. Currently applied techniques of medical imaging are being modified to enhance their prospects at the nano level. Moreover, nano level platforms are also being employed in the human body to enhance the imaging contrast and to track NPs in the body. Scientific approaches are being conducted in order to apply nanoscale techniques in stem cell transplantation and to diagnosis disease at earlier stages.

The emerging field of nanomedicine implies the applicability of nanotechnology in preventing and treating different types of diseases like cancer [193]. It has gained lot of interest in improvement of drug transportation and drug release. Certainly, pre-clinical nanomedicine research is still a flourishing area and it constructs a significant number of scientific approaches every year. To date, endorsed nanoplatforms for the clinical area are relatively very rare. Clinically available nanomedicines are currently confined to cancer-like diseases, but significant pre-clinical reports show that they can also be useful for other circumstances such as organ implantation, cardiovascular diseases etc. Nanoplatforms are explored to adapt immunity systems and are generating noteworthy outcomes and installing newer trends in the nanomedicine field. The rarity in nanomedicines translations may be attributed to the number of issues including manufacturing scaling ability, regulatory problems related to the deficiency in recognizing nanoformulations, their behaviour in the biological environment and the lack of patient selection. In this line, the importance of the imaging is very well appreciated at various footsteps alongside the nanomedicines expansion path as it may offer vital information in a non-destructive way.

The different imaging modalities such as MRI, CT, PET etc have transformed the field of medicine. These non-destructive modalities offer *in vivo* imaging of human anatomy and various biology related processes for diagnostics. However, among these modalities none of the techniques is ideal, as each technique has their own merits and demerits. In the line of advances in nanomedicines, the anatomy related techniques (CT and MRI), nuclear level techniques (PET and SPECT) and optical level techniques (fluorescent) are the main employed techniques for imaging *in vivo*. With the limitations of singular imaging modality, a combinational approach for two or more imaging techniques is progressively more favored to gain the best information. Usually, a multi-modality approach is a combination of two imaging tools which together gather and convey information in a complementary way, like anatomy related data and functional data such as CT–PET or MRI–PET. Radio-imaging techniques are non-destructive techniques used for imaging the various organs and tissue using radioisotopes, enhancement in dose forms for diagnosis and therapeutics of disease. Basics of different radio-imaging techniques are given in figure 3.30 [192].

The area of non-destructive diagnosis is progressing day by day as imaging techniques are advancing very fast. Due to computational power growth, currently available imaging modalities aim to provide comprehensive visualization starting from molecular level to cell level, organs, tissues and the entire biological scale [39]. The armory of techniques devoted to imaging has emerged in recent decades and now allows us to recognize and inspect biomedical profiles of patients by constructing the 2D and 3D images exclusive of destructive supervision of patient. Due to the

Type and Example Image	Description	Technique (Use of Radiation)	Applications	Cost	Current Use
Computed tomography (CT) 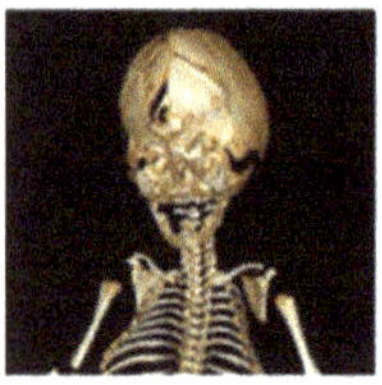	Uses X-rays to generate geometrically accurate 3D information about body structures. 2D cross-sectional (axial) images are first reconstructed using a computer, then reformatted to generate 2D images representing other planes or 3D surfaces or volumes. Also referred to as computed axial tomography (CAT).	Yes (yes)	• Whole body assessment • Trauma (e.g., spinal, thoracoabdominal, head), particularly skeletal trauma • Presence of pathological air or fluid collections • Identification of calcifications, stones • maging foreign objects (e.g., bullet, medical intervention) • Human identification • Skeletal remains, anthropology	$$	Often (less often in the USA)
Magnetic resonance imaging (MRI) 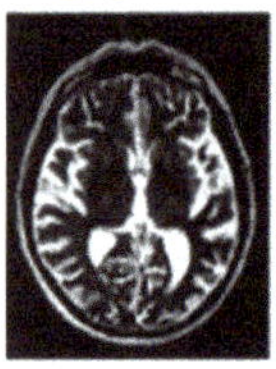	Imaging using a magnetic field, radio waves, and computational methods to produce geometrically accurate, detailed 2D or 3D images of soft tissues such as organs, fat, muscle, connective tissues, and body fluids.	Yes (no)	• Imaging soft tissues/organs in specific body regions • Trauma (e.g., spinal, thoracoabdominal, head), particularly soft tissue trauma • Assessing disease or congenital defects involving complex soft tissue structures (e.g., heart, brain) • Identification of pathological fluid or air collections • Fetal imaging	$$$	Rare
Magnetic resonance spectroscopy (MRS) 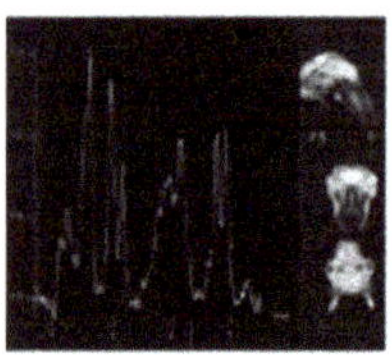	MRS characterizes chemical composition of the tissue.	Yes (no)	• Measuring metabolite levels in normal vs. abnormal tissue (e.g., tumors) • Most frequently applied to the brain • Assessing post-mortem chemical changes	$$$	Very rare
X-ray radiographs 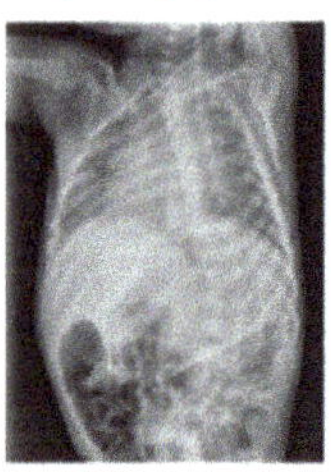	A single image prepared through radiation exposure. Dense objects, such as bone, block the radiation and appear white in an X-ray picture.	No (yes)	• Document fragments, fractures • Human identification	$	Routine, most often

Figure 3.30. Basics of different radio-imaging techniques (image reproduced with permission from [192]).

dissimilarity in the region-to-region contrasts, images display apparent description of the interior biology (anatomical), morphologies, and physiology related functions at the variant scale. Therefore, bioengineered images provide a base for detecting earlier stage pathological tests, estimation of the disease progress, stages of cancer, efficiency of the therapy etc, and they also assist in clinical level decisions for patient disease administration. Advanced and quick monitoring of cancer-like diseases by imaging modalities is a necessary and proficient non-destructive technique to lessen mortalities caused by insufficient information about the *in vivo* environment. To attain perceptible structures of the interior body by varying contrast between the normal and abnormal area, the contrast enhancing material, i.e. contrast agent, needs to be incorporated into the human body to increment the sensitivity and specific behaviour of the modalities to a target area. Through this approach, all the imaging modalities offer valuable information at their level and limitations. The preference of the technique is defined by the kind of information one wants to gain from the modalities. Analysis of the imaging modalities by stepwise approaches is a suitable approach to build a competent and pertinent diagnosis procedure. Figure 3.31 shows schematics for the stepwise guide to execute this diagnosis process.

Figure 3.32 shows the comparative classification of the imaging techniques. The criteria for the classification was chosen as comparatively less (bottom) to the most important (top) points to be considered in the case of diagnosis. Comparison of the imaging techniques alongside all criteria apparently shows that in comparison to the clinical level imaging technique, CT and MRI have superior execution because of the gathering of significant information from their superior resolutions. It was also observed that they are insensitive as compared to SPECT and PET, even though radiological contrast agents and magnetic formulation are safe. Moreover, none of them has in-depth penetrating limits, which means that biological entities might be absolutely visualized.

According to this classification, x-ray scanner and MRI are the broadly employed modalities and show superior proficiency as imaging instruments. Advancements in pre-clinical research have made these techniques extremely reachable and therefore

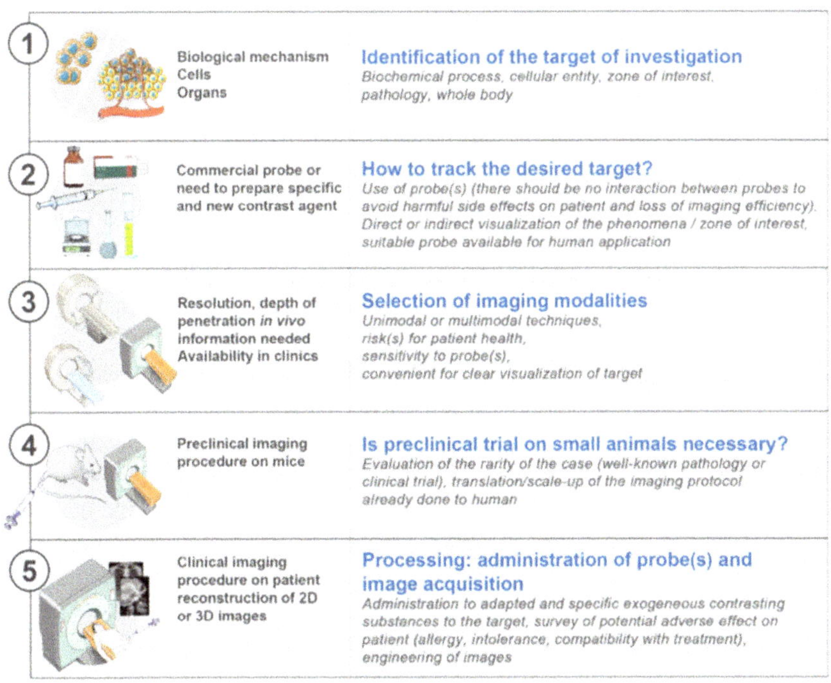
1
Biological mechanism
Cells
Organs
Identification of the target of investigation
Biochemical process, cellular entity, zone of interest, pathology, whole body
2
Commercial probe or need to prepare specific and new contrast agent
How to track the desired target?
Use of probe(s) (there should be no interaction between probes to avoid harmful side effects on patient and loss of imaging efficiency). Direct or indirect visualization of the phenomena / zone of interest, suitable probe available for human application
3
Resolution, depth of penetration in vivo information needed
Availability in clinics
Selection of imaging modalities
Unimodal or multimodal techniques, risk(s) for patient health, sensitivity to probe(s), convenient for clear visualization of target
4
Preclinical imaging procedure on mice
Is preclinical trial on small animals necessary?
Evaluation of the rarity of the case (well-known pathology or clinical trial), translation/scale-up of the imaging protocol already done to human
5
Clinical imaging procedure on patient reconstruction of 2D or 3D images
Processing: administration of probe(s) and image acquisition
Administration to adapted and specific exogeneous contrasting substances to the target, survey of potential adverse effect on patient (allergy, intolerance, compatibility with treatment), engineering of images

Figure 3.31. Schematics for the stepwise guide to execute radiological diagnosis process (the image is reproduced from [39], copyright 2019 with permission of Springer).

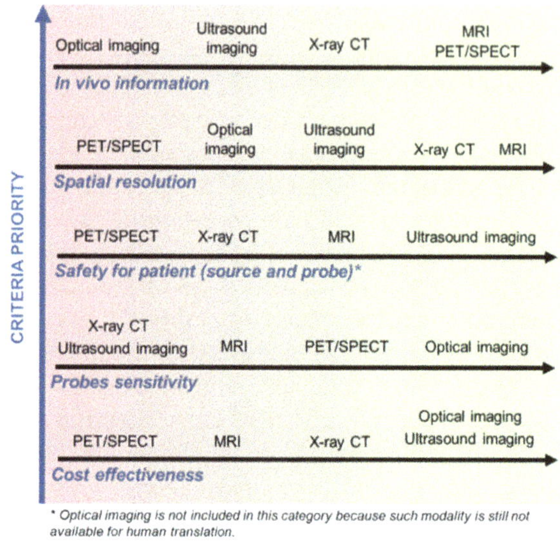

Figure 3.32. Comparative classification of the imaging techniques (the image is reproduced with permission from [39], copyright 2019 with permission of Springer).

increased their uses into the clinical level research. Though, once cannot make sure that which imaging modality will be more useful for the particular diseases. However, in multiple approaches, x-ray and MRI scanners are chosen as instruments or complementing devices for each other with greater efficacy to achieve diagnostics free from unclear information.

3.4 Nanomedicines and new generation imaging techniques

In the last two decades, many conventional biomedical imaging modalities have been demonstrated for regular pre-clinical and clinical practice. These imaging techniques like optical imaging, CT, ultrasound, MRI, PET, SPECT etc are being broadly employed to give superior performance in early diagnosis and therapies of cancer-like diseases. The molecular level imaging modalities differ from the conventional techniques in which biomarkers are employed to offer imaging of the targeted sites. It is requisite that these biomarkers should interface in a specific manner in the biological environment and provide imaging with respect to the molecular level change occurring at the desired site. Molecular level imaging candidates are endogenously activated molecules or exogenously activated probes employed for visualization, characterization, and quantification of the biological process within the living system.

Amongst all the molecular imaging techniques, none of the single imaging techniques is ideal to congregate all the requisites for biomedical applications. Consequently, the current inclination is in the direction of hybrid imaging techniques such as CT–PET, MRI–PET, CT–SPECT, OA–CT etc. Moreover, the combinational approach of MRI and ultrasound (US) is appealing as it predominantly offers accuracy for real-time supervision of high range ultrasound treatments. Therefore, the development of multi-modal imaging techniques for both MRI and US and a combination of these two offers synergistically activated benefits to present significant diagnosis information and therapeutic approaches. As it is exigent to combine dual-mode or multi-mode imaging techniques into a unique probe, this perception is certainly the most capable and suitable to tackle the present shortcomings of individual imaging techniques. Particularly, as nanoscale materials possess superior surface-to-volume ratio and multiple functional groups can be easily attached on the shells, it is achievable to utilize suitable alterations in structure and engineering alongside the attaching ligand conjugates to construct multifunctional nanomaterials for multi-modal imaging at molecular level. Currently, nanoscale materials based dual-mode or multi-mode imaging techniques or contrast enhancing candidates are being developed and employed for multi-modal imaging in living systems.

Even though different types of functionality, targeting ligand, imaging agents, and therapeutics payload can be integrated inside the structural construction of nanoscale materials or with conjugation onto the surfaces by various modifications as shown in figure 3.33, not each of the achievable alterations is required for individual nanoscale materials [141]. Particular imaging modalities or definite therapy purposes will direct one to the requisite approaches for structural design and surface functionalization, which leads to the most favorable performances in translational biomedical applications.

The utilization of nuclear level imaging modalities to study nanoscale therapeutics *in vivo* needs suitable radionuclide, nanocarrier and radiolabels strategy. Usually, radionuclides need to be compatible with the diagnosis technique employed, with PET and SPECT needing positron and gamma emitting radionuclides, respectively. Moreover, competent nuclear imaging modalities need radionuclide with superior specificity (i.e. decay constant of the material) and branching ratios (i.e. fractions of the decay event processed via decay mode and desired imaging). Considering these prerequisites, unsurprisingly there are roughly 1800

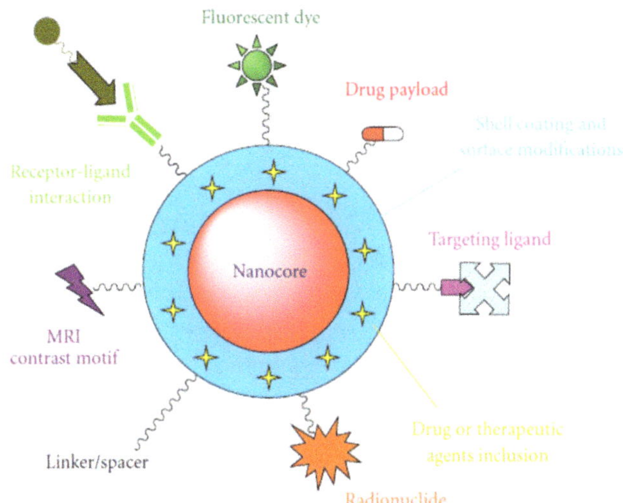

Figure 3.33. Schematics of the surface functionalized nanoparticles for molecular level imaging, drug delivery and therapy (images reproduced with permission from [140]).

radionuclides known but not many are used in routine pre-clinical and clinical level practice. Pre-clinical nuclear imaging modalities may assist in exploiting nanomedicines' *in vivo* response within the smaller and larger animal model by giving quantitative data related to the pharmacokinetics, biodistribution, targeting and drug transportation. Significantly, nuclear medical imaging offers the opportunity to execute this in a longitudinal way. The transportation period and tissue accumulation of nanoscale medicines are usually connected to the therapeutics effects. Thus, for the capability to establish nanoscale medicines in a quantitative way, pharmacokinetics and biological distribution play a promising role for competent progression and translations, as shown in figure 3.34.

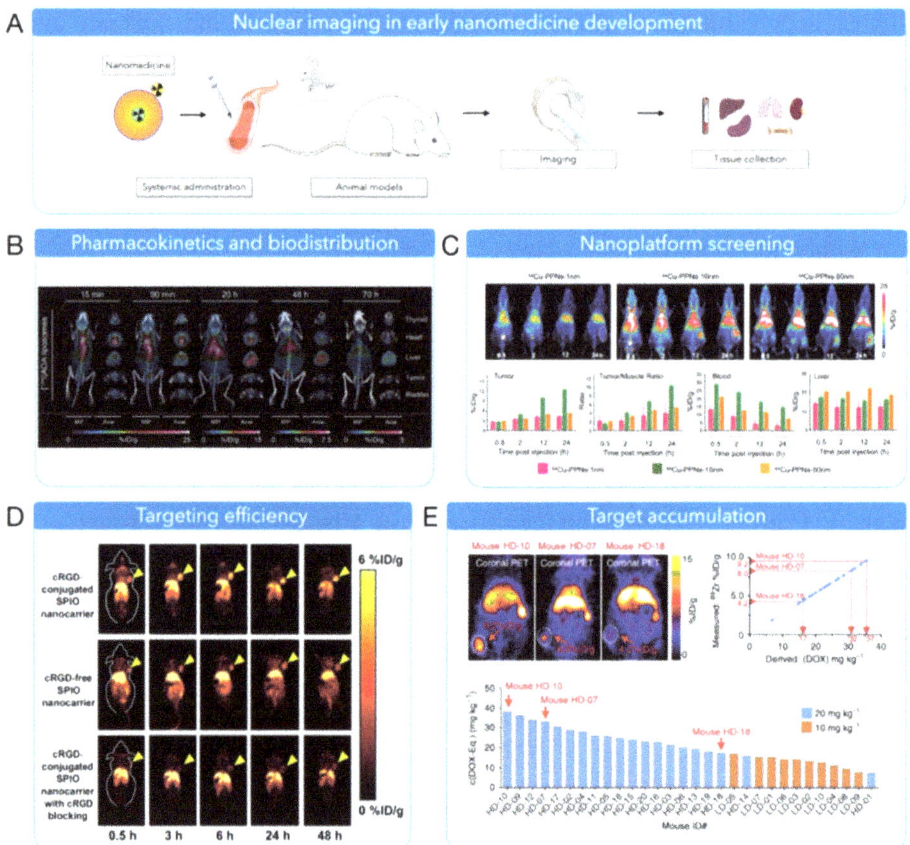

Figure 3.34. Nuclear imaging in basic nanomedicine research. (a) PET and SPECT have been extensively used in early nanomedicine development. Reprinted from [193], copyright (2011), with permission from Elsevier. (b) The pharmacokinetics and biodistribution of 124I-labeled liposomes were monitored longitudinally over 3 days by PET imaging. Reprinted with permission from [194]. (c) This kind of *in vivo* data can be integrated in screening procedures to select optimal formulation features. Reprinted with permission from [196], copyright 2018 John Wiley & Sons. (d) The effect of targeting ligands on doxorubicin-loaded iron oxide NPs was studied by PET imaging. Reprinted from [193], copyright (2011), with permission from Elsevier. (e) A nanotherapeutic's delivered dose in tumors can be determined using a PET nanoreporter approach. Reprinted from [197], copyright 2016 with permission of Springer.

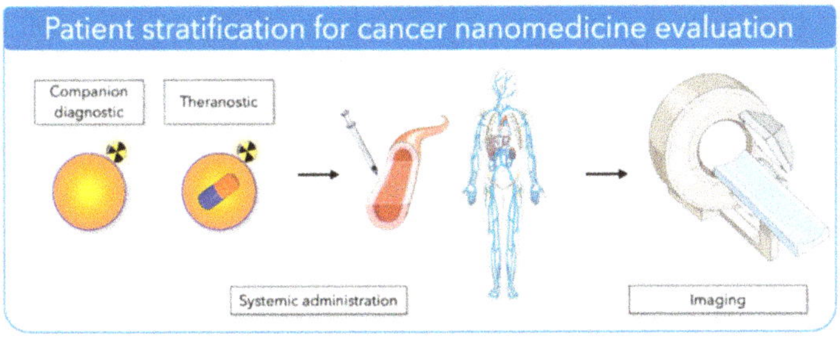

Figure 3.35. Schematic overview of patient stratification strategies for cancer nanomedicine evaluation. The tumor accumulation of companion diagnostic nanoparticles or theranostic nanomedicines can be determined using quantitative (nuclear) imaging techniques after systemic administration. Reprinted from [207], copyright (2020), with permission from Elsevier.

Although, nuclear level imaging modalities are decisively entrenched in pre-clinical level nanomedicine research, their character in clinical level practice is little marked [199]. This is notable by considering the fact that nuclear level imaging is non-destructive and may offer quantitative information predictable for nanomedicine therapeutics efficiency. Predominantly in the field of oncology, where clinical estimation of innovative targeting therapy is mainly provided by quantifying the biomarkers and companion diagnosis, it is astonishing that this is still not the standard practice in cancer nanoscale medicine execution. Most of the nanoscale medicines are being progressed for treatment of solid tumor as they rely on EPR effects for therapeutics efficiency. Even though it is very apparent that the EPR effects are very applicable in a pre-clinical level xeno-grafts model [200], it is persuasively exhibited in a human cancer patient with high inter- and intra-patient and tumors variability. Thus, in addition to the tissues and liquid biomarker, many more attempts are currently intended for the improvement of non-destructive imaging techniques to monitor the EPR profile in an individual patient (figure 3.35) [201]. Eventually, these approaches may be incorporated into the diagnosis and different stages of cancer or in the realm of therapeutics and will assist patients assortment and therapies outcomes prediction.

3.5 Conclusions

In this chapter, we have exemplified the different types of cancer imaging techniques and applications of nanoscale platforms in medical imaging techniques such as CT, PET, MRI, SPECT, optical and florescent etc. In comparison to the traditional contrasting agent, nanoscale platforms have shown enhanced signaling, target capability, and long circulating times in both *in vivo* and *in vitro* as well as in different models. The aid of nanoscale technology has made the imaging techniques more commanding than ever before and combined imaging strategies have revealed noteworthy assurance. The significant function of nanoscale imaging candidates includes diagnosis with therapy within the same platform. As a drug transportation agent, NPs have greater ability to accommodate different types of therapeutics agents to aim the location at the instant of medical imaging. In the last two decades, many therapeutics methods have been explored for integration in theranostics form, which incorporates chemo-therapies, photo-thermal therapies, radiation therapies, photodynamic therapies, immuno-therapies and gene therapies. To capitalize on clinical level translational research, all the properties of the nanoplatforms should be broadly studied, which incorporates their composition, formulation, shape, size, surface charge, dispersion properties, stabilities, incorporation routes, distributions, metabolism, clearances, and adverse effects on body.

In-depth studies for safe and efficient use of nanoscale platforms in well planned clinical studies will be a challenge and are much needed criteria for their advancement. At the current stage, most of the nano level contrasting candidates are still in trial phase. Although significant efforts have been attempted, not many nano level contrasting candidates have been assessed in human bodies. Current advancement in nanoscale research should be focused on improvisation of the target specification while reducing the toxic nature. Moreover, the significance of amplifying translational ability with a suitable animal model cannot be exaggerated, alongside knowing the pharmacokinetics outline of nanoplatforms in human bodies. Effectual advancement of the nanoplatforms for medical level imaging needs inter-disciplinary and multi-disciplinary research groups from physics, chemistry, biology, pharmacy, engineering and medicine backgrounds. In spite of all these issues, nanoscale platforms are promising for novel imaging modalities for a range of clinical level studies.

Acknowledgments

Author Sandeep B Somvanshi acknowledges Department of Science and Technology, Government of India for DST-INSPIRE Fellowship (IF170288).

References

[1] Wild C P 2019 The global cancer burden: necessity is the mother of prevention *Nat. Rev. Cancer* **19** 123–4

[2] Ferlay J, Colombet M, Soerjomataram I, Mathers C, Parkin D, Piñeros M, Znaor A and Bray F 2019 Estimating the global cancer incidence and mortality in 2018: GLOBOCAN sources and methods *Int. J. Cancer* **144** 1941–53

[3] Ferlay J, Ervik M, Lam F, Colombet M, Mery L, Piñeros M, Znaor A, Soerjomataram I and Bray F 2018 *Global Cancer Observatory: Cancer Today* (Lyon, France: International Agency for Research on Cancer)

[4] Kunjachan S, Ehling J, Storm G, Kiessling F and Lammers T 2015 Noninvasive imaging of nanomedicines and nanotheranostics: principles, progress, and prospects *Chem. Rev.* **115** 10907–37

[5] Louie A 2010 Multimodality imaging probes: design and challenges *Chem. Rev.* **110** 3146–95

[6] Janib S M, Moses A S and MacKay J A 2010 Imaging and drug delivery using theranostic nanoparticles *Adv. Drug Delivery Rev.* **62** 1052–63

[7] Fan Z, Fu P P, Yu H and Ray P C 2014 Theranostic nanomedicine for cancer detection and treatment *J. Food Drug Anal* **22** 3–17

[8] Crist R M, Dasa S S K, Liu C H, Clogston J D, Dobrovolskaia M A and Stern S T 2021 Challenges in the development of nanoparticle-based imaging agents: characterization and biology *Wiley Interdiscip. Rev.: Nanomed. Nanobiotech.* **13** e1665
[9] Arranja A G, Pathak V, Lammers T and Shi Y 2017 Tumor-targeted nanomedicines for cancer theranostics *Pharmacol. Res.* **115** 87–95
[10] De Jong M, Essers J and Van W M 2014 Weerden, Imaging preclinical tumour models: improving translational power *Nat. Rev. Cancer* **14** 481–93
[11] Baetke S C, Lammers T and Kiessling F Applications of nanoparticles for diagnosis and therapy of cancer *Br. J. Radiol.* **88** 20150207
[12] England C G, Hernandez R, Eddine S B Z and Cai W 2016 Molecular imaging of pancreatic cancer with antibodies *Mol. Pharm.* **13** 8–24
[13] Zhang Y, Jeon M, Rich L J, Hong H, Geng J, Zhang Y, Shi S, Barnhart T E, Alexandridis P and Huizinga J D 2014 Non-invasive multimodal functional imaging of the intestine with frozen micellar naphthalocyanines *Nat. Nanotechnol.* **9** 631–8
[14] Zhu X, Li J, Hong Y, Kimura R H, Ma X, Liu H, Qin C, Hu X, Hayes T R and Benny P 2014 99mTc-labeled cystine knot peptide targeting integrin αvβ6 for tumor SPECT imaging *Mol. Phar.* **11** 1208–17
[15] Cruz-Monserrate Z, Roland C L, Deng D, Arumugam T, Moshnikova A, Andreev O A, Reshetnyak Y K and Logsdon C D 2014 Targeting pancreatic ductal adenocarcinoma acidic microenvironment *Sci. Rep.* **4** 1–8
[16] Knoop K, Kolokythas M, Klutz K, Willhauck M J, Wunderlich N, Draganovici D, Zach C, Gildehaus F-J, Böning G and Göke B 2011 Image-guided, tumor stroma-targeted 131I therapy of hepatocellular cancer after systemic mesenchymal stem cell-mediated NIS gene delivery *Mol. Ther.* **19** 1704–13
[17] Ju Y, Dong B, Yu J and Hou Y 2019 Inherent multifunctional inorganic nanomaterials for imaging-guided cancer therapy *Nano Today* **26** 108–22
[18] Mahmoudi M, Serpooshan V and Laurent S 2011 Engineered nanoparticles for biomolecular imaging *Nanoscale* **3** 3007–26
[19] Willmann J K, Van Bruggen N, Dinkelborg L M and Gambhir S S 2008 Molecular imaging in drug development *Nat. Rev. Drug Discov.* **7** 591–607
[20] Harisinghani M G, Barentsz J, Hahn P F, Deserno W M, Tabatabaei S, van de Kaa C H, de la Rosette J and Weissleder R 2003 Noninvasive detection of clinically occult lymph-node metastases in prostate cancer *New Engl. J. Med.* **348** 2491–9
[21] Arruebo M, Fernández-Pacheco R, Ibarra M R and Santamaría J 2007 Magnetic nanoparticles for drug delivery *Nano Today* **2** 22–32
[22] Skotland T, Iversen T-G and Sandvig K 2010 New metal-based nanoparticles for intravenous use: requirements for clinical success with focus on medical imaging *Nanomed. Nanotechnol. Biol. Med.* **6** 730–7
[23] Welsher K, Sherlock S P and Dai H 2011 Deep-tissue anatomical imaging of mice using carbon nanotube fluorophores in the second near-infrared window *Proc. of the National Academy of Sciences* **108** 8943–8
[24] Ali-Boucetta H and Kostarelos K 2013 Carbon nanotubes in medicine & biology—therapy and diagnostics *Adv. Drug Delivery Rev.* **65** 1897–8
[25] Xu S and Chen H 2016 High-density mammalian cell cultures in stirred-tank bioreactor without external pH control *J. Biotechnol.* **231** 149–59

[26] Polyak A and Ross T L 2018 Nanoparticles for SPECT and PET imaging: towards personalized medicine and theranostics *Curr. Med. Chem.* **25** 4328–53

[27] Rahmim A and Zaidi H 2008 PET versus SPECT: strengths, limitations and challenges *Nucl. Med. Commun.* **29** 193–207

[28] Weber J, Beard P C and Bohndiek S E 2016 Contrast agents for molecular photoacoustic imaging *Nat. Methods* **13** 639–50

[29] Wang X, Pang Y, Ku G, Xie X, Stoica G and Wang L V 2003 Noninvasive laser-induced photoacoustic tomography for structural and functional *in vivo* imaging of the brain *Nat. Biotechnol.* **21** 803–6

[30] Li J, Huang J, Lyu Y, Huang J, Jiang Y, Xie C and Pu K 2019 Photoactivatable organic semiconducting pro-nanoenzymes *J. Am. Chem. Soc.* **141** 4073–9

[31] Mallidi S, Larson T, Tam J, Joshi P P, Karpiouk A, Sokolov K and Emelianov S 2009 Multiwavelength photoacoustic imaging and plasmon resonance coupling of gold nanoparticles for selective detection of cancer *Nano Lett.* **9** 2825–31

[32] Na H B, Song I C and Hyeon T 2009 Inorganic nanoparticles for MRI contrast agents *Adv. Mater.* **21** 2133–48

[33] Bi X, Ruan L, Liu Z, Li K, Ruan Y, Zheng W and Lin Q 2021 Quantitative analysis of magnetic cobalt particles with an optically pumped atomic magnetometer *Appl. Phys. Lett.* **118** 084101

[34] Evanics F, Diamente P, Van Veggel F, Stanisz G and Prosser R 2006 Water-soluble GdF_3 and GdF_3/LaF_3 nanoparticles physical characterization and NMR relaxation properties *Chem. Mater.* **18** 2499–505

[35] Hifumi H, Yamaoka S, Tanimoto A, Citterio D and Suzuki K 2006 Gadolinium-based hybrid nanoparticles as a positive MR contrast agent *J. Am. Chem. Soc.* **128** 15090–1

[36] Jun Y-w, Huh Y-M, Choi J-s, Lee J-H, Song H-T, Kim S, Yoon S, Kim K-S, Shin J-S and Suh J-S 2005 Nanoscale size effect of magnetic nanocrystals and their utilization for cancer diagnosis via magnetic resonance imaging *J. Am. Chem. Soc.* **127** 5732–3

[37] Tromsdorf U I, Bruns O T, Salmen S C, Beisiegel U and Weller H 2009 A highly effective, nontoxic T_1 MR contrast agent based on ultrasmall PEGylated iron oxide nanoparticles *Nano Lett.* **9** 4434–40

[38] Wang Y-X J 2015 Current status of superparamagnetic iron oxide contrast agents for liver magnetic resonance imaging *World J. Gastroenterol.* **21** 13400

[39] Wallyn J, Anton N, Akram S and Vandamme T F 2019 Biomedical imaging: principles, technologies, clinical aspects, contrast agents, limitations and future trends in nanomedicines *Pharm. Res.* **36** 78

[40] Kojima C, Umeda Y, Ogawa M, Harada A, Magata Y and Kono K 2010 X-ray computed tomography contrast agents prepared by seeded growth of gold nanoparticles in PEGylated dendrimer *Nanotechnology* **21** 245104

[41] Bonitatibus P J Jr, Torres A S, Goddard G D, FitzGerald P F and Kulkarni A M 2010 Synthesis, characterization, and computed tomography imaging of a tantalum oxide nanoparticle imaging agent *Chem. Commun.* **46** 8956–8

[42] Rabin O, Perez J M, Grimm J, Wojtkiewicz G and Weissleder R 2006 An X-ray computed tomography imaging agent based on long-circulating bismuth sulphide nanoparticles *Nat. Mater.* **5** 118–22

[43] De La Vega J C and Häfeli U O 2015 Utilization of nanoparticles as x-ray contrast agents for diagnostic imaging applications *Contrast Media Mol. Imag.* **10** 81–95

[44] Zhen X, Zhang C, Xie C, Miao Q, Lim K L and Pu K 2016 Intraparticle energy level alignment of semiconducting polymer nanoparticles to amplify chemiluminescence for ultrasensitive *in vivo* imaging of reactive oxygen species *ACS Nano* **10** 6400–9
[45] Miao Q, Xie C, Zhen X, Lyu Y, Duan H, Liu X, Jokerst J V and Pu K 2017 Molecular afterglow imaging with bright, biodegradable polymer nanoparticles *Nat. Biotechnol.* **35** 1102
[46] Seeni R Z, Yu X, Chang H, Chen P, Liu L and Xu C 2017 Iron oxide nanoparticle-powered micro-optical coherence tomography for *in situ* imaging the penetration and swelling of polymeric microneedles in the skin *ACS Appl. Mater. Interfaces* **9** 20340–7
[47] Shao D, Zhang X, Liu W, Zhang F, Zheng X, Qiao P, Li J, Dong W-f and Chen L 2016 Janus silver-mesoporous silica nanocarriers for SERS traceable and pH-sensitive drug delivery in cancer therapy *ACS Appl. Mater. Interfaces* **8** 4303–8
[48] Lane L A, Qian X and Nie S 2015 SERS nanoparticles in medicine: from label-free detection to spectroscopic tagging *Chem. Rev.* **115** 10489–529
[49] Chen P, Zheng Z, Zhu Y, Dong Y, Wang F and Liang G 2017 Bioluminescent turn-on probe for sensing hypochlorite *in vitro* and in tumors *Anal. Chem.* **89** 5693–6
[50] Li J-L, Tang B, Yuan B, Sun L and Wang X-G 2013 A review of optical imaging and therapy using nanosized graphene and graphene oxide *Biomaterials* **34** 9519–34
[51] He M, Huang P, Zhang C, Hu H, Bao C, Gao G, He R and Cui D 2011 Dual phase-controlled synthesis of uniform lanthanide-doped NaGdF4 upconversion nanocrystals via an OA/ionic liquid two-phase system for *in vivo* dual-modality imaging *Adv. Funct. Mater.* **21** 4470–7
[52] Farrera C, Torres Andón F and Feliu N 2017 Carbon nanotubes as optical sensors in biomedicine *ACS Nano* **11** 10637–43
[53] Murphy C J, Gole A M, Stone J W, Sisco P N, Alkilany A M, Goldsmith E C and Baxter S C 2008 Gold nanoparticles in biology: beyond toxicity to cellular imaging *Acc. Chem. Res.* **41** 1721–30
[54] Xu S, Cui J and Wang L 2016 Recent developments of low-toxicity NIR II quantum dots for sensing and bioimaging *TrAC, Trends Anal. Chem.* **80** 149–55
[55] Antaris A L, Chen H, Cheng K, Sun Y, Hong G, Qu C, Diao S, Deng Z, Hu X and Zhang B 2016 A small-molecule dye for NIR-II imaging *Nat. Mater.* **15** 235–42
[56] Lai T C, Bae Y, Yoshida T, Kataoka K and Kwon G S 2010 pH-sensitive multi-PEGylated block copolymer as a bioresponsive pDNA delivery vector *Pharm. Res.* **27** 2260–73
[57] Sun X, Cai W and Chen X 2015 Positron emission tomography imaging using radiolabeled inorganic nanomaterials *ACC. Chem. Res.* **48** 286–94
[58] Döge N, Hönzke S, Schumacher F, Balzus B, Colombo M, Hadam S, Rancan F, Blume-Peytavi U, Schäfer-Korting M and Schindler A 2016 Ethyl cellulose nanocarriers and nanocrystals differentially deliver dexamethasone into intact, tape-stripped or sodium lauryl sulfate-exposed *ex vivo* human skin-assessment by intradermal microdialysis and extraction from the different skin layers *J. Controlled Release* **242** 25–34
[59] Lu W, Huang Q, Ku G, Wen X, Zhou M, Guzatov D, Brecht P, Su R, Oraevsky A and Wang L V 2010 Photoacoustic imaging of living mouse brain vasculature using hollow gold nanospheres *Biomaterials* **31** 2617–26
[60] Smith B R and Gambhir S S 2017 Nanomaterials for *in vivo* imaging *Chem. Rev.* **117** 901–86
[61] Agdeppa E D and Spilker M E 2009 A review of imaging agent development *AAPS J.* **11** 286–99

[62] Olafsen T and Wu A M 2010 Antibody vectors for imaging *Seminars in Nuclear Medicine* (Amsterdam: Elsevier) pp 167–81

[63] Jiang L, Tu Y, Shi H and Cheng Z 2014 PET probes beyond 18F-FDG *J. Biomed. Res.* **28** 435

[64] Scott A M, Wolchok J D and Old L J 2012 Antibody therapy of cancer *Natl. Rev. Cancer* **12** 278–87

[65] Oliveira S, Heukers R, Sornkom J, Kok R J and en Henegouwen P M B 2013 Targeting tumors with nanobodies for cancer imaging and therapy *J. Controlled Release* **172** 607–17

[66] Vaneycken I, D'huyvetter M, Hernot S, De Vos J, Xavier C, Devoogdt N, Caveliers T and Lahoutte T 2011 Immuno-imaging using nanobodies *Curr. Opin. Biotechnol.* **22** 877–81

[67] Oliveira S, Van Dongen G A, Walsum M S-v, Roovers R C, Stam J C, Mali W, Van Diest P J and van Bergen en Henegouwen P M 2012 Rapid visualization of human tumor xenografts through optical imaging with a near-infrared fluorescent anti–epidermal growth factor receptor nanobody *Mol. Imaging* **11** 33–46

[68] Weissleder R and Mahmood U 2001 Molecular imaging *Radiology* **219** 316–33

[69] Hilderbrand S A and Weissleder R 2010 Near-infrared fluorescence: application to *in vivo* molecular imaging *Curr. Opin. Chem. Biol.* **14** 71–9

[70] Huang L, Gainkam L O T, Caveliers V, Vanhove C, Keyaerts M, De Baetselier P, Bossuyt A, Revets H and Lahoutte T 2008 SPECT imaging with 99m Tc-labeled EGFR-specific nanobody for *in vivo* monitoring of EGFR expression *Mol. Imaging Biol.* **10** 167–75

[71] Gainkam L O T, Keyaerts M, Caveliers V, Devoogdt N, Vanhove C, Van Grunsven L, Muyldermans S and Lahoutte T 2011 Correlation between epidermal growth factor receptor-specific nanobody uptake and tumor burden: a tool for noninvasive monitoring of tumor response to therapy *Mol. Imaging Biol.* **13** 940–8

[72] Hernot S, Unnikrishnan S, Du Z, Shevchenko T, Cosyns B, Broisat A, Toczek J, Caveliers V, Muyldermans S and Lahoutte T 2012 Nanobody-coupled microbubbles as novel molecular tracer *J. Controlled Release* **158** 346–53

[73] Stride E and Saffari N 2003 Microbubble ultrasound contrast agents: a review *Proc. of the Institution of Mechanical Engineers, Part H: Journal of Engineering in Medicine* **217** 429–47

[74] Ntziachristos V, Bremer C and Weissleder R 2003 Fluorescence imaging with near-infrared light: new technological advances that enable *in vivo* molecular imaging *Eur. Radiol.* **13** 195–208

[75] Solomon M, Liu Y, Berezin M Y and Achilefu S 2011 Optical imaging in cancer research: basic principles, tumor detection, and therapeutic monitoring *Med. Princ. Pract.* **20** 397–415

[76] Kijanka M, Warnders F-J, El Khattabi M, Lub-de Hooge M, van Dam G M, Ntziachristos V, de Vries L, Oliveira S and en Henegouwen P M B 2013 Rapid optical imaging of human breast tumour xenografts using anti-HER2 VHHs site-directly conjugated to IRDye 800CW for image-guided surgery *Eur. J. Nucl. Med. Mol. Imaging* **40** 1718–29

[77] Chen S, Liu J, Li Y, Wu X, Yuan Q, Yang R and Zheng J 2020 Hypoxia-responsive fluorescent nanoprobe for imaging and cancer therapy *TrAC, Trends Anal. Chem.* **131** 116010

[78] Chen H, Bi Q, Yao Y and Tan N 2018 Dimeric BODIPY-loaded liposomes for dual hypoxia marker imaging and activatable photodynamic therapy against tumors *J. Mater. Chem.* B **6** 4351–9

[79] Laxman K, Reddy B P K, Mishra S K, Robinson A, De A, Srivastava R and Ravikanth M 2020 Bioinspired carrier-free peptide conjugated BF_2-oxasmaragdyrin dye-based nano self-assemblies: a photostable NIR cancer theragnostic agent *NPG Asia Mater.* **12** 1–13
[80] Zhao L, Liu Y, Xing R and Yan X 2020 Supramolecular photothermal effects: a promising mechanism for efficient thermal conversion *Angew. Chem.* **132** 3821–9
[81] Fortin M-A, Petoral R M, Söderlind F, Klasson A, Engström M, Veres T, Käll P-O and Uvdal K 2007 Polyethylene glycol-covered ultra-small Gd_2O_3 nanoparticles for positive contrast at 1.5 T magnetic resonance clinical scanning *Nanotechnology* **18** 395501
[82] Na H B, Lee J H, An K, Park Y I, Park M, Lee I S, Nam D H, Kim S T, Kim S H and Kim S W 2007 Development of a T_1 contrast agent for magnetic resonance imaging using MnO nanoparticles *Angew. Chem.* **119** 5493–97
[83] Shilo M, Reuveni T, Motiei M and Popovtzer R 2012 Nanoparticles as computed tomography contrast agents: current status and future perspectives *Nanomedicine* **7** 257–69
[84] Sun X, Huang X, Zhao R, Chen B and Xie Q 2015 Meta-analysis: tobacco smoking may enhance the risk of acute pancreatitis *Pancreatology* **15** 286–94
[85] Nikam A N, Pandey A, Fernandes G, Kulkarni S, Mutalik S P, Padya B S, George S D and Mutalik S 2020 Copper sulphide based heterogeneous nanoplatforms for multimodal therapy and imaging of cancer: recent advances and toxicological perspectives *Coord. Chem. Rev.* **419** 213356
[86] Poulose A C, Veeranarayanan S, Mohamed M S, Nagaoka Y, Aburto R R, Mitcham T, Ajayan P M, Bouchard R R, Sakamoto Y and Yoshida Y 2015 Multi-stimuli responsive Cu_2S nanocrystals as trimodal imaging and synergistic chemo-photothermal therapy agents *Nanoscale* **7** 8378–88
[87] Pan D, Caruthers S D, Senpan A, Yalaz C, Stacy A J, Hu G, Marsh J N, Gaffney P J, Wickline S A and Lanza G M 2011 Synthesis of NanoQ, a copper-based contrast agent for high-resolution magnetic resonance imaging characterization of human thrombus *J. Am. Chem. Soc.* **133** 9168–71
[88] Lin M, Wang D, Li S, Tang Q, Liu S, Ge R, Liu Y, Zhang D, Sun H and Zhang H 2016 Cu (II) doped polyaniline nanoshuttles for multimodal tumor diagnosis and therapy *Biomaterials* **104** 213–22
[89] Zhang S, Zha Z, Yue X, Liang X and Dai Z 2013 Gadolinium-chelate functionalized copper sulphide as a nanotheranostic agent for MR imaging and photothermal destruction of cancer cells *Chem. Commun.* **49** 6776–78
[90] Liu R, Jing L, Peng D, Li Y, Tian J and Dai Z 2015 Manganese (II) chelate functionalized copper sulfide nanoparticles for efficient magnetic resonance/photoacoustic dual-modal imaging guided photothermal therapy *Theranostics* **5** 1144
[91] Chen L-J, Sun S-K, Wang Y, Yang C-X, Wu S-Q and Yan X-P 2016 Activatable multifunctional persistent luminescence nanoparticle/copper sulfide nanoprobe for *in vivo* luminescence imaging-guided photothermal therapy *ACS Appl. Mater. Interfaces* **8** 32667–74
[92] Zhao Z, Xu K, Fu C, Liu H, Lei M, Bao J, Fu A, Yu Y and Zhang W 2019 Interfacial engineered gadolinium oxide nanoparticles for magnetic resonance imaging guided micro-environment-mediated synergetic chemodynamic/photothermal therapy *Biomaterials* **219** 119379
[93] Jin Y, Li Y, Yang X and Tian J 2019 Neuroblastoma-targeting triangular gadolinium oxide nanoplates for precise excision of cancer *Acta Biomater.* **87** 223–34

[94] Li J, You J, Dai Y, Shi M, Han C and Xu K 2014 Gadolinium oxide nanoparticles and aptamer-functionalized silver nanoclusters-based multimodal molecular imaging nanoprobe for optical/magnetic resonance cancer cell imaging *Anal. Chem.* **86** 11306–11
[95] Wu M, Xue Y, Li N, Zhao H, Lei B, Wang M, Wang J, Luo M, Zhang C and Du Y 2019 Tumor-microenvironment-induced degradation of ultrathin gadolinium oxide nanoscrolls for magnetic-resonance-imaging-monitored, activatable cancer chemotherapy *Angew. Chem.* **131** 6954–9
[96] Wang F, Wen L, Liu J, Peng W, Meng Z, Chen Q, Wang Y, Ke B, Guo Y and Mi P 2020 Albumin nanocomposites with MnO_2/Gd_2O_3 motifs for precise MR imaging of acute myocardial infarction in rabbit models *Biomaterials* **230** 119614
[97] Shen Z, Fan W, Yang Z, Liu Y, Bregadze V I, Mandal S K, Yung B C, Lin L, Liu T and Tang W 2019 Exceedingly small gadolinium oxide nanoparticles with remarkable relaxivities for magnetic resonance imaging of tumors *Small* **15** 1903422
[98] Cai W, Zhang Y, Wang J, Wang Z, Tian Y, Liu H, Pan H, Fu L, Chen W and Wu C 2020 Engineering the surface of Gd_2O_3 nanoplates for improved T1-weighted magnetic resonance imaging *Chem. Eng. J.* **380** 122473
[99] Zeng Y, Li H, Li Z, Luo Q, Zhu H, Gu Z, Zhang H, Gong Q and Luo K 2020 Engineered gadolinium-based nanomaterials as cancer imaging agents *Appl. Mater. Today* **20** 100686
[100] Shen Z, Liu T, Yang Z, Zhou Z, Tang W, Fan W, Liu Y, Mu J, Li L and Bregadze V I 2020 Small-sized gadolinium oxide based nanoparticles for high-efficiency theranostics of orthotopic glioblastoma *Biomaterials* **235** 119783
[101] Cho M, Sethi R, Lee S S, Benoit D N, Taheri N, Decuzzi P and Colvin V L 2014 Gadolinium oxide nanoplates with high longitudinal relaxivity for magnetic resonance imaging *Nanoscale* **6** 13637–45
[102] Loh K P, Ho D, Chiu G N C, Leong D T, Pastorin G and Chow E K H 2018 Clinical applications of carbon nanomaterials in diagnostics and therapy *Adv. Mater.* **30** 1802368
[103] Zhang L, Liu R, Peng H, Li P, Xu Z and Whittaker A K 2016 The evolution of gadolinium based contrast agents: from single-modality to multi-modality *Nanoscale* **8** 10491–510
[104] Wang X, Valiev R R, Ohulchanskyy T Y, Ågren H, Yang C and Chen G 2017 Dye-sensitized lanthanide-doped upconversion nanoparticles *Chem. Soc. Rev.* **46** 4150–67
[105] Das P, Fatehbasharzad P, Colombo M, Fiandra L and Prosperi D 2019 Multifunctional magnetic gold nanomaterials for cancer *Trends Biotechnol.* **37** 995–1010
[106] Saleem J, Wang L and Chen C 2018 Carbon-based nanomaterials for cancer therapy via targeting tumor microenvironment *Adv. Healthcare Mater.* **7** 1800525
[107] Yang Y, Chen S, Li H, Yuan Y, Zhang Z, Xie J, Hwang D W, Zhang A, Liu M and Zhou X 2018 Engineered paramagnetic graphene quantum dots with enhanced relaxivity for tumor imaging *Nano Lett.* **19** 441–8
[108] Panich A M, Salti M, Goren S D, Yudina E, Aleksenskii A, Vul A Y and Shames A I 2019 Gd (III)-grafted detonation nanodiamonds for MRI contrast enhancement *J. Phys. Chem. C* **123** 2627–31
[109] Chen H, Qiu Y, Ding D, Lin H, Sun W, Wang G D, Huang W, Zhang W, Lee D and Liu G 2018 Gadolinium-encapsulated graphene carbon nanotheranostics for imaging-guided photodynamic therapy *Adv. Mater.* **30** 1802748
[110] Manus L M, Mastarone D J, Waters E A, Zhang X-Q, Schultz-Sikma E A, MacRenaris K W, Ho D and Meade T J 2010 Gd (III)-nanodiamond conjugates for MRI contrast enhancement *Nano Lett.* **10** 484–9

[111] Yang W, Wu X, Dou Y, Chang J, Xiang C, Yu J, Wang J, Wang X and Zhang B 2018 A human endogenous protein exerts multi-role biomimetic chemistry in synthesis of paramagnetic gold nanostructures for tumor bimodal imaging *Biomaterials* **161** 256–69

[112] Kulkarni S, Pandey A and Mutalik S 2020 Liquid metal based theranostic nanoplatforms: application in cancer therapy, imaging and biosensing *Nanomed. Nanotechnol. Biol. Med.* **26** 102175

[113] Ghai A, Singh B, Hazari P P, Schultz M K, Parmar A, Kumar P, Sharma S, Dhawan D and Mishra A K 2015 Radiolabeling optimization and characterization of ^{68}Ga labeled DOTA–polyamido-amine dendrimer conjugate–animal biodistribution and PET imaging results *Appl. Radiat. Isot.* **105** 40–6

[114] Fernández-Barahona I, Muñoz-Hernando M, Pellico J, Ruiz-Cabello J and Herranz F 2018 Molecular imaging with ^{68}Ga radio-nanomaterials: shedding light on nanoparticles *Appl. Sci.* **8** 1098

[115] Wang C, Zhao N, Huang Y, He R, Xu S and Yuan W 2020 Coordination of injectable self-healing hydrogel with Mn–Zn ferrite@ mesoporous silica nanospheres for tumor MR imaging and efficient synergistic magnetothermal-chemo-chemodynamic therapy *Chem. Eng. J.* **401** 126100

[116] Liu Y, Li J, Chen M, Chen X and Zheng N 2020 Palladium-based nanomaterials for cancer imaging and therapy *Theranostics* **10** 10057

[117] Nie L, Chen M, Sun X, Rong P, Zheng N and Chen X 2014 Palladium nanosheets as highly stable and effective contrast agents for *in vivo* photoacoustic molecular imaging *Nanoscale* **6** 1271–6

[118] Chen M, Chen S, He C, Mo S, Wang X, Liu G and Zheng N 2017 Safety profile of two-dimensional Pd nanosheets for photothermal therapy and photoacoustic imaging *Nano Res.* **10** 1234–48

[119] Chen M, Tang S, Guo Z, Wang X, Mo S, Huang X, Liu G and Zheng N 2014 Core–Shell Pd@ Au nanoplates as theranostic agents for in-vivo photoacoustic imaging, ct imaging, and photothermal therapy *Adv. Mater.* **26** 8210–6

[120] Chen M, Guo Z, Chen Q, Wei J, Li J, Shi C, Xu D, Zhou D, Zhang X and Zheng N 2018 Pd nanosheets with their surface coordinated by radioactive iodide as a high-performance theranostic nanoagent for orthotopic hepatocellular carcinoma imaging and cancer therapy *Chem. Sci.* **9** 4268–74

[121] Guo Z, Chen M, Peng C, Mo S, Shi C, Fu G, Wen X, Zhuang R, Su X and Liu T 2018 pH-sensitive radiolabeled and superfluorinated ultra-small palladium nanosheet as a high-performance multimodal platform for tumor theranostics *Biomaterials* **179** 134–43

[122] Liu Y, Ai K and Lu L 2012 Nanoparticulate x-ray computed tomography contrast agents: from design validation to *in vivo* applications *ACC. Chem. Res.* **45** 1817–27

[123] Dou Y, Guo Y, Li X, Li X, Wang S, Wang L, Lv G, Zhang X, Wang H and Gong X 2016 Size-tuning ionization to optimize gold nanoparticles for simultaneous enhanced CT imaging and radiotherapy *ACS Nano* **10** 2536–48

[124] Popovtzer R, Agrawal A, Kotov N A, Popovtzer A, Balter J, Carey T E and Kopelman R 2008 Targeted gold nanoparticles enable molecular CT imaging of cancer *Nano Lett.* **8** 4593–6

[125] Wang H, Zheng L, Peng C, Shen M, Shi X and Zhang G 2013 Folic acid-modified dendrimer-entrapped gold nanoparticles as nanoprobes for targeted CT imaging of human lung adencarcinoma *Biomaterials* **34** 470–80

[126] Yang Y, Chen M, Wang B, Wang P, Liu Y, Zhao Y, Li K, Song G, Zhang X B and Tan W 2019 NIR-II driven plasmon-enhanced catalysis for a timely supply of oxygen to overcome hypoxia-induced radiotherapy tolerance *Angew. Chem. Int. Ed.* **58** 15069–75

[127] Ni D, Bu W, Ehlerding E B, Cai W and Shi J 2017 Engineering of inorganic nanoparticles as magnetic resonance imaging contrast agents *Chem. Soc. Rev.* **46** 7438–68

[128] Lee N and Hyeon T 2012 Designed synthesis of uniformly sized iron oxide nanoparticles for efficient magnetic resonance imaging contrast agents *Chem. Soc. Rev.* **41** 2575–89

[129] Mi P, Cabral H, Kokuryo D, Rafi M, Terada Y, Aoki I, Saga T, Takehiko I, Nishiyama N and Kataoka K 2013 Gd-DTPA-loaded polymer–metal complex micelles with high relaxivity for MR cancer imaging *Biomaterials* **34** 492–500

[130] Zhu X, Chi X, Chen J, Wang L, Wang X, Chen Z and Gao J 2015 Real-time monitoring *in vivo* behaviors of theranostic nanoparticles by contrast-enhanced t1 imaging *Anal. Chem.* **87** 8941–8

[131] Zhao H, Zhao L, Wang Z, Xi W, Dibaba S T, Wang S, Shi L and Sun L 2019 Heterogeneous growth of palladium nanocrystals on upconversion nanoparticles for multimodal imaging and photothermal therapy *J. Mater. Chem.* B **7** 3652–60

[132] Zhao P, Jin Z, Chen Q, Yang T, Chen D, Meng J, Lu X, Gu Z and He Q 2018 Local generation of hydrogen for enhanced photothermal therapy *Nat. Commun.* **9** 1–12.

[133] Bharathiraja S, Bui N Q, Manivasagan P, Moorthy M S, Mondal S, Seo H, Phuoc N T, Phan T T V, Kim H and Lee K D 2018 Multimodal tumor-homing chitosan oligosaccharide-coated biocompatible palladium nanoparticles for photo-based imaging and therapy *Sci. Rep.* **8** 1–16.

[134] Zhu W, Chen M, Liu Y, Tian Y, Song Z, Song G and Zhang X 2019 A dual factor activated metal–organic framework hybrid nanoplatform for photoacoustic imaging and synergetic photo-chemotherapy *Nanoscale* **11** 20630–7

[135] Zhou G, Wang Y S, Jin Z, Zhao P, Zhang H, Wen Y and He Q 2019 Porphyrin–palladium hydride MOF nanoparticles for tumor-targeting photoacoustic imaging-guided hydrogenothermal cancer therapy *Nanoscale Horizons* **4** 1185–93

[136] Song M, Liu N, He L, Liu G, Ling D, Su X and Sun X 2018 Porous hollow palladium nanoplatform for imaging-guided trimodal chemo-, photothermal-, and radiotherapy *Nano Res.* **11** 2796–808

[137] Guo Z *et al* 2018 pH-sensitive radiolabeled and superfluorinated ultra-small palladium nanosheet as a high-performance multimodal platform for tumor theranostics *Biomaterials* **179** 134–43

[138] Chen M, Tang S, Guo Z, Wang X, Mo S, Huang X, Liu G and Zheng N 2014 Core–Shell Pd@Au nanoplates as theranostic agents for in-vivo photoacoustic imaging, CT imaging, and photothermal therapy *Adv. Mater.* **26** 8210–16

[139] Yang Y, Chen M, Wang B, Wang P, Liu Y, Zhao Y, Li K, Song G, Zhang X-B and Tan W 2019 NIR-II driven plasmon-enhanced catalysis for a timely supply of oxygen to overcome hypoxia-induced radiotherapy tolerance *Angew. Chem. Int. Ed.* **58** 15069–75

[140] Liu Z, Kiessling F and Gätjens J 2010 Advanced nanomaterials in multimodal imaging: design, functionalization, and biomedical applications *J. Nanomater.* **2010** 894303

[141] Josephson L, Kircher M F, Mahmood U, Tang Y and Weissleder R 2002 Near-infrared fluorescent nanoparticles as combined MR/optical imaging probes *Bioconj. Chem.* **13** 554–60

[142] Moore A, Medarova Z, Potthast A and Dai G 2004 *In vivo* targeting of underglycosylated MUC-1 tumor antigen using a multimodal imaging probe *Cancer Res.* **64** 1821–7

[143] Veiseh O, Sun C, Gunn J, Kohler N, Gabikian P, Lee D, Bhattarai N, Ellenbogen R, Sze R and Hallahan A 2005 Optical and MRI multifunctional nanoprobe for targeting gliomas *Nano Lett.* **5** 1003–8

[144] Yoon T J, Yu K N, Kim E, Kim J S, Kim B G, Yun S H, Sohn B H, Cho M H, Lee J K and Park S B 2006 Specific targeting, cell sorting, and bioimaging with smart magnetic silica core–shell nanomaterials *Small* **2** 209–15

[145] Lee J H, Jun Y, Yeon S I, Shin J S and Cheon J 2006 Dual-mode nanoparticle probes for high-performance magnetic resonance and fluorescence imaging of neuroblastoma *Angew. Chem. Int. Ed.* **45** 8160–2

[146] Huh Y M, Lee E S, Lee J H, Jun Y, Kim P H, Yun C O, Kim J H, Suh J S and Cheon J 2007 Hybrid nanoparticles for magnetic resonance imaging of target-specific viral gene delivery *Adv. Mater.* **19** 3109–12

[147] Choi J-s, Jun Y-w, Yeon S-I, Kim H C, Shin J-S and Cheon J 2006 Biocompatible heterostructured nanoparticles for multimodal biological detection *J. Am. Chem. Soc.* **128** 15982–3

[148] Yoo M K, Kim I Y, Kim E M, Jeong H-J, Lee C-M, Jeong Y Y, Akaike T and Cho C S 2007 Superparamagnetic iron oxide nanoparticles coated with galactose-carrying polymer for hepatocyte targeting *J. Biomed. Biotechnol.* **2007** 094740

[149] Lin Y-S, Wu S-H, Hung Y, Chou Y-H, Chang C, Lin M-L, Tsai C-P and Mou C-Y 2006 Multifunctional composite nanoparticles: magnetic, luminescent, and mesoporous *Chem. Mater.* **18** 5170–2

[150] Lu C-W, Hung Y, Hsiao J-K, Yao M, Chung T-H, Lin Y-S, Wu S-H, Hsu S-C, Liu H-M and Mou C-Y 2007 Bifunctional magnetic silica nanoparticles for highly efficient human stem cell labeling *Nano Lett.* **7** 149–54

[151] Zhang C, Wängler B, Morgenstern B, Zentgraf H, Eisenhut M, Untenecker H, Krüger R, Huss R, Seliger C and Semmler W 2007 Silica-and alkoxysilane-coated ultrasmall superparamagnetic iron oxide particles: a promising tool to label cells for magnetic resonance imaging *Langmuir* **23** 1427–34

[152] Zhang C, Jugold M, Woenne E C, Lammers T, Morgenstern B, Mueller M M, Zentgraf H, Bock M, Eisenhut M and Semmler W 2007 Specific targeting of tumor angiogenesis by RGD-conjugated ultrasmall superparamagnetic iron oxide particles using a clinical 1.5-T magnetic resonance scanner *Cancer Res.* **67** 1555–62

[153] Xie J, Chen K, Lee H-Y, Xu C, Hsu A R, Peng S, Chen X and Sun S 2008 Ultrasmall c (RGDyK)-coated Fe_3O_4 nanoparticles and their specific targeting to integrin $\alpha v\beta 3$-rich tumor cells *J. Am. Chem. Soc.* **130** 7542–3

[154] Huang G, Zhang C, Li S, Khemtong C, Yang S-G, Tian R, Minna J D, Brown K C and Gao J 2009 A novel strategy for surface modification of superparamagnetic iron oxide nanoparticles for lung cancer imaging *J. Mater. Chem.* **19** 6367–72

[155] Guthi J S, Yang S-G, Huang G, Li S, Khemtong C, Kessinger C W, Peyton M, Minna J D, Brown K C and Gao J 2010 MRI-visible micellar nanomedicine for targeted drug delivery to lung cancer cells *Mol. Pharm.* **7** 32–40

[156] Liu Y, Yuan H, Fales A M, Register J K and Vo-Dinh T 2015 Multifunctional gold nanostars for molecular imaging and cancer therapy *Front. Chem.* **3** 51

[157] Liu Y, Chang Z, Yuan H, Fales A M and Vo-Dinh T 2013 Quintuple-modality (SERS-MRI-CT-TPL-PTT) plasmonic nanoprobe for theranostics *Nanoscale* **5** 12126–31

[158] Fales A M, Yuan H and Vo-Dinh T 2014 Development of hybrid silver-coated gold nanostars for nonaggregated surface-enhanced Raman scattering *J. Phys. Chem.* C **118** 3708–15

[159] Shukla R, Bansal V, Chaudhary M, Basu A, Bhonde R R and Sastry M 2005 Biocompatibility of gold nanoparticles and their endocytotic fate inside the cellular compartment: a microscopic overview *Langmuir* **21** 10644–54
[160] Libutti S K, Paciotti G F, Byrnes A A, Alexander H R, Gannon W E, Walker M, Seidel G D, Yuldasheva N and Tamarkin L 2010 Phase I and pharmacokinetic studies of CYT-6091, a novel PEGylated colloidal gold-rhTNF nanomedicine *Clin. Cancer Res.* **16** 6139–49
[161] Link S and El-Sayed M A 1999 Spectral properties and relaxation dynamics of surface plasmon electronic oscillations in gold and silver nanodots and nanorods *J. Phys. Chem.* B **103** 8410–26
[162] Durr N J, Larson T, Smith D K, Korgel B A, Sokolov K and Ben-Yakar A 2007 Two-photon luminescence imaging of cancer cells using molecularly targeted gold nanorods *Nano Lett.* **7** 941–5
[163] von Maltzahn G, Centrone A, Park J H, Ramanathan R, Sailor M J, Hatton T A and Bhatia S N 2009 SERS-coded gold nanorods as a multifunctional platform for densely multiplexed near-infrared imaging and photothermal heating *Adv. Mater.* **21** 3175–80
[164] Gao X, Yang L, Petros J A, Marshall F F, Simons J W and Nie S 2005 *In vivo* molecular and cellular imaging with quantum dots *Curr. Opin. Biotechnol.* **16** 63–72
[165] Burke A, Ding X, Singh R, Kraft R A, Levi-Polyachenko N, Rylander M N, Szot C, Buchanan C, Whitney J and Fisher J 2009 Long-term survival following a single treatment of kidney tumors with multiwalled carbon nanotubes and near-infrared radiation *Proc. Natl. Acad. Sci.* **106** 12897–902
[166] Liu Z, Fan A C, Rakhra K, Sherlock S, Goodwin A, Chen X, Yang Q, Felsher D W and Dai H 2009 Supramolecular stacking of doxorubicin on carbon nanotubes for *in vivo* cancer therapy *Angew. Chem. Int. Ed.* **48** 7668–72
[167] Poland C A, Duffin R, Kinloch I, Maynard A, Wallace W A, Seaton A, Stone V, Brown S, MacNee W and Donaldson K 2008 Carbon nanotubes introduced into the abdominal cavity of mice show asbestos-like pathogenicity in a pilot study *Nat. Nanotechnol.* **3** 423
[168] Weissleder R, Stark D D, Engelstad B L, Bacon B R, Compton C C, White D L, Jacobs P and Lewis J 1989 Superparamagnetic iron oxide: pharmacokinetics and toxicity *Am. J. Roentgenol.* **152** 167–73
[169] Bulte J W and Kraitchman D L 2004 Iron oxide MR contrast agents for molecular and cellular imaging *NMR Biomed.* **17** 484–99
[170] Hudgins P A, Anzai Y, Morris M R and Lucas M A 2002 Ferumoxtran-10, a superparamagnetic iron oxide as a magnetic resonance enhancement agent for imaging lymph nodes: a phase 2 dose study *Am. J. Neuroradiol.* **23** 649–56
[171] Brown M 2003 PDT: light at the end of the tunnel? *Drug Discov. Today* **17** 767–68
[172] Roy I, Ohulchanskyy T Y, Pudavar H E, Bergey E J, Oseroff A R, Morgan J, Dougherty T J and Prasad P N 2003 Ceramic-based nanoparticles entrapping water-insoluble photosensitizing anticancer drugs: a novel drug–carrier system for photodynamic therapy *J. Am. Chem. Soc.* **125** 7860–5
[173] Jain T K, Roy I, De T K and Maitra A 1998 Nanometer silica particles encapsulating active compounds: a novel ceramic drug carrier *J. Am. Chem. Soc.* **120** 11092–5
[174] Shalviri A, Foltz W D, Cai P, Rauth A M and Wu X Y 2013 Multifunctional terpolymeric MRI contrast agent with superior signal enhancement in blood and tumor *J. Controlled Release* **167** 11–20

[175] Abbasi A Z, Prasad P, Cai P, He C, Foltz W D, Amini M A, Gordijo C R, Rauth A M and Wu X Y 2015 Manganese oxide and docetaxel co-loaded fluorescent polymer nanoparticles for dual modal imaging and chemotherapy of breast cancer *J. Controlled Release* **209** 186–96

[176] Mao D, Wu W, Ji S, Chen C, Hu F, Kong D, Ding D and Liu B 2017 Chemiluminescence-guided cancer therapy using a chemiexcited photosensitizer *Chem.* **3** 991–1007

[177] Li H, Sun J, Zhu H, Wu H, Zhang H, Gu Z and Luo K 2020 Recent advances in development of dendritic polymer-based nanomedicines for cancer diagnosis *Wiley Interdiscip. Rev. Nanomed. Nanobiotechnol.* e1670

[178] Cook A B and Perrier S 2020 Branched and dendritic polymer architectures: functional nanomaterials for therapeutic delivery *Adv. Funct. Mater.* **30** 1901001

[179] El-Betany A M, Kamoun E A, James C, Jangher A, Aljayyoussi G, Griffiths P, McKeown N B and Gumbleton M 2020 Auto-fluorescent PAMAM-based dendritic molecules and their potential application in pharmaceutical sciences *Int. J. Pharm.* **579** 119187

[180] Jin M, Zhang Y, Gao G, Xi Q, Yang Y, Yan L, Zhou H, Zhao Y, Wu C and Wang L 2018 MRI Contrast agents based on conjugated polyelectrolytes and dendritic polymers *Macromol. Rapid Commun.* **39** 1800258

[181] Li C, Wang J, Lu X, Ge H, Jin X, Guan Q, Pan R, Li P, Cai W and Zhu X 2020 Hydrogen peroxide-response nanoprobe for CD44-targeted circulating tumor cell detection and H_2O_2 analysis *Biomaterials* **255** 120071

[182] Tan S, Yang H, Xue S, Qiao J, Salarian M, Hekmatyar K, Meng Y, Mukkavilli R, Pu F and Odubade O Y 2020 Chemokine receptor 4 targeted protein MRI contrast agent for early detection of liver metastases *Sci. Adv.* **6** eaav7504

[183] Filippi M, Nguyen D-V, Garello F, Perton F, Bégin-Colin S, Felder-Flesch D, Power L and Scherberich A 2019 Metronidazole-functionalized iron oxide nanoparticles for molecular detection of hypoxic tissues *Nanoscale* **11** 22559–74

[184] Han Y, Zhou X, Qian Y, Hu H, Zhou Z, Liu X, Tang J and Shen Y 2019 Hypoxia-targeting dendritic MRI contrast agent based on internally hydroxy dendrimer for tumor imaging *Biomaterials* **213** 119195

[185] Yi X, Xu M, Zhou H, Xiong S, Qian R, Chai Z, Zhao L and Yang K 2018 Ultrasmall hyperbranched semiconducting polymer nanoparticles with different radioisotopes labeling for cancer theranostics *ACS Nano* **12** 9142–51

[186] Qiu J, Hameau A, Shi X, Mignani S, Majoral J P and Caminade A-M 2019 Fluorescent phosphorus dendrimers: towards material and biological applications *ChemPlusChem* **84** 1070–80

[187] Cong H, Wang K, Zhou Z, Yang J, Piao Y, Yu B, Shen Y and Zhou Z 2020 Tuning the brightness and photostability of organic dots for multivalent targeted cancer imaging and surgery *ACS Nano* **14** 5887–900

[188] Ma Y, Mou Q, Wang D, Zhu X and Yan D 2016 Dendritic polymers for theranostics *Theranostics* **6** 930

[189] Masao O *et al* 2017 Asia–Pacific clinical practice guidelines on the management of hepatocellular carcinoma: a 2017 update *Hepatol. Int.* **11** 317–70

[190] Arami H, Teeman E, Troksa A, Bradshaw H, Saatchi K, Tomitaka A, Gambhir S S, Häfeli U O, Liggitt D and Krishnan K M 2017 Tomographic magnetic particle imaging of cancer targeted nanoparticles *Nanoscale* **9** 18723–30

[191] Xu X, Liu K, Wang Y, Zhang C, Shi M, Wang P, Shen L, Xia J, Ye L and Shi X 2019 A multifunctional low-generation dendrimer-based nanoprobe for the targeted dual mode MR/CT imaging of orthotopic brain gliomas *J. Mater. Chem.* B **7** 3639–43

[192] Jones N, Ropero-Miller J, Waltke H, McLeod-Henning D, Weiss D and Barcus H 2016 *Proc. of the Int. Forensic Radiology Research Summit (Amsterdam, May 10–11)*

[193] Yang X, Hong H, Grailer J J, Rowland I J, Javadi A, Hurley S A, Xiao Y, Yang Y, Zhang Y and Nickles R J 2011 cRGD-functionalized, DOX-conjugated, and 64Cu-labeled superparamagnetic iron oxide nanoparticles for targeted anticancer drug delivery and PET/MR imaging *Biomaterials* **32** 4151–60

[194] Engudar G, Schaarup-Jensen H, Fliedner F P, Hansen A E, Kempen P, Jølck R I, Kjaer A, Andresen T L, Clausen M H and Jensen A I 2018 Remote loading of liposomes with a 124I-radioiodinated compound and their *in vivo* evaluation by PET/CT in a murine tumor model *Theranostics* **8** 5828

[195] Masao C *et al* 2016 PET predicts the efficacy of anti-cancer nanotherapy *Nat. Commun.* **7** 1–8

[196] Yu B, Wei H, He Q, Ferreira C A, Kutyreff C J, Ni D, Rosenkrans Z T, Cheng L, Yu F and Engle J W 2018 Efficient uptake of ^{177}Lu-Porphyrin-PEG nanocomplexes by tumor mitochondria for multimodal-imaging-guided combination therapy *Angew. Chem. Int. Ed.* **57** 218–22

[197] Pérez-Medina C, Teunissen A J, Kluza E, Mulder W J and van der Meel R 2020 Nuclear imaging approaches facilitating nanomedicine translation *Adv. Drug Delivery Rev.* **154–155** 123–41

[198] Man F, Lammers T and de Rosales R T 2018 Imaging nanomedicine-based drug delivery: a review of clinical studies *Mol. Imaging Biol.* **20** 683–95

[199] Petersen G H, Alzghari S K, Chee W, Sankari S S and La-Beck N M 2016 Meta-analysis of clinical and preclinical studies comparing the anticancer efficacy of liposomal versus conventional non-liposomal doxorubicin *J. Controlled Release* **232** 255–64

[200] van der Meel R, Sulheim E, Shi Y, Kiessling F, Mulder W J and Lammers T 2019 Smart cancer nanomedicine *Nat. Nanotechnol.* **14** 1007–17

[201] Lee H, Shields A F, Siegel B A, Miller K D, Krop I, Ma C X, LoRusso P M, Munster P N, Campbell K and Gaddy D F 2017 ^{64}Cu-MM-302 positron emission tomography quantifies variability of enhanced permeability and retention of nanoparticles in relation to treatment response in patients with metastatic breast cancer *Clin. Cancer Res.* **23** 4190–202

[202] Fales A M, Yuan H and Vo-Dinh T 2011 Silica-coated gold nanostars for combined SERS detection and singlet oxygen generation: a potential nanoplatform for theranostics *Langmuir* **27** 12186

[203] Fales A M, Yuan H and Vo-Dinh T 2013 Cell-penetrating peptide enhanced intracellular Raman imaging and photodynamic therapy *Mol. Pharm.* **10** 2291–8

[204] Yuan H, Fales A M, Khoury C G, Liu J and Vo-Dinh T 2013 Spectral characterization and intracellular detection of Surface-Enhanced Raman Scattering (SERS)-encoded plasmonic gold nanostars *J. Raman Spectrosc.* **44** 234–9

[205] Liu Y, Yuan H, Kersey F R, Register J K, Parrott M C and Vo-Dinh T 2015 Plasmonic gold nanostars for multi-modality sensing and diagnostics *Sensors* **15** 3706–20

[206] Huang H-C, Barua S, Sharma G, Dey S K and Rege K 2011 Inorganic nanoparticles for cancer imaging and therapy *J. Controlled Release* **155** 344–57

[207] Pérez-Medina C, Abdel-Atti D, Tang J, Zhao Y, Fayad Z A, Lewis J S, Mulder W J and Reiner T 2016 Nanoreporter PET predicts the efficacy of anti-cancer nanotherapy *Nat. Commun.* **7** 1–8

Chapter 4

Synergy between nanomedicine and tumor imaging

Sandeep B Somvanshi and Nanasaheb D Thorat

The emerging area of nanomedicine has marked a supreme breakthrough in diagnostics and therapy of different kinds of disease including cancer. The exceptional and noteworthy features of nanoscale materials such as higher surface area, superior chemical stability, the capability of accommodating different kind of drugs, tailored surfaces etc provide many benefits as compared to their bulk form. Moreover, nanomedicines with synergistic combinations for imaging and treatment monitoring have displayed growing implications in cancer therapies as they offer superior efficacy in clinical level practice. The diagnostics and therapeutics potentials of these synergistic approaches have gained substantial interest for next generation anti-cancer therapies. In particular, recent advancements in novel nanomedicine employing both diagnosis and therapeutic strategy with therapy monitoring have produced optimism for effectual and achievable cancer treatment. The present chapter gives a brief overview of the synergistic approaches employed within nanomedicines and tumor imaging. Initially, recent trends and the different imaging techniques for cancer are introduced along with a brief account of the multifunctional nanoplatforms for cancer diagnosis. Further, the different kinds of imaging nanoplatforms for therapy monitoring and image-guided nanomedicine animal models and clinical implications are discussed.

4.1 Introduction

Cancer is one of the leading global diseases which caused around 10 million deaths in 2020 and the mortalities are still increasing day by day [1]. According to the World Health Organization (WHO), this trend will reach up to ~29 million new cancer patients and ~16 million new mortalities per year by 2040 [2]. Cancer is a type of disease in which cells grow in an uncontrolled and abnormal way. The main causes behind cancer are exterior things such as unhealthy diet, tobacco

doi:10.1088/978-0-7503-3675-8ch4 © IOP Publishing Ltd 2022

consumption, infected organisms and interior things such as hormonal growth, immune system and inherent genetic mutation. The currently available treatment methods of cancer consist of chemotherapies, radiotherapies, immunotherapies and hormonal therapies [3, 4]. Recently, the incredible impact of nanoscale cancer technology is in the area of combinational therapies with image-guided monitoring. By tailoring the different features of nanomaterials like physicochemical properties, biological properties such as toxicity, immunity and circulating period can be easily modulated. The upcoming trends are to utilize the shapes, sizes and surface properties of nanomaterials to improve cellular uptakes, circulation time, immunity responses and body clearances in order to advance cancer therapeutics.

In recent years, nanomedicine has evolved as a chief area in the realm of medicine which merges the knowledge and information of medicine, physics, pharmaceutics, chemistry and materials science. This may lead to the establishment of a globalized nanomedicine marketplace, which is estimated to reach new milestones in the realm of medicine. A schematic of conventional and nanomedicine based cancer treatment is shown in figure 4.1. Different kinds of nanoscale materials have been significantly employed for various biomedical applications like bioimaging, drug delivery, biosensing, tissue engineering, anti-bacterial, anti-oxidant and magnetic hyperthermia. The different biomedical applications of nanoscale materials are summarized in figure 4.2.

The companionable features between nanoscale sizes and the biological system, integrated with the ability to tailor their physical and chemical properties with detailed characterization, facilitates the expressive rise of nanoscale materials as an exceptional tool for numerous biomedical applications (figure 4.3). These nanoscale materials engineered with multi-functionalities offer superior potential for customized approaches in disease administration and therapeutics, and can significantly advance the diagnosis and treatment of different cancer diseases. Bioimaging is deemed to be one of the most utilized techniques in the area of biomedical healthcares. Through the exceptional surface properties, nanoscale platforms could

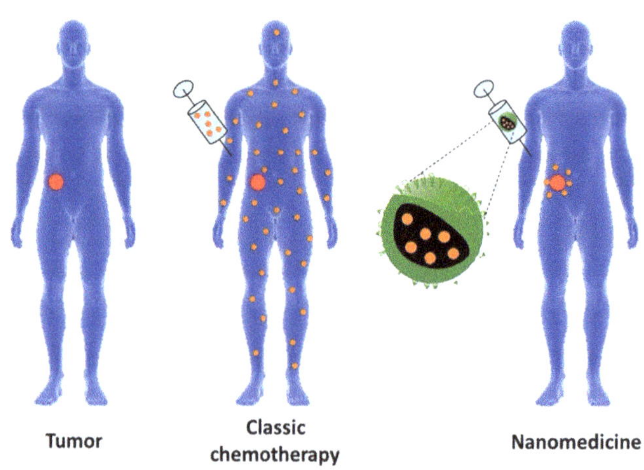

Figure 4.1. Schematics of conventional and nanomedicine based cancer treatment (image reproduced from [5], copyright (2021), with permission from Elsevier).

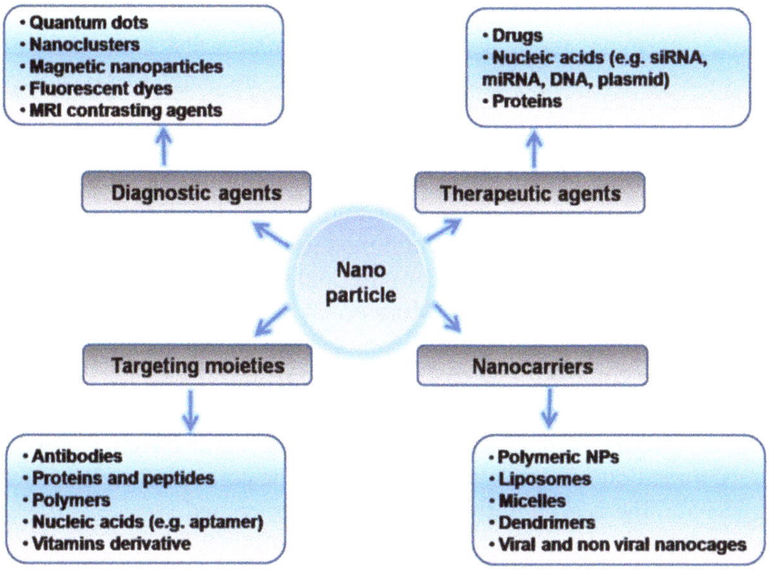

Figure 4.2. Biomedical applications of nanoscale materials (image reproduced from [6], copyright (2017), with permission from Elsevier).

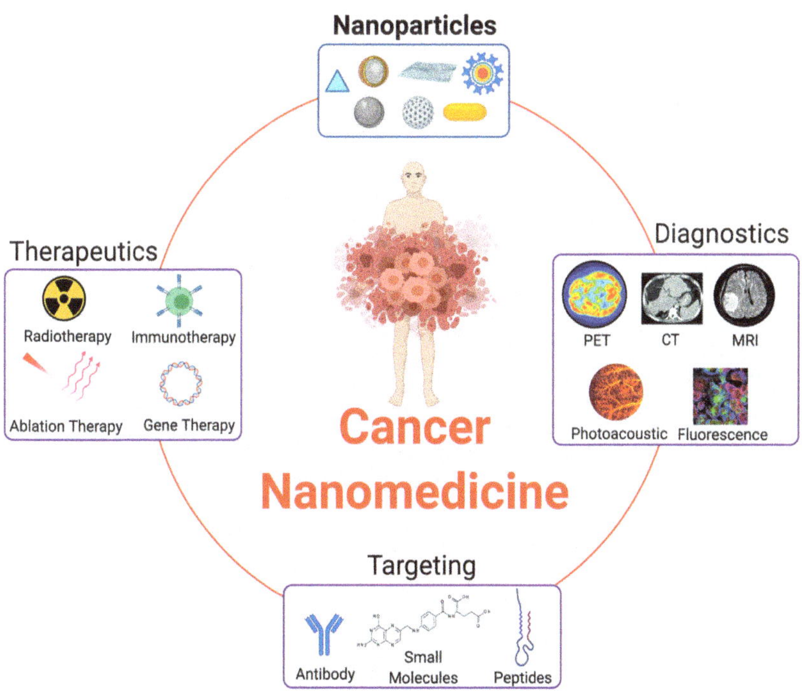

Figure 4.3. Schematics of the cancer nanomedicine (image reproduced with permission from [7] CC BY 4.0).

offer contrasting augmentation in different imaging modalities for earlier detection and diagnosis, screening, and image-guided cancer treatments. These imaging modalities cover optical, radiological, magnetic resonance imaging (MRI) and computed tomography (CT). The prospect of commencing two or more modalities within the same nanoplatforms with minimum interface makes these nanoscale platforms appealing and beneficial. These kinds of nanoscale platforms can effectively function as multimodal contrasting agent for imaging and provide harmonizing information for precise diagnostics. Combining for a multimodal approach, nanoscale materials are also being fabricated to accompany conventionally used therapeutics like surgeries, chemotherapies, radiotherapies etc. Multimodal and multifunctional therapy are advancing along with advances in technologies. The singular nanosystem that is able to provide contrast augmentation for different imaging modality may offer more correct and detailed information of the physiology and anatomy of diseases. Integration of imaging with therapeutics attains safe and effectual approaches as sufficient accumulation inside the tumor tissue can be controlled and its effect on the tumor targets and the nearby normal cells can be supervised.

Even though the field of nanomedicines is comparatively new, this research area is evolving quickly and is being extensively employed in the area of biomedicine and other areas of routine life. In the realm of medicine, the nanoscale material presents one of the outstanding approaches for diagnosis and therapeutics purpose along with theranostics. Figure 4.4 shows different nanostructured material employed in

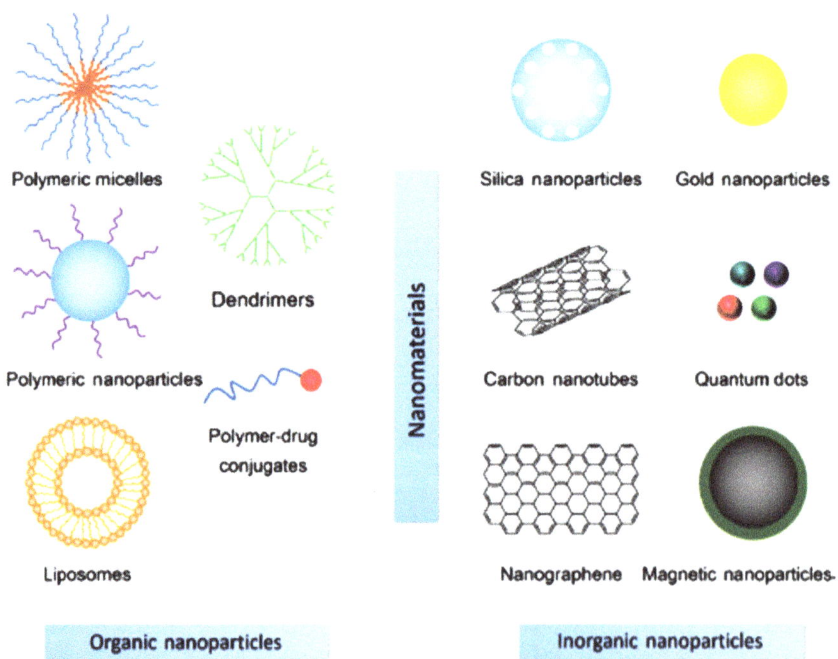

Figure 4.4. Types of nanostructured materials employed in nanomedicine (image reproduced with permission from [8], copyright 2017 Walter de Gruyter GmbH, Berlin/Boston).

nanomedicine including liposome, dendrimer, polymer nanoparticle, micelle, nanocrystals, metallic and inorganic nanomaterials such as silica nanoparticles, gold nanoparticles, quantum dots, carbon nanotubes, magnetic nanoparticles, graphene nanomaterials etc. The therapeutics output of nanoscale materials are robustly dependent on the chemical compositions, and other properties such as surface chemistry (charges and hydrophilic behavior), physical properties (sizes and shapes) and surface functionalisation (figure 4.5). To conquer the anomalous physiology of the tumor tissues, nanoscale medicine offers advantages of advanced permeability and EPR effects to advance drug accumulation inside the tumors, therefore reaching the therapeutics drug amount. Prerequisites of promising nanoscale systems for cancer therapeutics are constantly emerging, as the resolutions of the unachieved requisites therapeutics goal and demands the contribution of new perceptions to develop precise medicinal tools. The design and functionalizing of nanoscale materials differ enormously and the number of prospective applications is increasing day by day, so present trends in nanoscale medicine point towards tailor-made nanoscale devices. However, it is significant to perceive that nanoscale medicine based therapeutics is not an ideal tool, as it has a lot of issues to tackle. Nanoscale medicines have evolved as a promising approach against cancer and thus the number of research articles on cancer nanomedicine is increasing day by day (figure 4.6). Currently, there are around 110 clinical trials ongoing which involve the applications of nanoscale technologies for cancer therapeutics according to the National Institute of Health (NIH 2020). The list of some clinically approved biomedical nanoscale devices for cancer therapeutics are summarized in table 4.1. The list of biomedical nanoscale systems that are in clinical trials for cancer therapeutics are summarized in table 4.2.

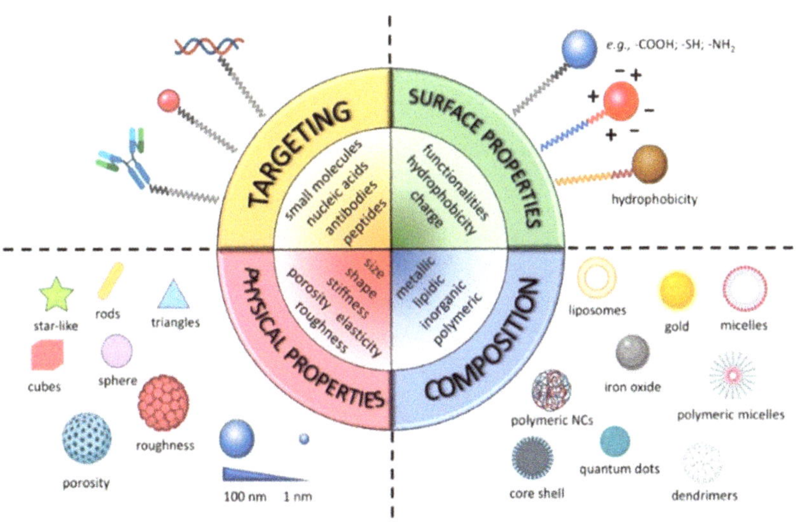

Figure 4.5. Tailor-made physicochemical properties of nanoscale materials (image is reproduced with permission from [9] CC BY 4.0).

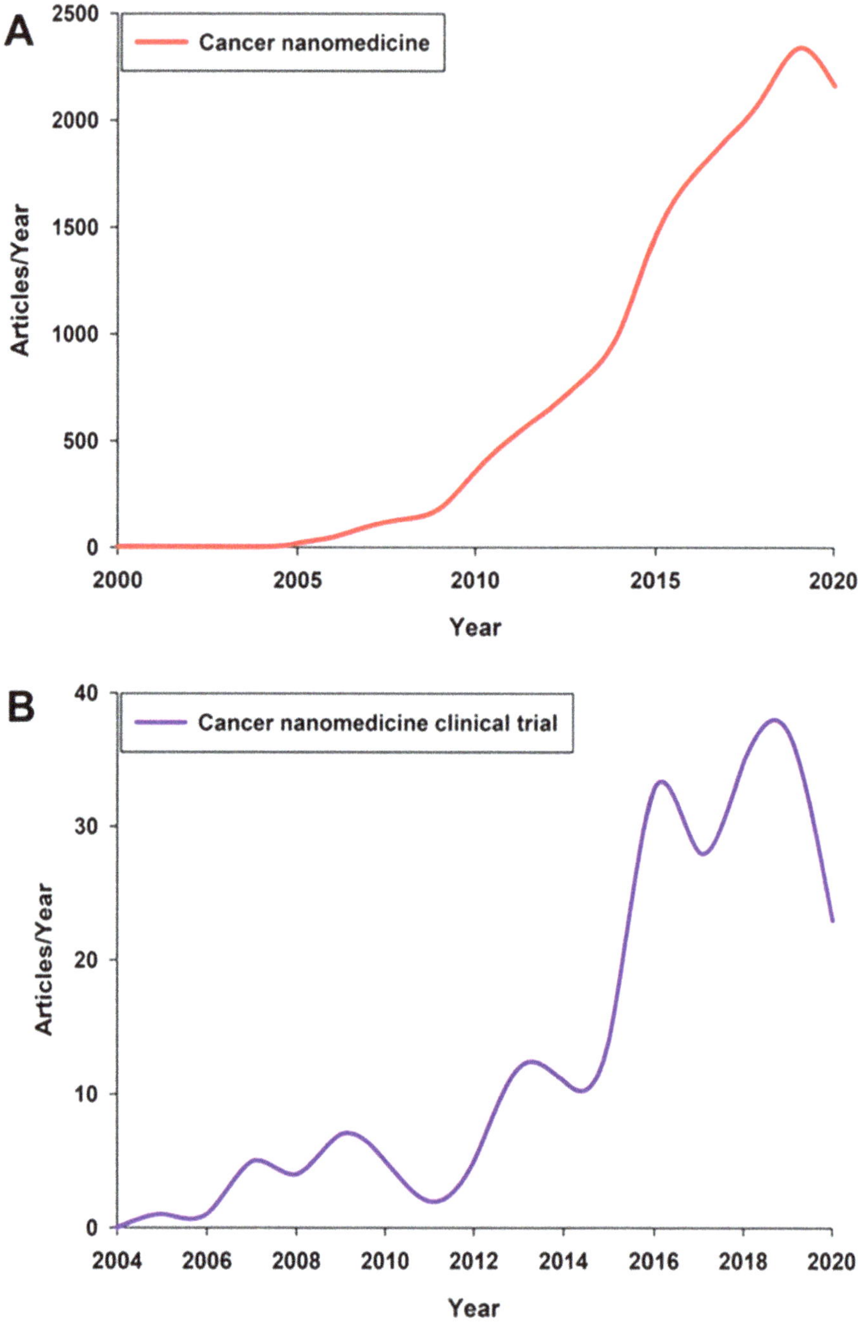

Figure 4.6. Research articles published up to 2020 referring to terms (a) 'Cancer nanomedicine' (b) 'Cancer nanomedicine clinical trial' (image reproduced with permission from [5], copyright (2021), with permission from Elsevier).

Table 4.1. Examples of clinically approved biomedical nanodevices for cancer therapy (table reproduced with permission from [5], copyright (2021), with permission from Elsevier).

Product	Type	Chemotherapeutic agent	Size (nm)	Indication	Approved by	Biologic license application
Adagen®	Polymeric nanoparticle	Bovine pegademase	n/a	Severe combined immunodeficiency (SCID)	FDA	019,818
Bexxar®	Antibody-radioactive element conjugate	Iodine-131	n/a	Non-Hodgkin's lymphoma	FDA	125,011
DaunoXome®	Liposome	Daunorubicin	45	AIDS-related Kaposi's sarcoma, metastatic ovarian cancer, metastatic breast cancer, multiple myeloma	FDA	050,704
DepoCyt®	Liposome	Cytarabine	n/a	Lymphomas or leukemia with meningeal spread add neoplastic meningitis	FDA	21–041
Eligard®	Polymeric nanoparticle	Leuprolideacetate	n/a	Prostate cancer	FDA	021,731
Kadcyla®	Antibody-drug conjugate	DM1	n/a	Metastatic breast cancer	FDA	125427/0
Marqibo®	Liposome	Vincristine	163	Acute lymphoid leukemia	FDA	202,497
Mepact®	Liposome	Mifamurtide	n/a	Osteosarcoma	EMA	EMEA/H/C/000802
Myocet®	Liposome	Doxorubicin	150	Breast	EMA	EMEA/H/C/000297
Mylotarg®	Antibody-drug conjugate	Calicheamicin	n/a	Acute myeloid leukemia.	FDA	761,060
Onivyde®	Liposome	Irinotecan	n/a	Pancreatic cancer	FDA	207,793
Ontak®	Fusion protein	Denileukindiftito	n/a	Cutaneous T-cell lymphoma	FDA; EMA	103767; EU/3/01/075
Vyxeos®	Liposome	Daunorubicin and cytarabine	n/a	Acute Myeloid Leukemia	FDA	209,401
Zevalin®	Antibody-radioactive element conjugate	Yttrium-90	n/a	Non-Hodgkin's lymphoma	FDA; EMA	125019; EMEA/H/C/000547

Table 4.2. Examples of biomedical nanosystems in clinical trials for cancer therapy (table reproduced with permission from [5], copyright (2021), with permission from Elsevier).

Type of nanomaterial	Product	Chemotherapeutic agent	Indication	Status	Clinical trial reference
Dendrimer	AZD4320	AZD4320	Advanced solid tumors; lymphoma; multiple myeloma; hematologic malignancies	Phase I	NCT04214093
Gold nanoparticle	Aurimmune	TNF	Solid tumor	Phase I	NCT00356980
Liposome	CPX1	Irinotecan	Colorectal cancer	Phase II	NCT00361842
	LE-SN38	Sn-38	Neoplasms	Phase II	NCT00046540
	Lipoplatin™	Cisplatin	Non-small cell lung cancer; breast cancer; gastric cancer	Phase III	NCT02702700
	LNDDP	Cisplatin	Malignant mesothelioma	Phase II	NCT00004033
	2B3–101	Doxorubicin	Glioma	Phase I, II	NCT01386580
Polymeric conjugate	XMT1001	Camptothecin	Small cell lung cancer; non-small cell lung cancer	Phase I	NCT00455052
	Cpc634	Docetaxel	Ovarian cancer	Phase II	NCT03742713
	CRLX101-Olaparib	Olaparib	Urothelial cancer; small cell lung cancer; non-small cell lung cancer; prostate cancer	Phase I; Phase II	NCT02769962
Polymeric micelle	Nk105	Paclitaxel	Breast cancer nor metastatic recurrent	Phase III	NCT01644890
	Nanoxel® M	Docetaxel	Head and neck squamous cell carcinoma	Phase II	NCT02639858
	Lipusu®	Paclitaxel	Breast cancer	Phase IV	NCT02142790
	Nanoplatin	Gemcitabine	Locally advanced and metastatic pancreatic cancer	Phase I; Phase II	NCT00910741
	E7389-e044–112	Eribulin-lf	Solid tumors	Phase I	NCT01945710
	Nc6004	Cisplatin	Head and neck cancer	Phase II	NCT03771820
	Paclical	Paclitaxel	Ovarian cancer	Phase III	NCT00989131
Targeted minicell	TargomiRs	miRNA mimic	Malignant pleural mesothelioma; non-small cell lung cancer	Phase I	NCT02369198

For characterization of biological processes within living systems, it is necessary to pursue biological level events without removal of the tissue and cells of interest, i.e., to supervise processes in the natural environment without troubling the living systems under observation. Thus, imaging modalities employed in this area are non-destructive and utilize various properties of tissues, sometimes integrated with imaging probes as the source of contrast enhancer. The imaging modalities may offer spatial resolutions sufficient to monitor the biological events in tissues over a time period without interrupting them. This type of imaging aids in recognising the pathological movements, progress and undergoing mechanisms of various diseases and therefore provides the potentiality for earlier diagnosis and supervision of treatment.

Molecular level imaging modalities have promising applications in the area of translational research. By visualizing the biological process at the sites of diseased tissue, scientists are able to set up and expand explicit biomarkers, which can be employed in diagnosis, drug discovery and therapeutics. Figure 4.7 displays a schematical representation of the usual molecular level imaging studies. It is initiated with the exploration of the pathology of the biological events for cancer disease. The second step belongs to the identification of the target specification towards the biological event, like an overview of the cell receptor or intra-cellular protein. The third step belongs to the identification or synthesis of the molecular level probes, specially target oriented. These molecular probes can be integrated with the

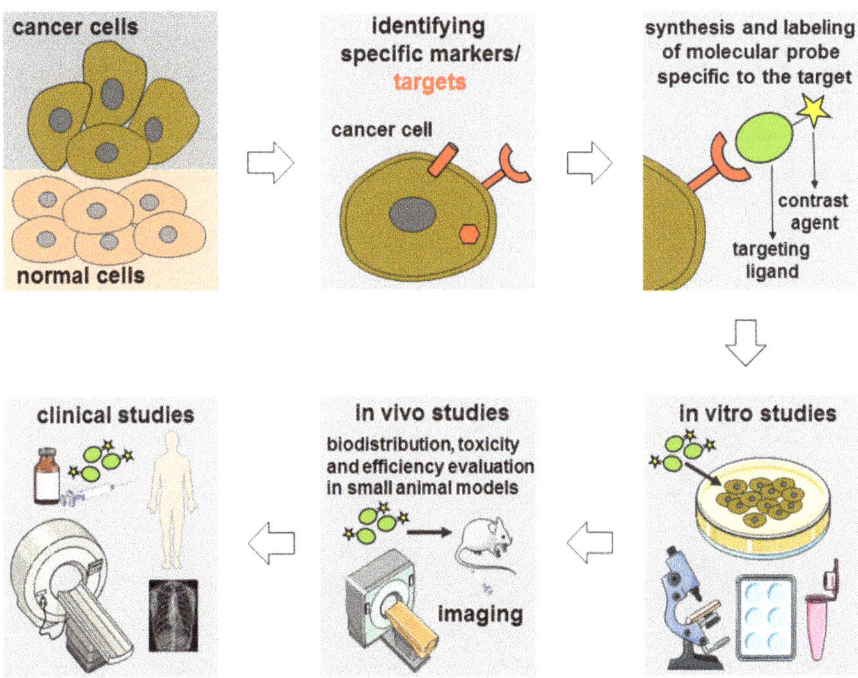

Figure 4.7. Schematic demonstration of imaging modalities in translational research (all the images are reproduced with permission from [10] CC BY 4.0).

contrasting agents, so they can be employed as tracers and can be easily visualized in *in vivo* and *in vitro* study. The molecular probes need to be tested *in vitro* to evaluate their interfaces, specific nature, and toxic nature. After successful evaluation *in vitro*, these probes need to be tested *in vivo* (inside the small animal) to evaluate their activities in biological surroundings. After checking the pharmacokinetic and pharmacodynamics behaviour, these molecular probes can be easily translated from pre-clinical practice to clinical practice.

The employment of small animals models in pre-clinical research enables evaluation of the biodistribution, pharmacokinetic and biological response (probable toxicities, side effects etc) of the prospective contrasting agent and drug. *In vivo* assessment of the molecular probe in small animal models can be executed by the various non-destructive imaging techniques, like optical imaging, CT, positron emission tomography (PET), MRI, single-photon emission computed tomography (SPECT), ultrasound imaging, photoacoustic imaging etc. Many of these imaging techniques are utilized in clinical practice, as shown in figure 4.8, which made pre-clinical evaluations to some extent a consistent prediction for outcomes in human trials. Optical and photoacoustic imaging modalities are frequently employed in the pre-clinical stage, chiefly because of the limitation in penetrating depths. These imaging techniques are appropriate in humans only for superficial tissue examination. On the other hand, there are some constraints for all these imaging techniques in terms of sensitivity and spatial resolutions. For this cause, the combination or integration of imaging techniques such as CT–PET, fluorescence molecular tomography (FMT)–CT or MRI–PET are needed which may offer detailed information for the desired site of the tumor.

The applications of nanomedicine have plentiful benefits such as higher drugs accommodating capability, enhanced drug water solubility and increased blood half-life of the drug in comparison to the administrations of the individual drug. Moreover, owing to the sizes of nanoscale systems, they have lower penetrating depth and extravasations in healthy tissues, which avoids their accretion inside the healthy organ. The mechanisms related to the nanomedicine accumulations and extravasations at the disease location are usually referred to as passive targeting,

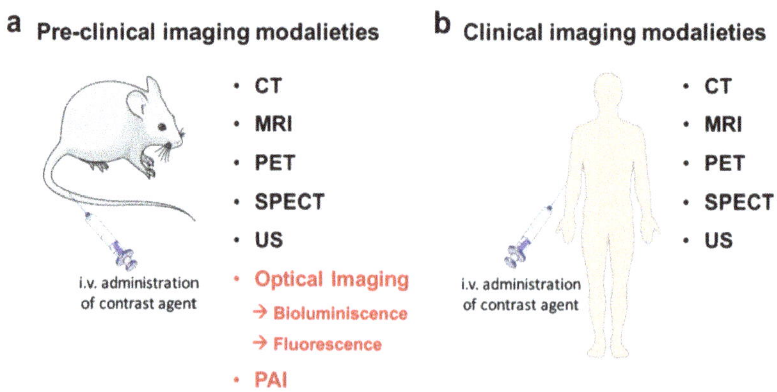

Figure 4.8. Imaging techniques employed in pre-clinical (a) and clinical (b) cancer treatments (all the images are reproduced with permission from [10] CC BY 4.0).

which are mainly based on EPR effects. As the nanomedicine is taken inside the tumor region, it possibly enters the cell via nonspecific endocytosis or may liberate the chemotherapeutics payloads at the internal spaces where the drug can be diffused and attain the tumor cell. Comparative schematics of the properties, pharmacokinetics and biodistribution of chemotherapeutics and nanomedicine is shown in figure 4.9.

Recently, different kinds of nanoscale materials have emerged as promising tools in cancer therapy and diagnostics, because of their multifunctional properties and interstitial properties which aids effectual diagnostics, imaging, and therapies. However, nanomaterial synthesized via chemical routes possesses numerous issues connected to the toxic nature, costs and efficacy. In recent decades, nanoscale technologies have been extensively employed in the field of diagnostics and treatments of different types of disease like cancer, infectious diseases, neurological disease, cardiovascular disease, diabetic disease etc. In consideration of the constraints in conventionally used therapeutics, many scientists and nanotechnologists have focused their interest on designing and developing different kinds of nanomaterials which include liposomes, metallic nanomaterials, lipid-based nanomaterials etc (figure 4.10). It is worth noting that nanoscale materials have significantly advanced the field of diagnosis and treatment of different kinds of cancer due to the nano level sizes, tailor-made properties, accessible surface chemistry, improved drug accommodation, ease in penetrating ability, and enhanced stability within the tumor site. Alongside, the outstanding biocompatible nature, biodegrading ability, multifunctionality in bioimaging, biosensing, diagnosis and therapy, has augmented the potentiality of these nanoscale materials in different biomedical applications. Table 4.3 summarizes different types of nanotheranostics

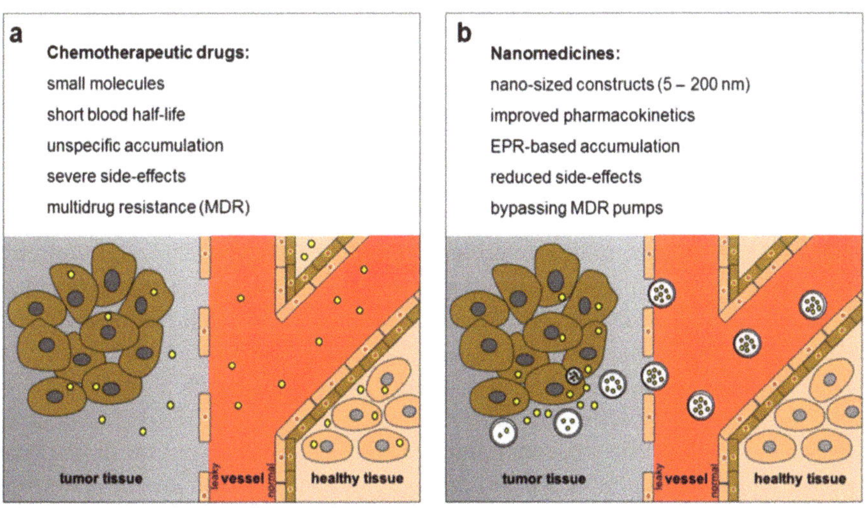

Figure 4.9. Comparative schematics of chemotherapeutic drug and nanomedicines with their biodistribution in normal and cancer tissue (all the images are reproduced with permission from [10] CC BY 4.0).

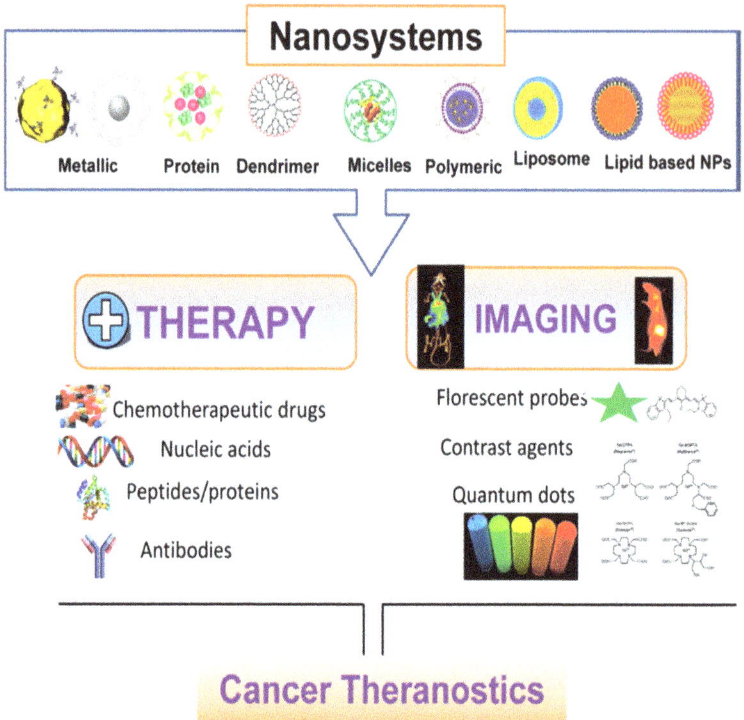

Figure 4.10. Schematic representation of nanoscale systems for cancer theranostics (image reproduced with permission from [11] CC BY 4.0).

which are approved by FDA or are currently under clinical trial. Although presently available nanotheranostics agents in clinical trials are rare, soon their use will increase with expressive rates in consideration with the current advances.

The area of nanoscale medicine is advancing cancer therapeutics and displaying immense potential for the future of medicine. Currently, many of the researchers are reporting inclusive accounts of investigable and marketable products, which are receiving FDA endorsement for utilization in clinical level practice based on the types of intervention. Additionally, efforts are progressing with nanoscale materials in integration with multimodal imaging techniques. These multimodal abilities are advancing and revolutionizing in novel strategies to improve cancer diagnostics and treatment, offering a wide spectra of novel techniques, which might significantly enhance the diagnosis and generate precise therapeutics intervention with improved efficacy. Insight acquired from recent decades related to research in tumor biological behavior and nano-biotechnology are requisite components of advanced imaging approaches. The capability to image tumor responses to intervention in an accurate and precise manner play an important and crucial role in design and implantation of effectual therapeutics, as shown in figure 4.11. Non-destructive imaging modalities need to be optimized at pre-clinical and clinical level phases. Moreover, as depicted

Table 4.3. Nanotheranostics systems in clinical stage of development (table reproduced with permission from [11] CC BY 4.0).

Nanosystem	Description	Cancer type	Sponsor/Agency	Clinical Trial ID/Phase
Silica nanoparticles	For real-time imaging of lymph node metastasis	Colon, head and neck, breast cancer	Memorial Sloan Kettering Cancer Center	NCT02106598Phase 1 and 2
Polysiloxane Gd-nanoparticles	To assessing the MTD of AGuIX-NP along with cisplatin and radiation in cervical cancer patients	Advanced cervical cancer	Gustave Roussy,NCI, France	NCT03308604Phase 1
Liposomes	Evaluating immunogenic chemotherapy combined with Ipilimumab and Nivolumab in patients with metastatic luminal B breast cancer	Breast cancer	Oslo University Hospital	NCT03409198Phase 2B
Carbon nanoparticles	Use of carbon nanoparticles for primary and lymph nodes tumors isolation and mapping in the laparoscopic surgery	Colorectal tumor	Aiguo, Lu	NCT03350945Not Applicable
Protein-based nanoparticles	To perceive the side effects and MTD of EphB4-HSA fusion protein with chemotherapy in patients with solid tumors	Solid tumors	Vasgene Therapeutics, Inc.	NCT02495896Phase 1
Hafnium oxide (HfO2) nanoparticle	To find MTD of NBTXR3 which is, activated by radiation, Brachytherapy	Prostate cancer	Nanobiotix	NCT02805894Phase 1
Polymeric nanoparticles	To estimate MTD, safety, PK, PD of AZD2811 with/without azacitidine in patients with relapsed AML	Acute myeloid leukaemia	AstraZeneca	NCT03217838Phase 1
Gold nanoparticles	To estimate the efficacy of NU-0129, (nucleic acids prepared on the exterior of a spherical gold nanoparticle)	Glioblastoma	Northwestern UniversityNational Cancer Institute (NCI)	NCT03020017Early Phase 1
Polymeric nanoparticles	To study the anti-cancer effect of CetuximabNanoparticles.	Colon cancer	Ahmed A H Abdellatif	NCT03774680Phase 1
Polymeric nanoparticles	Open-label PET study with [89Zr]-Df-CriPec® docetaxel in patients with solid tumors.	Solid tumor	Cristal TherapeuticsVU University Medical Center	NCT03712423Phase 1
Polymeric nanoparticles	To evaluate anti-tumor activity CRLX101 plus enzalutamide in prostate cancer patients who already treated with enzalutamide.	Prostate cancer	National Cancer Institute (NCI)	NCT03531827Phase 2

(*Continued*)

Table 4.3. (*Continued*)

Nanosystem	Description	Cancer type	Sponsor/Agency	Clinical Trial ID/Phase
Micelles	To evaluate the efficacy and safety of Docetaxel Micellein Recurrent or Metastatic HNSCC	Head and neck squamous cell carcinoma	Samyang Biopharmaceutical Corporation	NCT02639858Phase 2
Liposomes	To study the distribution profile and radiation dosimetry of 188Re-BMEDAliposomes	Tumors	Nuclear Energy Research Institute of Taiwan	NCT02271516Phase 1
Liposomes	To study the MTD of EphA2 siRNA-encapsulated liposomes, evaluate efficacy in the tumor cell, which we cannot be cured by treatment	Solid tumors	M.D. Anderson Cancer CenterNational Cancer Institute (NCI)	NCT02191878Phase 3
Protein-based nanoparticles	To determine the MTD of ABI-009 and evaluate safety and anti-tumor activity	Bladder cancer	National Cancer Institute, Aadi, LLC	NCT02009332,Phase 1
Protein-based nanoparticles	To evaluate the activity of ONTAK in cutaneous T-cell Lymphoma (CTCL)	CTCL	Eisai Inc. TMC, Ligand pharmaceuticals, NCI.	NCT00211198Phase 4
PSMA-targeted polymeric nanoparticles	A Study of BIND-014 efficacy in various lung cancer patients	Squamous cell, NSCLC	BIND Therapeutics	NCT02283320Phase 2
Protein-based nanoparticles	To find MTD for rapamycin loaded albumin with standard chemotherapy in solid tumors	Solid tumors	National Cancer Institute Children's Oncology group	NCT02975882Phase 1
PSMA-conjugates	To determine the activity of Lu-PSMA vs cabazitaxel in prostate cancer	Prostate cancer	ANUPCTG, ANSTO, PCFA, ARTnet, and Movember Foundation	NCT03392428Phase 2
CCK2 receptor targeting 111In peptide conjugates	Radioactivity uptake of 111In-CP04 in tumor and other tissues	Thyroid carcinoma	Paola Anna Erba	NCT03246659Phase 1
67Cu-Peptide conjugates	MTD study of 64Cu-SARTATE	Neuroblastoma	Clarity Pharmaceuticals Ltd	NCT04023331Phase 1 and 2
Iron oxide nanoparticles (SPIONs)	To find the feasibility of using SPIONs—Ferumoxytol in MRI analysis	Head and neck cancer	M.D. Anderson Cancer Center	NCT01895829Phase 1
Lipid-based nanoparticles	To study proposes targeted delivery cytotoxic drugs, viaformulated LTSL activated by using focused ultrasound (FUS)	Liver tumors	University of Oxford	NCT02181075Phase1
Gold nanoparticles	To evaluate the PTT efficacy of PEGylated AuroShell suspension	Primary and metastatic lung tumors	Nanospectra Biosciences, Inc.	NCT01679470

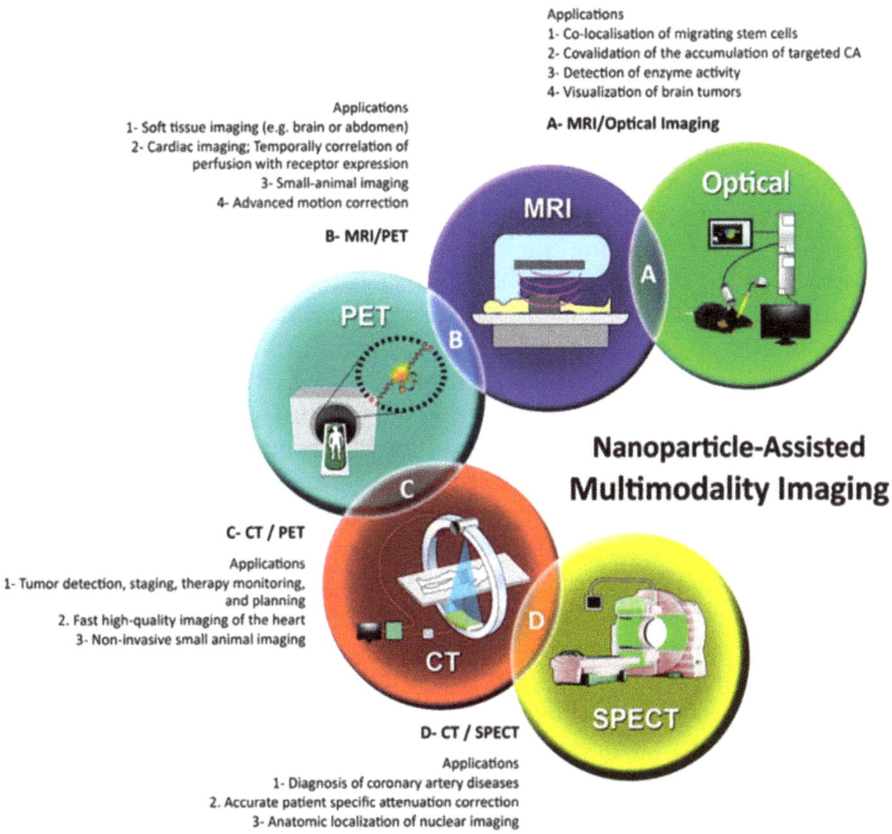

Figure 4.11. Schematic representation of nanoparticle-based multimodality imaging (image reproduced from [12], copyright 2011 with permission from Elsevier).

in figure 4.11, multimodal imaging permits combinational approaches in these imaging modalities while controlling the exceptional benefits of each of them correspondingly. The explicit benefits will differ across the techniques and mostly depend on the applications, which range from basic level research to clinical level research and the types of imaging information needed.

Nanoscale multifunctional materials play an important role in designing and developing smart technology and imaging candidates by combination of multiple moieties into a singular nanosystem. These multifunctional nanoscale materials may have benefits for imaging, pharmacokinetics, *in vivo* targeting and responses to the biological event. There is immense potential for specifically created hybrid molecular probes with functionalization of varying targeted moieties as smaller molecules, peptides, aptamers or antibodies. Moreover, expressive advancement in the multi-dimensional image modalities with integration of co-delivery of therapeutics agent or diagnosis tracer has facilitated improved non-destructive detections of patho-logical profiles. This may give rise to a specifically observed area of interest with information which ranges from anatomy to sub-cellular scale, and aids in identifying the imaging based cancer biomarker and molecular level signature. To attain utmost clinical benefits from these strategies, the supervision and treatment strategies need optimization subjective to the cancer types and can be modified dependent on individual responses.

Nanoscale medicine holds potential to advance anti-cancer therapeutics. Conventionally, nanoscale medicines are employed for the modulation of the biodistribution and targeting site accumulations of appropriately transported chemotherapeutics, thus enhancing the balance between efficiency and toxicity. In pre-clinical stages, nanoscale medicines usually increase tumor cell inhibition and prolong survival as compared to the freely administered drug, but in the clinical phase patients benefit only by nanoscale medicines due to reduction in side effects. In spite of recently approved nanomedicines like liposome-based materials, the successive rates of clinical level translations remain comparatively low. In light of this, the unusual imbalance between ongoing pre-clinical investigations reporting the advancement of more complexing nanoscale medicines, and the comparatively smaller number of nanoscale medicines that are approved for clinical applications, this has become the point of intensive debate. In terms of clinical translations, the prime issue is to select accurate drugs and the appropriate combinational regime, and to utilize them in suitable disease indications and an appropriate number of patients. To ensure that we begin to tackle the exact translation issues, we must identify the key strategies, to direct nanoscale medicines' clinical level designs and ensuring the apparent therapeutics advantages to the patient. From this viewpoint, 'SMART' cancer nanoscale medicines were conceptualized as an umbrella term for realistic and rational strategy for the advancement and refinement of cancer therapeutics (figure 4.12). Relying on the tumor sites, grades and stages, cancer can be treated with the combinational approaches of surgeries, chemotherapies, immunotherapies etc. Remarkably, on the other hand, clinical level trials with nanoscale medicines are usually developed for estimation in singular therapy stages. This makes it complicated to compare nanodrugs towards standards in terms of efficiency and, notably, they are not utilized in an optimal way for some of the inherent abilities of nanoscale medicines formulation. Certainly, nanoscale medicines combine in a good manner with conventional chemotherapeutics, they can easily accommodate various drugs within a single platform and they easily interface with an exterior stimulus in an effective manner as compared to drugs in free conditions. Nanoscale medicines rely more on vascular perfusions and permeability of smaller molecules drugs and this feature benefits from utilizing pharmacokinetics and physically controlled combinational therapeutics. Secondly, nanoscale medicines deliver a superior amount of drug at the tumor site and remain at the tumor site for longer time and thus it is beneficial to affect physically controlled combinational therapeutics. Lastly, nanoscale medicines can be developed to give a response to the local physically applied trigger in a specific manner by induction of the drug liberation. These characteristics should be utilized more significantly to construct more effectual anti-cancer combinational therapeutics (figure 4.13).

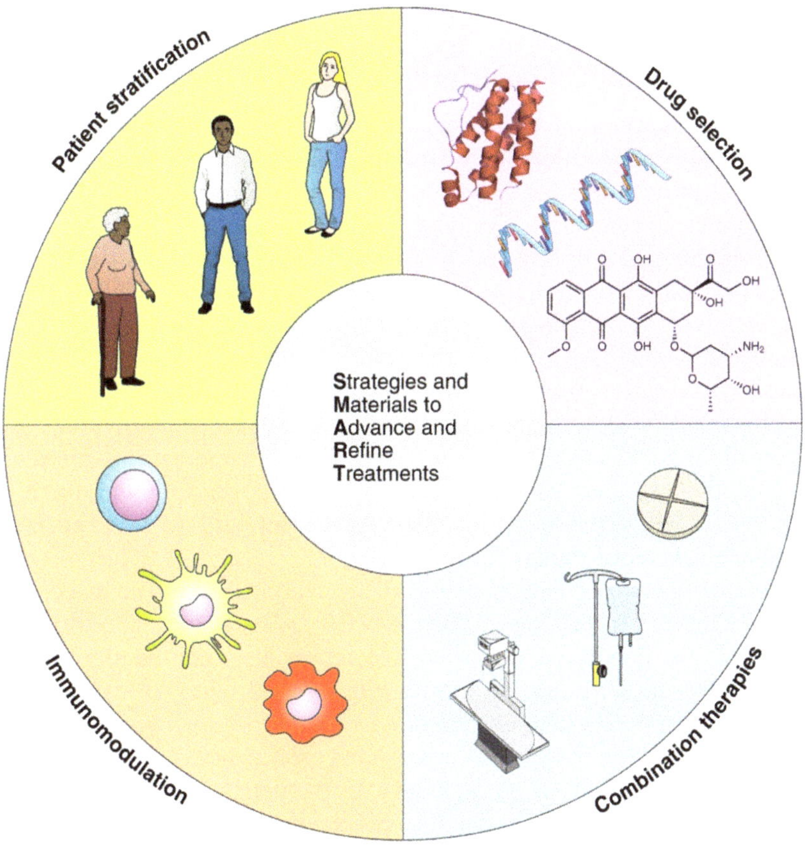

Figure 4.12. Smart strategies and materials to advance and refine cancer nanomedicine treatments (images reproduced from [13], copyright 2019 with permission of Springer).

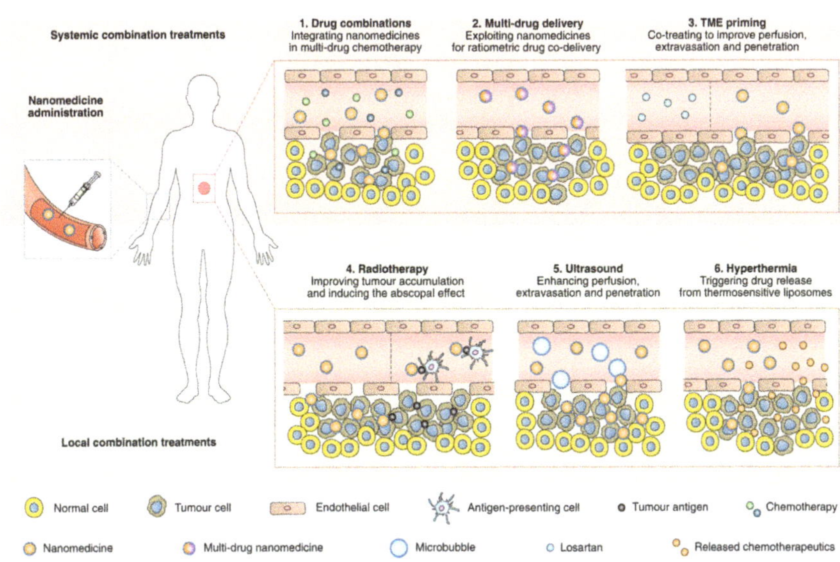

Figure 4.13. Smart cancer nanomedicine based combination therapies (image reproduced from [13], copyright 2019 with permission of Springer).

4.2 Multifunctional nanoplatforms for cancer diagnosis

The detection of cancer at an early stage is connected with the patient's prognosis as it enables timely intervention, at an earlier stage, to avert cancer cell growth. However, it is not the regular scenario, as cancer is ordinarily diagnosed after its growth and reaches the detection level, which is easier to visualize. For such situations, imaging can be utilized to verify the diagnostics, and it may require biopsies to be acquired from the suspected cancer tumor to be verified in histology or cytology technique to authenticate whether the cell is cancer affected or not. The other issue in complication of cancer diagnosis is the heterogeneous nature inside the cancer lesion. Cancerous cells normally present with pre-cancer cells and also even with healthy cells like immuno-cells. This heterogeneous nature may obstruct estimation of samples at the cell or molecule level. In the case of molecule level estimations, the gathered samples need to be homogenous, and therefore the attendance of healthy tissues inside the sample can lead to false decrement or increment at the level of the tested molecule.

The aims of the cancer detection are: (i) detection of the pre-cancer change or detection of cancer at earlier stages when very few cells are starting to transform into cancer cells, in the conditions of non-visible cancer also, i.e. the aim is to achieve greater sensitivity in detection; (ii) monitoring of the progress of cancers and their responses to therapy. The diagnostics of cancers mainly involves screening of the biomarker, utilization of imaging to observe the cancer or its early development, or detection of the biomarker inside the biopsy of the patient (figure 4.14). Nanoscale technologies have the potential to enhance cancer diagnostics by improving both the screening and imaging modalities (figure 4.15) via utilization of nanoscale materials and nanoscale fabrications that may generate a newer diagnosis platform with superior features for earlier detection of cancer. Moreover, the miniaturizing of

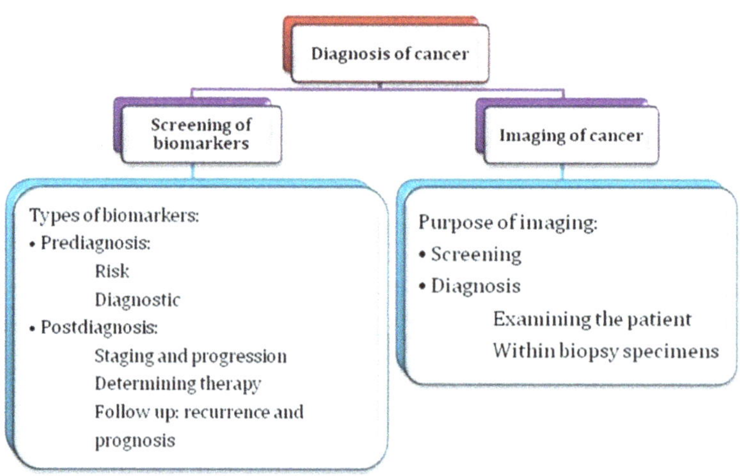

Figure 4.14. Steps involved in diagnosis of cancer (image reproduced from [14], copyright (2020), with permission from Elsevier).

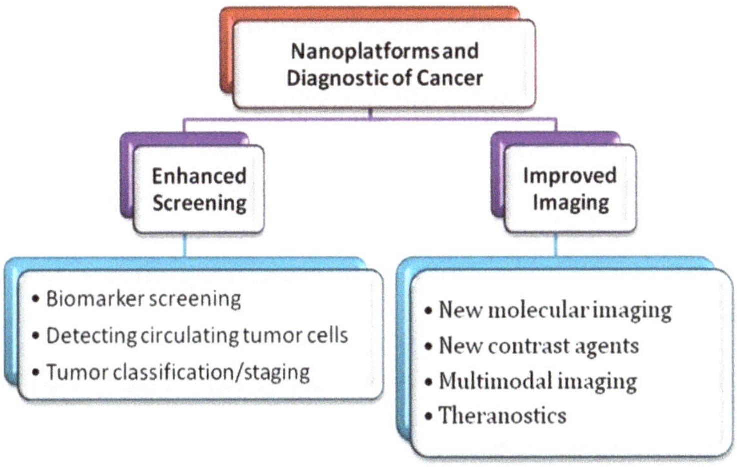

Figure 4.15. Contribution of nanoplatforms for advancement of cancer diagnostics (image reproduced from [14], copyright (2020), with permission from Elsevier).

nanomaterials eliminates the distress of destructiveness for the patient, especially the distress that is connected to the endoscopic level technique. The range of nanoscale materials that are being employed in the area of diagnostics of cancer includes quantum dot, carbon nanotube, fullerene, metal organic framework, gold nanomaterials, silver nanomaterials, zinc oxides, liposome, polymeric nanomaterials, dendrimer etc. These nanoscale materials have desired features which can promote their use for screening and imaging of the cancer growth. The special feature includes size and shape tuning along with superior surface-to-volume ratio. The high surface-to-volume ratio enables the functionalization of these nanomaterials with different targeting and imaging agents, i.e. it becomes multifunctional. For instance, surface functionalizing with specifically opted moiety, which can be recognized and bind to the explicit biomarker, enables their utilization for specific targeting. In parallel, these nanoscale materials can be functionalized with multiple imaging candidates alongside the therapeutics. An additional benefit of nanoscale materials is that they can produce signals of their own which can be used in biosensing. Such features lead to improved imaging modalities that were not achievable in the absence of nanoscale materials. For instance, metal nanoscale materials enable the use of surface plasmonic resonance microscopes as they enhance the light scattering for *in vitro* imaging.

Metal nanoscale materials like silver, aluminium and gold may improve fluorescent yield in imaging and can be referred to as metallic nanoparticles improved fluorescent imaging, mainly relying upon nanoparticles' size and surface features. Moreover, metal nanoparticles like gold and silver act as amplifiers to generate stronger Raman spectra which can be used in surface-enhanced Raman spectroscopy based imaging, which allows deeper tissue penetration. For example, deeper tissue imaging like photoacoustic imaging enables the use of non-ionizing near infrared radiation, which results in generation of the ultrasound wave that is gathered and convertible to an electric signal. For this purpose, photoacoustic imaging employs carbon nanotubes and nanoshells in preference to the other nanoscale materials. Other deep tissue imaging modality utilizes gold nanoscale structures as its luminescence can be sensed by utilizing two-photon luminescence in imaging modality of the cancers. All the above mentioned imaging techniques have been enhanced for biomedical imaging due to the extraordinary properties of nanoscale materials.

As these nanoscale materials are multifunctional, they may accommodate or integrate other imaging moieties. This offers additional advantages, as two or more imaging techniques can be employed at the same time, thus it can be referred to as multimodality or multiplexing imaging. This type of imaging merges multiple imaging techniques to acquire the information related to cancers like localizing of the tumor, metastatic and molecular level information. Other benefits of the multifunctional approach is that both the imaging and therapeutic agent can be accommodated inside the nanoplatforms, it enables the diagnostics and therapeutics together, allows monitoring of the patient's responsiveness to treatment via imaging and it may be known as theranostic.

In recent years, multifunctional nanoscale platforms have gained significant interest in the area of cancer diagnosis and therapeutics. Different types of multifunctional nanoplatforms with the integration of a variety of functionalizations for longer circulation time, targeting ability, stimuli-responsive sensitivities, intracellular level drug transportation for therapeutics and imaging are offering the capability to kill tumor cells with no or less adverse effects by providing improved contrasting for imaging of the tumor site and supervision of the outcome of the nanoplatforms and real-time therapy monitoring.

Although nanoscale technologies have not yet been employed in clinical practice for cancer diagnostics, they are already in the global market in a range of biomedical tests and screenings, such as gold-based nanoparticles in home pregnancy tests. In the diagnostics of cancer, nanoscale platforms have been applied to capturing the cancer biomarkers like cancer-related proteins, DNA of the circulated tumor, circulated tumor cell, and exosomes. The indispensable benefit of employing nanoscale materials for cancer diagnosis relies on their superior surface area as compared to their bulk counterparts. Due to the surface properties, nanoscale materials can be embedded in molecule, peptide, aptamer, and any other moiety (figure 4.16). This moiety can bind to identify cancer molecules. Upon introducing different binding ligands to cancerous cells, the multivalent effect can be attained, which may improve the specific nature and sensitivity of the assays. Nanoscale materials based diagnosis techniques have been developed as a potential tool for real-time, expedient and economically cheaper cancer diagnostics and detection. Figure 4.17 represents the summarization of the current progression in nanoplatform based applications in cancer diagnostics. In the last decade, many attempts have been made to advance nanoplatform based cancer diagnostics. As compared to the presently obtainable cancer diagnosis, a range of nanoscale based materials that have displayed development in terms of selectivity and sensitivity offer exclusively newer capacity that cannot be achieved with conventional strategies. This

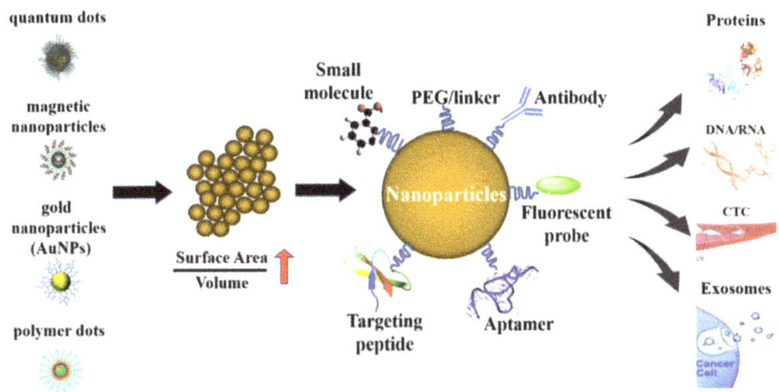

Figure 4.16. Schematics of functionalization of nanoparticles (image reproduced from [15] (2019) CC BY 4.0, with permission of Springer).

advancement will enhance the survival rates in cancer patients by providing earlier detection. Moreover, this advancement can be employed to supervise the growth of cancer cells and their response to treatment, which can contribute to developing superior strategies for cancer treatment. In the past years, superior advancement has been made in the area of nanoplatform based cancer diagnostics. Even though only a few nanoplatforms are being promoted in clinical level practice, with close collaborations between physicists, chemists, biologists, nanotechnologists, doctors and other allied researchers, nanoplatforms based cancer diagnostics is set to move into clinical practice in the upcoming years.

In view of the clinical translation, it is the therapeutic approach (i.e. types of cancers, biological architectures at the cell or molecule level and condition of the disease and patients) that confers the directional and endpoint objective of flawless coordinated diagnosis and therapeutics of multifunctional nanoplatforms, which is called 'theranostics'. On the other hand, though there are numerous studies toward advancements of multifunctional nanoplatforms, a low number of investigations have productively been translated into clinical level practice exclusively for diagnostic purpose by utilizing inorganic nanoscale materials for imaging and biosensing. Macro level molecules with spherical structure (for example liposome, dendrimer and micelle) may deceive or accommodate the diagnosis and therapeutics agent and improve solubility and the blood circulating period, while shielding them from quicker elimination and biodegradation. Multifunctional nanoplatforms can entrap anti-cancer agents like doxorubicin and paclitaxel, which may be coupled with the moieties like antibodies, aptamers, and imaging probes like gold nanoparticles and quantum dots. Such conjugations can result in enhanced accumulations of drugs inside tumor tissues, i.e. the well known EPR effect, as resulting in leaked vascular surroundings speedily raising neoplasm.

Advancement in nanoscale technologies has significantly influenced cancer diagnosis and therapeutics. Different types of nanoscale materials are being developed as contrast agents and therapeutics with optimal efficacy. The loading

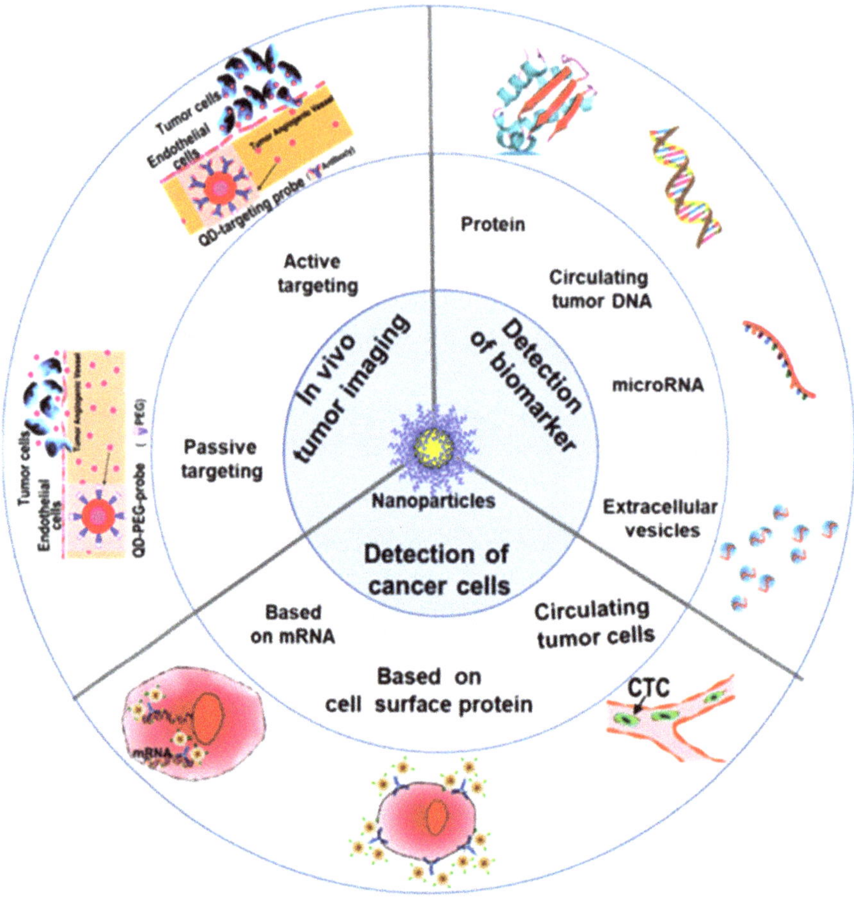

Figure 4.17. Schematical representation of nanotechnology applications in cancer diagnosis (image reproduced from [15] (2019) CC BY 4.0, with permission of Springer).

of the contrasting agents and drug onto the surface of nanoscale materials has numerous benefits like enhanced drugs solubility, longer circulation period, enhanced pharmacokinetics and pharmacodynamics, continuously optimized drug release, and fewer adverse effects in comparison with the freely transported drug [16]. Moreover, these nanoplatforms protect the drug or contrasting agent from quick clearance and show an enhanced blood circulation period to overcome physiological barriers with enhanced presence of the therapeutics drugs. Thus, numerous attempts have been made for investigations of the different multifunctional nanoplatforms for cancer therapeutics. Recently, many researchers have concentrated their attention on the design and development of nanoscale medicine to fulfil the growing demands of proficient cancer treatment.

In the category of nanoscale materials, metal organic frameworks (MOFs) are broadly investigated materials due to their exceptional properties like higher surface area, controlled size distribution, tailor-made framework, and enhanced biocompatible behaviour. In comparison to the conventional porous nanoscale materials, MOFs with tailor-made pore sizes and physical/chemical properties are outstanding candidates for bioapplications in cancer therapeutics. The benefits of MOFs in bioapplications are: (i) tuned compositions which include metallic buildings block and organic linker, which are able to integrate periodically with an arranged functional group; (ii) larger pore volumes and higher surface area which could convey greater potentiality for loading of the contrast agents and therapeutic drugs and adsorptions in the pores channel; (iii) outstanding pore frameworks and tuned pore sizes which offer enabled control of drug release and loadable kinetics; (iv) easily altered surfaces and outstanding biodegradation which could lessen the toxic nature and enhance the therapeutics efficiency; (v) the crystalline nature of MOFs facilitate characterization of the structure and may effectively permit superior drug loading and release. With these merits, MOFs with exceptional porous nature and distinguished surface features have been established as outstanding agents for bioapplications. However, the urgent outstanding issue is how to benefit from MOFs in cancer therapeutics. Figure 4.18 shows a schematical representation of MOFs-mediated multifunctional nanoplatforms for cancer treatment. Synergistically developed MOFs in nanoscale form for cancer therapeutics have been extensively investigated by many researchers and notable demand of MOF for cancer treatment strategy was also undertaken.

Zhang *et al* recently developed multifunctional nanoplatforms of porphyrin-based MOFs for synergistically activated cancer therapeutics (figure 4.19) [17]. This

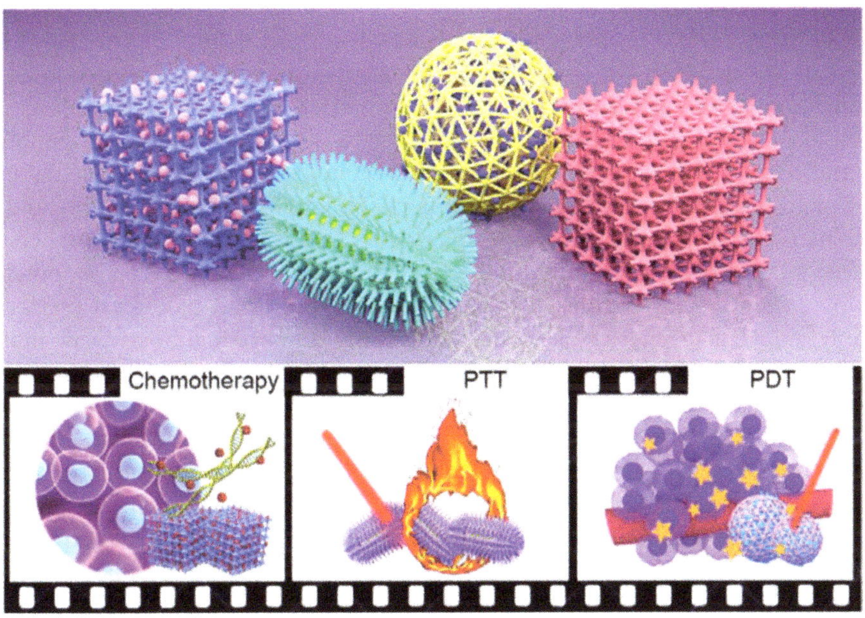

Figure 4.18. Schematical representation of MOFs-mediated multifunctional nanoplatforms for cancer treatment (image reproduced with permission from [16], copyright 2018 John Wiley & Sons).

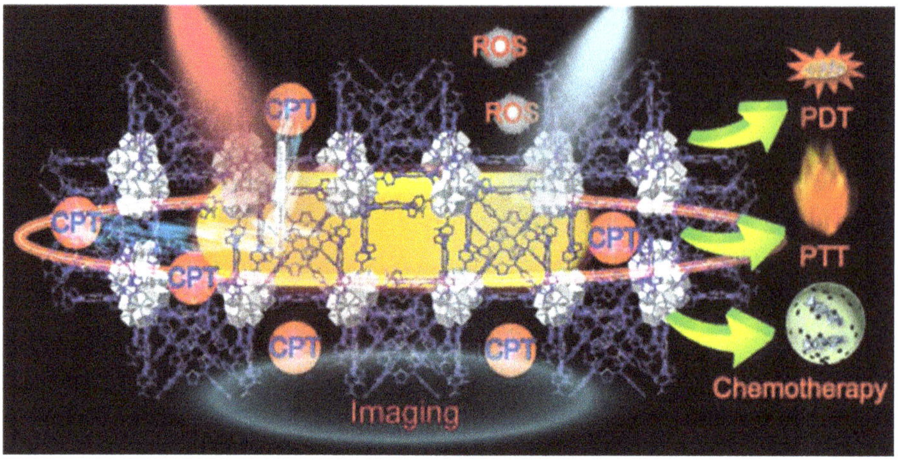

Figure 4.19. Schematical representation of multifunctional nanoplatforms of porphyrin-based MOFs (AuNR@MOFs) loaded Camptothecin (CPT) for synergistic cancer therapeutics (image reproduced with permission from [17], copyright 2018 John Wiley & Sons).

multifunctional nanoscale platform was developed by the control of porphyrin MOF growth on the surfaces of gold nanorods. The porphyrin MOF shells can be utilized for the loading of contrast agent for diagnosis and therapeutics drugs within this core–shell type nanocomposite. The cores of the gold nanorods exhibit proficient photothermal effect under near infrared light exposure, which can offer release of the therapeutics drug for improved chemotherapeutics. Moreover, this nanoplatform showed that chemotherapeutics drugs like camptothecin can also be loaded onto the MOF for synergistically controlled effects for destruction of the cancer tumor and suppressing cancer reappearance.

Self-assembly of organic and inorganic hybrids is a dominant class of nanoscale material which exhibits potential physicochemical and biological features, making it superior for cancer diagnostics and treatment. By employing self-assembly and the different types of organic–inorganic hybrids as buildings blocks, researchers are capable of performing a multitude of hybrid nanoplatforms. These potential nanoplatforms display a constructive interface of nano and biological properties, while retaining their physicochemical functionality. In particular, nanoscale materials prepared via self-assembly of organic and inorganic hybrid building blocks have displayed plenty of potential benefits in laboratories and pre-clinical level practice, leading to their profitable application for cancer diagnostics and treatment. From this perspective, employing self-assembly for the fabrication of the organic–inorganic nanoplatforms may not only integrate the inherent properties of heterogeneously active building blocks, but also profoundly acquire newer physicochemical and biological functionalities via supramolecular interfaces between them. The fabrication approach and clinical level benefits of self-assembly based nanoplatforms are being rigorously and extensively investigated by many researchers. Table 4.4 lists some of the self-assembled organic nanoplatforms for

Table 4.4. List of some self-assembled organic nanoplatforms currently used in clinical trials (table reproduced with permission from [19], copyright (2017) American Chemical Society.).

Platform type	Trade name	Formulation	Indication	Clinical benefits
		Liposomes		
	DaunoXome	Liposomal daunorubicin	Breast cancer, advanced HIV-associated Kaposi sarcoma, acute nonlymphocytic leukemia, ovarian cancer, multiple myeloma	Enhanced drug deposition in tumor, decreased side effects, also capable of escaping multidrug resistance
	Myocet	Liposomal doxorubicin	Used together with cyclophosphamide for the first-line treatment of metastatic breast cancer in adult women	Decreased cardiotoxicity and enhanced *in vivo* retention
	Doxil/Caelyx	PEGylated liposomal doxorubicin	HIV-associated kaposi sarcoma, ovarian cancer, breast cancer, multiple myeloma	Increased circulation stability and reduced cardiotoxicity
	Marqibo	Liposomal vincristine	Leukemia, Hodgkin disease, non-Hodgkin lymphomas, Wilms' tumor, rhabdomyosarcoma, neuroblastoma	Long circulation half-life, enhanced tumor accumulation, sustained drug release and reduced neurotoxicity
	Mepact	Liposomal mifamurtide	Osteosarcoma	Longer plasma half-life
	Halaven	Liposomal eribulin mesylate	Breast cancer, liposarcoma	Relatively wide therapeutic window and favorable pharmacokinetics
		Micelles		
	Genexol-PM	PEGylated micellar paclitaxel	Breast cancer, small cell lung cancer	Permitting much higher doses to be used and enhanced tumor distribution
		Supramolecular protein-drug formulation		
	Abraxane	Albumin-bound paclitaxel	Breast cancer, pancreatic cancer, non-small-cell lung cancer	Reduced toxicity, increased circulation time

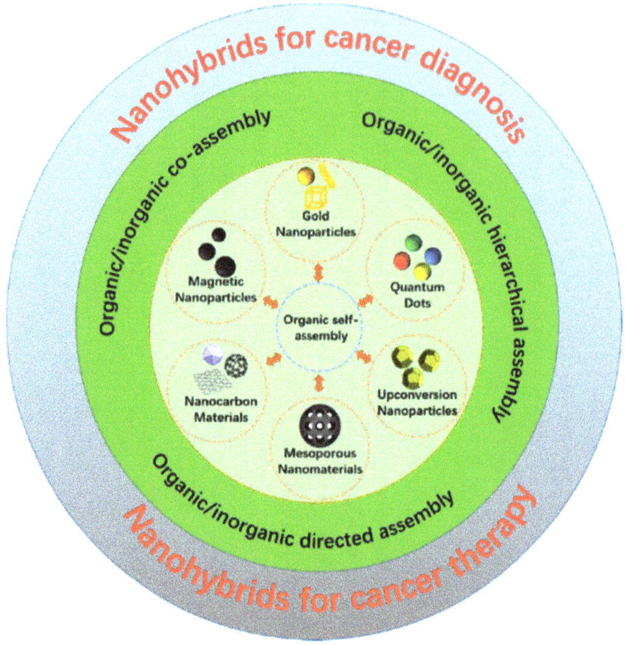

Figure 4.20. Schematics of multifunctional organic self-assembly for cancer theranostics (image reproduced with permission from [18], copyright (2017) American Chemical Society.).

cancer diagnostics and treatment in clinical practice. As depicted in figure 4.20, self-assembled organic nanoplatforms (exhibiting their functionalities with derivatives) can be employed for the manufacturing of self-assembled nanomedicines. The key benefit of these organic building blocks can be fabricated economically and in pure form while possessing tuned biological features. On the whole, multifunctional organic/inorganic self-assembled building blocks can be very significant in a broader assay of cancer diagnostics and detection. With quick advancements in tumor pathology and perception of the interface at molecular and nano levels, naturally available biomacromolecules are gradually being employed for manufacture of self-assembly based nanoplatforms, which can fetch potentiality benefit the cancer patient.

Multifunctional phototheranostics has been potentially applied in the area of cancer diagnostics and therapeutics due to its extraordinary properties and applications. In multifunctional phototheranostics, photo-triggered nanoscale materials are employed with surface functionalization to offer diagnosis and therapy simultaneously. At present, with the advancement of therapeutics efficiency the presently available treatment in the clinic, scientists and technologists are devoted to developing a substitute approach for cancer imaging and therapeutics, which should be safer, validated and cost effective. In the phototheranostic strategies the less or non-toxic agent is triggered by exposing it to light radiation to provoke cell demise exclusive of damage to healthy cells. Alongside, with the speedy advancement of nanoscale technologies in recent years, phototheranostic nanomedicines have also gained a lot of interest, which aims to constantly refine their performance. Furthermore, with the advancement of nanoscale technology in recent decades, combinational phototherapeutics and nanomedicines, coined as phototheranostics nanomedicines have attained significant interest, which aims at the refinement of phototheranostic efficiency. To achieve superior understanding of phototheranostics nanomedicines, some of the therapeutics principles and associated phototherapeutic agents are illustrated in figure 4.21. Li *et al* [19] have designed and developed an organic multifunctional phototheranostics nanoscale system comprising semiconducting polymer nanoparticle (SPN) coated with membrane of triggered fibroblast, for multimodal image-guided cancer theranostics. As depicted in figure 4.22, AF-SPN showed specifically targeted effects on cancer-related fibroblast, enhancing the tumors accretion of nanoscale particles in the tumor's tissue. Alongside, combinational photothermal and photodynamic therapies aided by AF-SPN lead to a dramatic anti-tumor efficiency. As depicted in figure 4.23, Zhang *et al* [20] developed perflurooctyl bromide (PFOB) base on liposome for oxygen transportation to the tumor tissue. In the course of improving tumor hypoxia, phototheranostic action with greater translation capacity, affixed in the lipids layer, can be notably augmented.

Nanoscale Fe_3O_4 magnetic materials are being broadly investigated as nanoplatforms for cancer nanomedicines, due to superior biocompatible nature, different physical/chemical features and compatibility at the biological scale. Signified as maghemites and magnetites, the different iron oxide base magnetic nanoplatforms are being designed for cancer diagnostics and therapeutics. The advancement of nanoscale technologies has expanded the class of iron oxide nanoplatforms. Different wet chemical fabrication techniques are being employed to prepare the iron oxide cancer nanomedicine, which include chemical coprecipitation, thermal decompositions, hydrothermal processes, sol–gel methods etc. Among these methods, the thermal decompositions technique is elaborated broadly and utilized for fabrication of iron oxide nanoplatforms with precise control on size and shape. This controlled synthesis is of great interest for nanoscale medical application as the physical/chemical properties and nanoscale biointeractions of nanomedicine strongly depends on their structures. Surface functionalization is one of the prime issues which can influence the complete performance of the cancer nanomedicine. Usually, surface functionalization of iron oxides may be done all through or subsequent to preparation with different strategies including chemical graft, physical absorptions, biorecognitions, wrappings and one-pot synthesis methods. In view of the functionality, the introduction of the coating layer or functional group at the surface of iron oxide may guard the inside magnetic cores from the oxidizing process, enhance their stabilities and biocompatibility in biological surroundings, enhance the tumor targeting efficacy and accretion, or bring supplementary functionality inside nanoscale platforms.

Iron oxide nanoscale materials had been significantly employed in the cancer diagnosis process for imaging of initial stage tumors and cancer-related immunocells. Owing to the extraordinary properties of iron oxide nanoscale materials, they have been applied in some pre-clinical and clinical level cancer nanomedicines. Although there are many improvements in MRI imaging modalities and contrast enhancing, a singular imaging technique is not able to offer inclusive information of

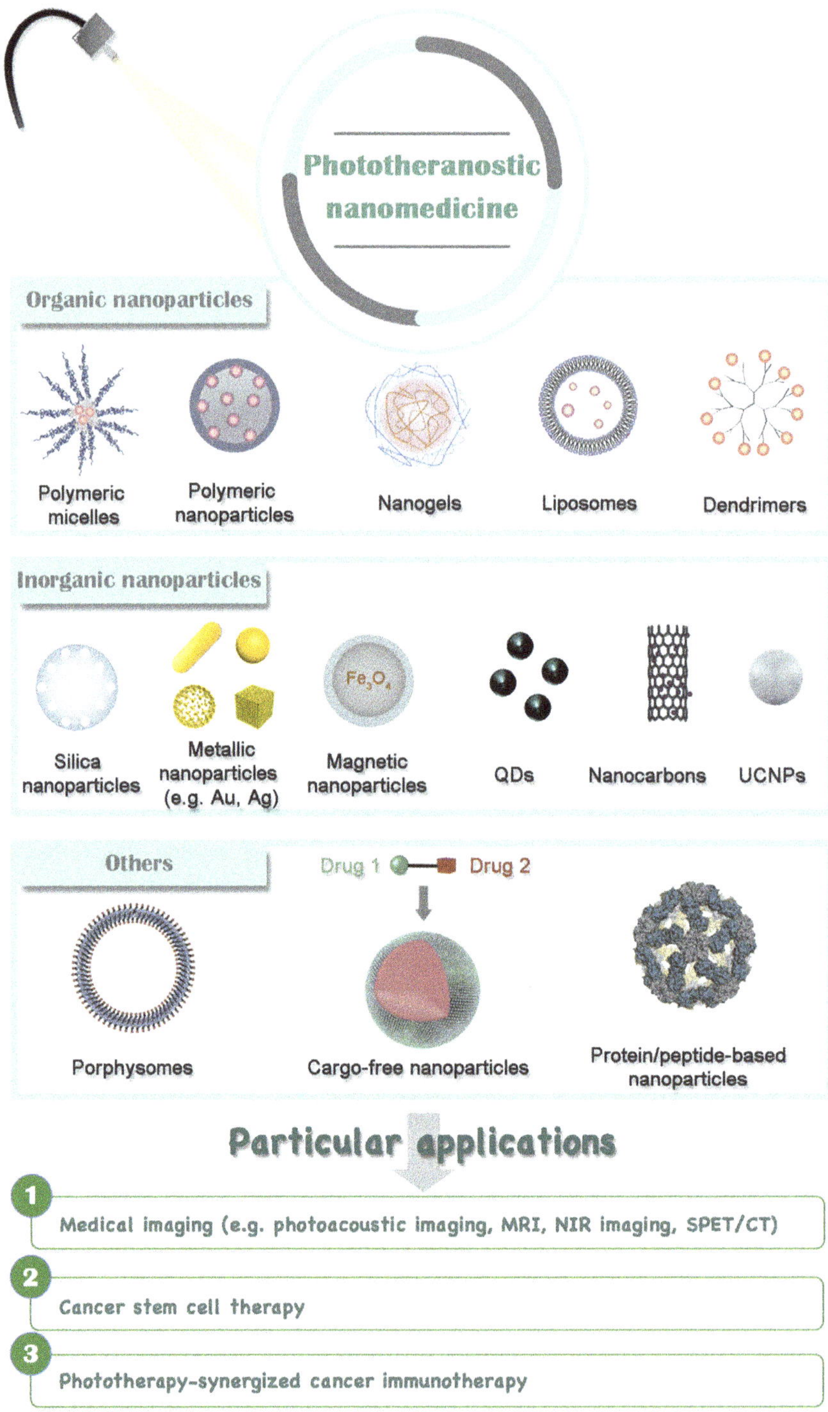

Figure 4.21. Schematical representation of phototheranostic nanomedicines (image reproduced from [21], copyright 2020 with permission from Elsevier).

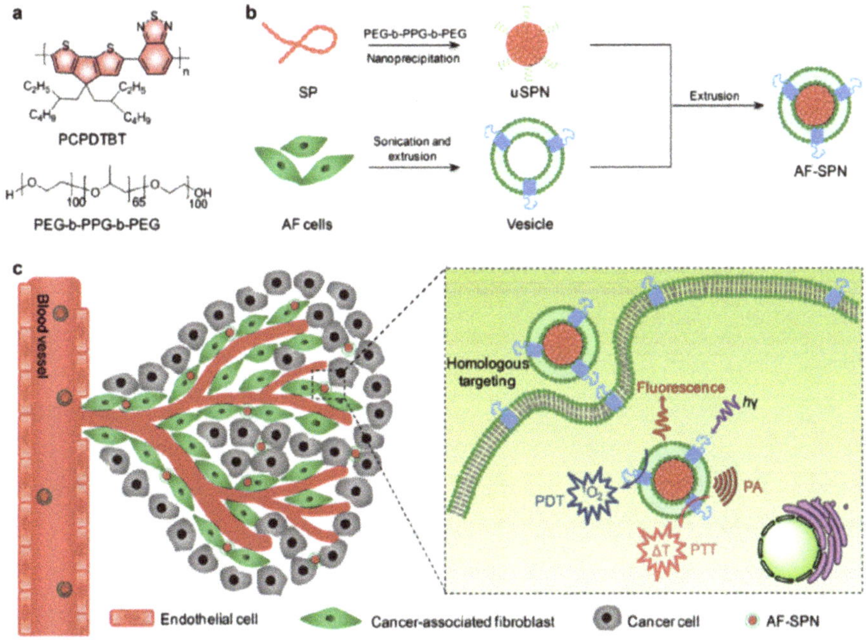

Figure 4.22. Schematical representation of an organic multifunctional phototheranostics nanosystem for multimodal image-guided cancer theranostics, including chemical structure of a variety of components (images reproduced with permission from [19], copyright (2018) American Chemical Society; [21], copyright 2020 with permission from Elsevier).

lesions. Instantaneous acquisition of T_1 and T_2 signal has been followed to gain corresponding information from the tumor tissue. Recently, Lu *et al* [22] investigated iron oxides nanoplatforms which are assembled with the assistance of pH-responded i-motif DNA. After exposure to the acidic tumors microenvironment, the nanoscale materials are disassembled, which leads to noteworthy decrement in the relaxivity ratios (r_2/r_1), which switch from T_2 to T_1 contrasting (figure 4.24(a)). These smarter nanoplatforms are being employed in detection of earlier stages smaller hepatic-cellular carcinomas in a xenografts animal models (figure 4.24(b)). For instance, superparamgnetic iron oxide materials with decoration of the nerve bind peptides (NP41) are being employed to detect nerve densities in prostate cancer, displaying strong magnetic particle imaging signals as compared to the pristine iron oxide nanoplatforms (figure 4.24(c)) [23]. Remarkably, magnetothermal therapies can be combined with magnetic particle imaging to build superparamgnetic iron oxide materials based theranostics platforms. This pioneering investigation was demonstrated by Tay and coworkers [24]. Firstly, the therapeutics plans were laid out with the supervision of quantitative magnetic particle imaging. Consequently, magnetic particle imaging gradient employed spatial localizations of nano-magnetic hyperthermia to the chosen region for precise treatment (figure 4.24(d)). This theranostics platform addresses the key challenges in traditional magnetothermal therapies, i.e. difficulties in localizations of hyperthermic heat to the targeted lesion

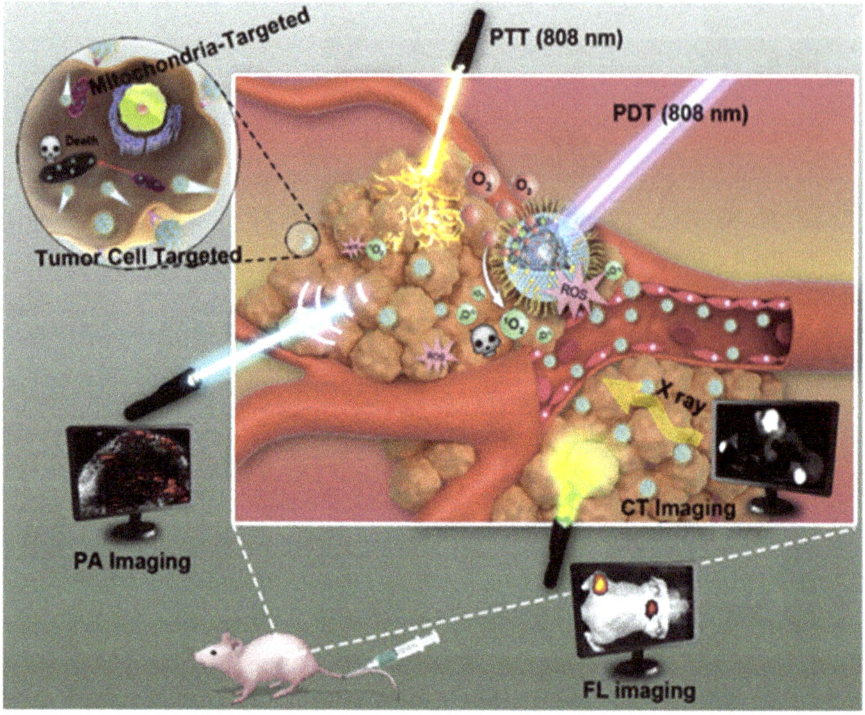

Figure 4.23. Schematical representation of the multifunctional nano red blood cells for performance in triple image-guided cancer phototherapy (images reproduced with permission from [20], copyright 2018 John Wiley & Sons; [21], copyright 2020 with permission from Elsevier).

devoid of collateral damage to normal cells, especially the clearing organ. These significant heating effects were then further noted in nanoparticles internalized cancer cells and tumor-containing mouse models (figure 4.24(e)). Furthermore, the therapeutics effects can be further enhanced by cooperating with the programmable death ligands (figure 4.24(f)).

Despite significant research progress in iron oxide based cancer nanomedicines, clinical translation is currently progressing slowly and there are still numerous issues that need to be tackled. Firstly, simple synthesis approaches and uniform product of iron oxide nanoparticles are not routinely accomplished concurrently. The synthesis of surface functionalized iron oxide nanoparticles with preferred performance constantly needs a multifaceted synthesis process or carefully observed reactions circumstances. Thus, development of handy, repetitive, and facile synthesis approaches will facilitate commercialization of iron oxide based nanomedicines. Secondly, taking note of the clinical demands for earlier detection of cancer, the spatial resolutions of iron oxide based bioimaging requires further improvements for smaller cancer cells cluster or for singular cell screening. Thirdly, the morphology and size of the iron oxide nanoplatforms influences both magnetically activated responses and hydrodynamic performance *in vivo*. The features of iron oxide nanoplatforms should be cautiously chosen and optimized for successful

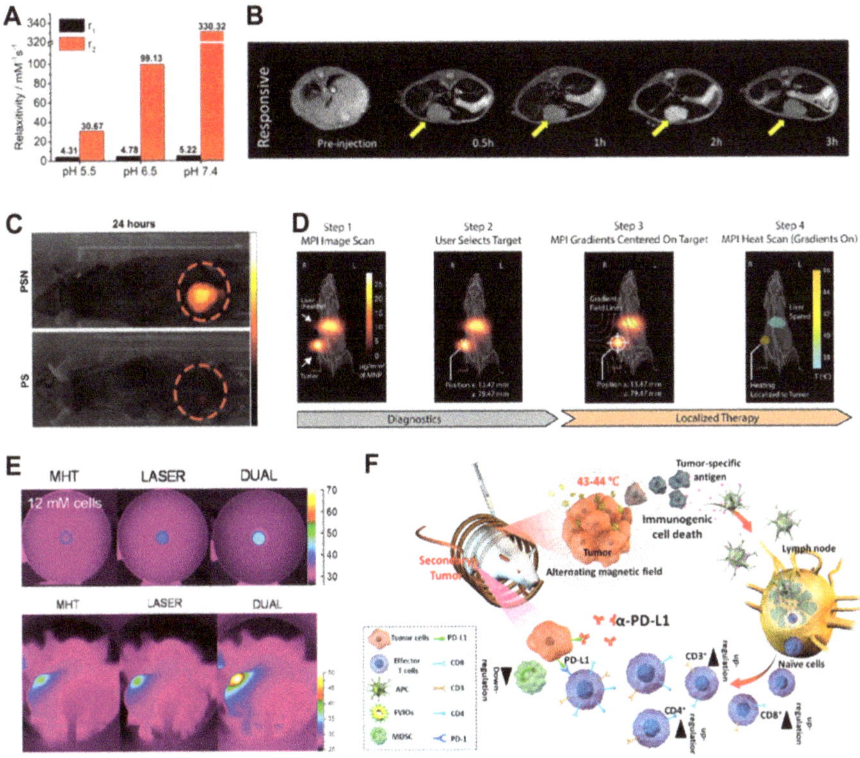

Figure 4.24. Multifunctional magnetic iron oxide based nanoplatforms for cancer diagnostic and therapy (images A and D reproduced with permission from [25], copyright (2018) American Chemical Society; image B reprinted from [21], copyright (2020), with permission from Elsevier; image C reprinted with permission from [23], copyright (2018) American Chemical Society; image E reprinted with permission from [25], copyright (2016) American Chemical Society).

magnetically activated targeting. Lastly, there are lot of hidden issues in cancer biology related nanomedicine. Superior understanding of tumor heterogeneity and nanoscale biology interfaces is needed to overcome the different biology related hurdles in nanomedicines based cancer diagnostics and therapies. We anticipate that constant developments in this multidisciplinary field will convey more iron oxide based nanoplatforms closer to clinical level practice and contribute toward the battle against cancer.

Because of the extraordinary sensitivity (up to the pico level) and quantitative behaviour, radionuclides dependent imaging considers the typical modalities for molecular level imaging. Moreover, compared to optical imaging there is no tissue penetration. However, the disadvantage of nuclear level imaging is that the resolution of PET or SPECT is not much higher. Even with internal higher contrasting sensitivity of the nuclear imaging modality, the developments of targeting nanoscale materials agent have been comparatively inadequate. The applications of radionuclide have been exposed particularly in the supervision of nanotherapeutic transportation inside the solid tumor. Different kinds of nanoparticles are being studied for the advancement of the targeting nuclear imaging agent. Additionally, interests is increasing in development of multimodal contrasting agent for utilization in corresponding imaging modalities like PET/ optical, MRI/PET, SPECT/MRI etc. In some of the conditions, multimodal imaging enables the utilization of optical technique through therapeutics interventions. Recently, a dextran coated superparamagnetic iron oxide nanoscale material labeled with ^{64}Cu and near infrared fluorophores was utilized to display the utilities of combined fluorescent molecular tomography and PET for imaging tumors linked to macrophages (figure 4.25) [27, 28].

Chitosan is a valuable candidate that in the lead of suitable nanoplatforms modifications can offer multifunction ability for cancer imaging and therapeutics. Yoon and coworkers employed two dissimilar formulations strategies of surface-altered chitosan based nanoplatforms to accommodate doxorubicin, hydrophobic chemotherapeutics or complexing Bcl-2 siRNA for genome therapies while containing imaging agent on the surface of nanoplatforms (figure 4.26) [29]. In this theranostics approach, Yoon *et al* consecutively delivered Bcl-2 siRNA-nanoplatforms and DOX-nanoplatforms to tackle the drugs resistances in cancer environment by anti-apoptotic mechanism parallel to the triggered apoptosis. Doxorubicin administering can eventually provoke the up regulation of anti-apoptotic protein, such as BCL-2, as a cell level protection mechanism and averts chemotherapeutic efficiency. DOX-nanoplatforms were devised by chemical conjugation of the hydrophobic moieties like 5-beta-cholanic acids on hydrophilic chitosan backbones, and doxorubicin was accommodated inside the core of prepared nanoplatforms by dialysis in water/DMSO. Also, siRNA-nanoplatforms were devised by thiolating glycol chitosans as the initial precursor materials. The utilization of glycol coated nanoplatforms conferred extensively various kinds of molecule with similar inherent physical and chemical properties and facilitated bioengineered therapeutics strategies. Theranostics, where the multifunctional nature plays an important role in

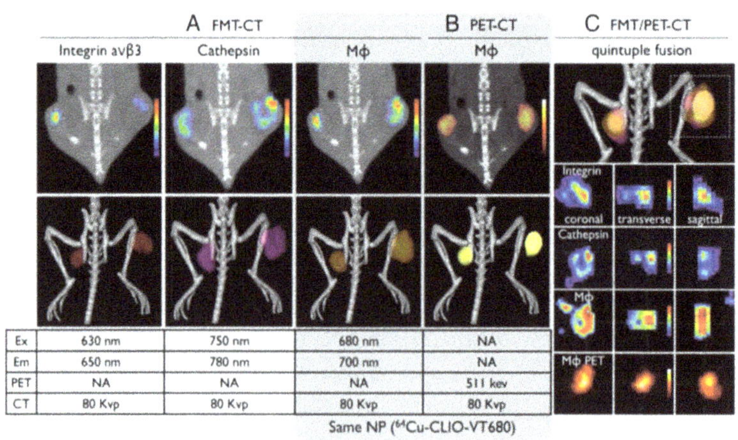

Figure 4.25. Multimodal imaging with hybrid PET-optical dextran nanoparticle enables visualization of tumor biomarker expression (images reproduced with permission from [28]).

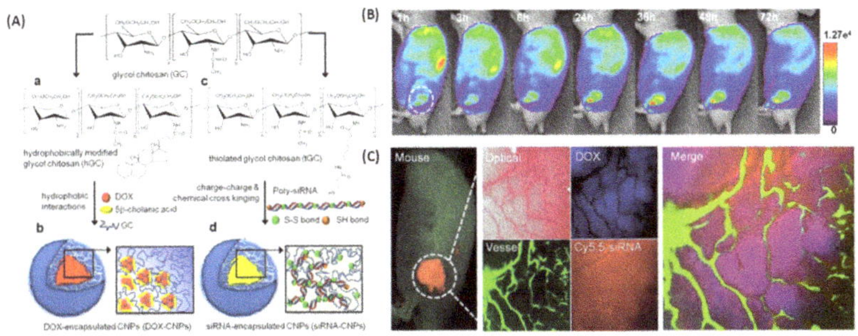

Figure 4.26. Multifunctional glycol chitosan nanoplatforms for near infrared fluorescent imaging and drug delivery of hydrophobic drugs and siRNA (images reproduced with permission from [29], copyright 2014, The Authors, with permission of Springer).

utilizing similar drug transporters with desired *in vivo* behaviors for imaging and therapy, can assist in pre-clinical and clinical level practice. Usually, in theranostics nanomedicines, the researcher utilizes singular types of nanoplatforms to achieve a multifunctional role.

4.3 Nanoplatforms for therapy monitoring using imaging techniques

Cancer theranostics is a unique perception which signifies the integration of imaging and therapies. It is a revolutionary new field of medicine but mainly connected with conventional imaging and therapeutics. It embraces the various methods to attain inclusive diagnostics, *in vivo* molecular level imaging and a personalized therapeutic regime. In recent years, the trend is for attacking this effort with upcoming material and nanoscale technologies, in the effort to design and develop ideal nanoplatforms and strategies to overcome realistic issues in clinical practice. In attempts to tackle these key obstacles in cancer therapeutics, the different nanoplatforms are being significantly exposed for cancer diagnosis and therapeutics. A nanoplatform holds superior potentiality in cancer diagnosis and therapy. Provided with refined nanostructures and superior surface areas, nanoscale materials can encapsulate the different kinds of diagnosis and therapeutics agents via chemical conjugations or physical encapsulations. Furthermore, nanoscale materials are recognized as targeting a tumor by passive accretion or active target approach. By combination of their abilities to hold different cargoes and to target tumors, they can utilized for targeting cancer diagnosis and therapeutics to attain higher quality images depicting tumor sites and to attain improved therapeutics efficiency devoid of severe toxicity to the healthy cell. For this cause, theranostics nanoplatforms for both diagnosis and therapeutics functionality are being extensively studied as advanced nanocarrier systems.

As cancer is one of the extremely variant and compliant diseases, different types of treatment options need to be chosen relying on patient characteristics and disease progress. A cancer nanomedicine researcher hopes that theranostics nanoplatforms offer different therapeutic approaches that are convenient for individual patients and thus result in enhanced prognosis. Moreover, theranostics nanoplatforms can supervise therapeutics efficiency following the treatment which can accelerate the clinical level therapeutics decisions.

A nanoparticles based theranostics system exploits different types of nanoplatforms, for example magnetic nanoparticles, carbon nanotubes, gold nanostructure, polymeric nanoparticles, silica nanoparticles etc. Fascinatingly, some of the types of nanoparticles, for example gold nanoshells or nanorods or carbon nanotube absorbs light energies and then scatters or emits specific type of diagnosis and therapeutics signal, for example, ultrasound, Raman or fluorescent signal. These types of nanomaterials can function as theranostics nanoplatforms on their own, whereas, usually, nanoscale platforms are altered with supplementary diagnosis and therapeutics agents so as to function as theranostics nanomaterials. Nanoscale platforms can be tagged chemically or physically with radionuclides, contrasting agents, optical imaging agents etc. Concurrently, the anti-cancer agent which includes a hydrophobic chemical drug, peptide, protein, or genetically active drug are physically accommodated inside or chemically integrated on the surface of nanoscale materials.

The multifaceted progress of nanoscale carriers from the point of administration to the tumor site has revealed the need to design and develop strategies that enable *in vivo* screening of the injected drugs delivery system. Non-destructive imaging techniques are capable of offering *in vivo* screening of nanoscale materials in relation to their pharmacokinetic profile, biodistributions, tumors dispositions, drug release and therapeutics efficiency (figure 4.27). The labeling of nanomedicines formulation with imaging agent results in a theranostics platform that has different benefits and applications. Moreover, considering the above described point that EPR effects are extremely varyable, nanomedicines based chemotherapeutics are only effectual in a particular subclass of patient and thus theranostics nanomedicine that can be employed in a non-destructive way and significantly evaluates tumor targeting efficacy is much needed. The gained imaging information can then be utilized to pre-select the appropriate patient with adequate higher tumor accretion of nanomedicines for subsequent treatment, thus supplying the individual medicine.

Different types of imaging modality are presently accessible viz. MRI, CT, PET, SPECT, optical imaging, ultrasound etc. These modalities have their individual benefits and drawbacks in terms of spatial and temporal resolution, sensitivity in probe detection and signal penetration depth, and the choice of suitable imaging technique depends on the type of information desired. For example, optical imaging is often employed for *in vivo* imaging of smaller animal model due to their safe nature, timely manner, and economy. However, it is impractical to image deeper tissue or larger living systems. This can be tackled by employing radionuclides based imaging modalities like PET and SPECT, which offer deeper tissue penetration power and sensitivity. But PET and SPECT have comparatively reduced spatial resolution and lack of anatomy related information. To gather anatomy related information, they are frequently integrated or coupled with CT or MRI, which enables sensitivity and higher resolution soft as well as harder tissues visualization. In a similar fashion, optical imaging also benefits from such combined imaging

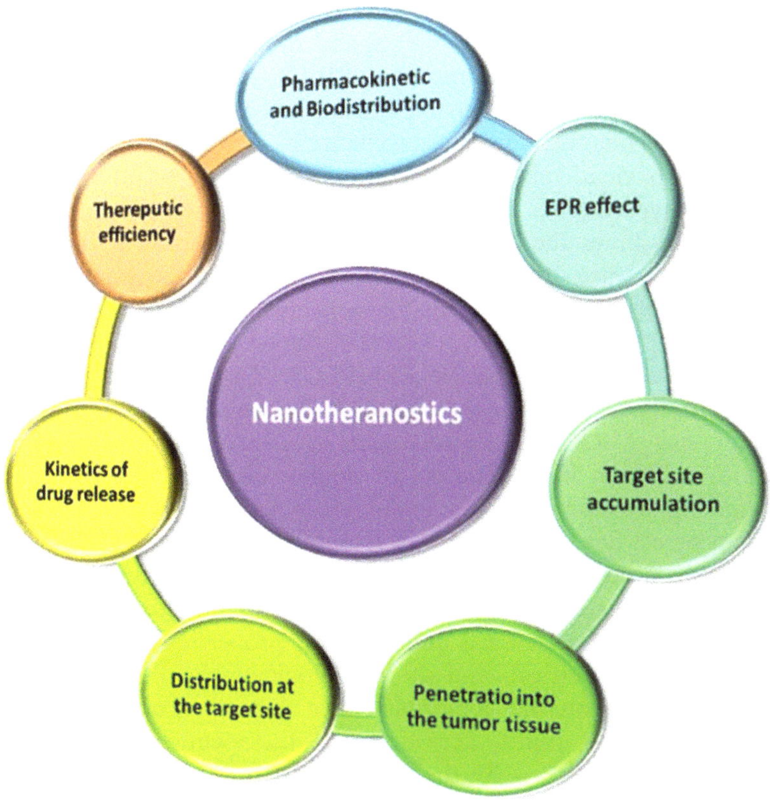

Figure 4.27. Applications of nanotheranostics. By combination of both the diagnosis and therapeutics features inside the singular nanomedicines system, significant characteristics of tumor targeting with drug deliverance can be visualized and monitored (image reproduced with permission from [30], copyright (2010) American Chemical Society).

protocol. In most pre-clinical situations, optical imaging is not able to correctly allocate the probes signals to the animal organ and subsequently only provides moderate useful feedback on nanomedicine biodistributions. When coupled with CT, organs of interest can be targeted and the anatomy related information gathered from CT can be integrated with the fluorescence signals gained from optical imaging, thus providing more precise biodistribution evaluation. In addition to the utilization of *in vivo* imaging for supervision of target sites accretion, imaging and especially MRI can be employed to supervise payload release. The MRI signals are extremely reliant upon the accessibility of free diffused H_2O molecules near the probe, discrete MRI signals are produced when paramagnetic MRI contrasting agents are available at the various locations, which are encapsulated in or attached over the core of liposome, associated with the encapsulating versus relapsing drug payload. This strategy was explored to supervise drug release from intravenous way administration with temperature sensed liposome. For instance, the attempt has been made to administer drugs in an intravenous way with sensitive liposome co-loaded with the MRI contrasting agents along with doxorubicin to rat model. Two groups of animals are utilized, control and animal, in which a tumor is heated with higher intensities focusing ultrasound (HIFU), and the release of MRI probes in the tumor activated by HIFU enable heating to be supervised by MRI. Groups given hyperthermic treatment displayed a change in T_1 in tumor tissues as a result of heating enabled payload release. Other groups given temperature dependent liposome without hyperthermic treatments showed minimum payload release at the tumor site. This shows the potentiality of utilizing imaging in non-destructive supervised drug release from nanomedicine platforms. Imaging may also be employed to support in evaluation, whether actively targeted tumor actually benefits attaining superior tumor efficacy. Recently, superparamgnetic iron oxide was co-loaded with poly lactic-co-glycolic acid (PLGA) functionalized with arginylglycylaspartic acid (RGD) to enable quantifying and visualizing accretion of NPs in the tumor employing MRI and electron spin resonance. There was an eightfold increment of accretion in the tumors of doubly targeting NPs comparative to passive targeting of NPs.

Notable progress has been made in development of nanomedicines, which have outcomes in advanced pharmacokinetics, in high tumor accretion, in superior antitumor efficiency and reduced adverse effects. Tumor targeting efficacy of nanomedicine depends on the physical and chemical properties of nanoscale carriers (sizes and surface properties), and the pathological/physiological nature of the targeted tissues. But there are numerous issues to be overcome to attain general consensus on how this tumor accretion and therapeutics efficiency of nanomedicine can be exaggerated by the physical and chemical features. Presently, nanomedicine utilized in clinics mostly relies on passive targeting, that is the EPR effect. Many attempts need to be practiced for superior understanding of the *in vivo* behaviour of passive and active targeting nanomedicine, and nanoscale formulations that can be outwardly activated to liberate the content at the targeted sites. Although functionalization with targeted ligand enhances the cell uptake of nanomedicine *in vitro*, *in vivo* tumor accretion frequently does not increase. In spite of a large number of investigations employed on active targeting NPs, many did not make it to the clinical level. Thus, the additional value of including targeted moiety is still a crucial topic and needs to be further studied. However, actively targeting nanomedicines are specifically valuable for the deliverance of biotherapeutics and for combinational therapies (with pharmacologically activated ligand). Moreover, the imaging needs to be coupled in an intensive manner in nanomedicines treatment to specifically facilitate the patient pre-selection in order to advance clinical level translations. Since tumor and metastatic are extremely responsive to therapeutics efficiency of nanomedicine, they have notable intra-individual differences. Advancing imaging strategies to supervise tumor accretion and therapeutics efficiency of nanomedicine will realize pre-selection of the patient who has higher tumor accretion and efficiency of injecting nanomedicine, which will help in treatment of the appropriate patient nanomedicine, and prohibit non-responders who can go for other treatments modality. By integration of imaging features in nanomedicine formulation, theranostics nanomedicines have superior

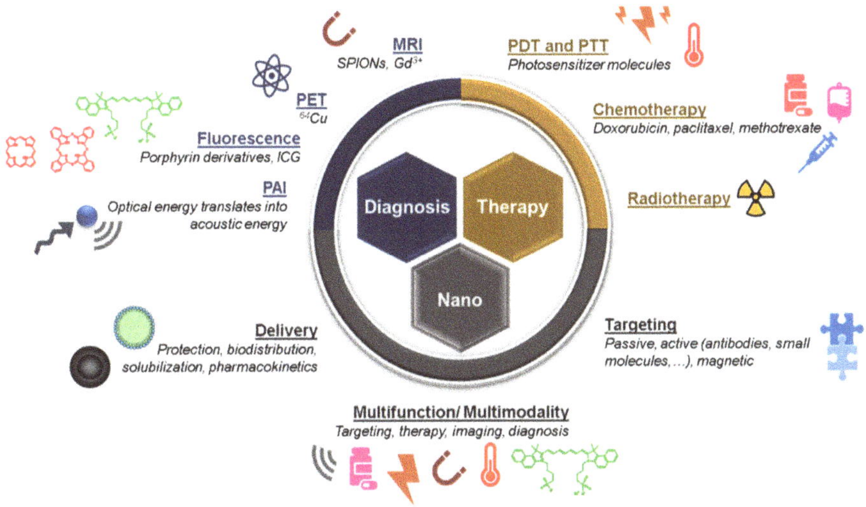

Figure 4.28. Schematical representation of triple features in theranostics nanoplatform, namely nano-sized particles, therapeutics, and diagnosis agent (image reproduced with permission from [31]).

potentiality to attain more suitable clinical level benefit. The features of nano-theranostics are summarized in figure 4.28.

Nuclear level nanomedicine imaging is broadly studied as a progressed diagnosis tool and includes the interpretation of radionuclides in the human body, detection of the emitted gamma ray and production of image that offer detailed radionuclide distributions and physiological characterizations of the organ and tissue. Different nanoscale imaging agents are being developed showing the dual-mode performance as both the diagnosis and therapeutics tool. However, some of the nanoscale materials show lower distribution and cells penetrating depth, and therefore, their non-desirable pharmacokinetics need improvement. Different novel strategies are being utilized in order to improve their pharmacokinetics and biodistributions. Radiopharmacy is an interdisciplinary and multidisciplinary scientific field and liable to advancement, formulations, preparations, quality controls and administrating of radiopharmaceuticals. Radiopharmaceuticals are the drug encapsulating radionuclide and pharmaceuticals part, utilized for the diagnostics and treatment of different cancer-like diseases. The pharmaceutical parts are chosen depending on the preferred localizing in particular organs, which is desirable for imaging or partaking in the physiological functions of the organs. After selection, the pharmaceutical parts labeled with the appropriate radionuclides and localization in the organs may be sensed with different imaging modalities. Different nanotheranostics based on polymer NPs are being developed and radiolabeled with present radionuclide by utilizing different strategies intended for the diagnostics and treatment of the disease. Linkable molecules like chelators agent are bound to radionuclides and NPs to improve their stability. The properties of shorter media and lower half-life of radionuclides, their radioactivity decay and chemical structures can affect their significant applications in clinical trials. Thus, radiopharmaceuticals should be chosen with proper care. For instance, radiopharmaceuticals that emit gamma rays and beta particles have theranostics features. They serve as both the diagnosis and therapeutics facility to evaluate physiology and anatomy related information in tissue. The proper choice of radionuclides plays a significant role for targeted nanotheranostics to the desirable tumor site. If alpha, beta and gamma emitting radionuclides are employed to radio label the NPs, then they attain theranostic properties. These emitter radionuclides also induce the visualizing of the cell functions and the supervision of the molecular processes inside the cell. Radio labeling of nanoscale materials has been broadly employed as a potential diagnosis approach in nuclear nanomedicine imaging. Different radiolabeled nanoscale materials are being designated and developed for imaging tumors and other lesions due to the proficiency characteristics. Inorganic nanoscale platforms like gold, silver, silica etc based nanoscale materials or organic NPs as polymer, carbon nanomaterials and liposomes are being explored as a multifunctional nanotheranostics.

Real-time screening and tracking of the drug release profile is basically significant to avoid side effects or ineffective treatment in personalized medicinal treatment. However, the advancement of non-destructive drugs presenting the platforms still remains exigent. Ding *et al* [32] reported novel synthesis of MRI contrasting agents for drug release tracking (SMART) which coupled the photothermal cores and paramagnetic drug loaded shells with thermal valves in hybrid structures. Via near infrared photothermal effects originated from inner cores of Au–Cu9s5, exploded release of drug loading inside the mesoporous silica shells was achieved. The associated utilization of phase-changed materials averts premature drug release and regulates heat effects, which keeps local temperatures below 45 °C, and enables synergistic chemotherapy and mild hyperthermic effect *in vitro* and *in vivo*. Moreover, drug release from a SMART platform facilitates proton accessing ability to the paramagnetic ion decorated in the mesoporous channel, which enhances longitudinal T_1 relaxations rates and showing positive signals co-relations to the quantity of releasing drugs, which enables non-destructive real-time supervision of drug release events. This study shows the potentiality of developed MRI nanophores like SMART for real-time screening and supervision of drug delivery for precise theranostics application. Figure 4.29 represents the work principle of SMART for real-time supervision of drug release. This SMART nanoplatform mainly exhibits functional components. The inside core is the heating engine depending on gold and copper chalcogenide nanohybrids developed, which produces heat by exposing it to near infrared radiation, activates drug release and sensitizes the chemotherapeutics. Au ions present in nanohybrids enhance the photothermal and photodynamic effects of copper chalcogenide, while copper chalcogenide facilitates the hepatobiliary clearance of gold, making Au-Cu9D5 NPs a superior candidate as biodegradable inorganic nanomedicines. Further, MSN shells cover the inherent cores, which serve as the transporter for drugs and gate keeping molecules in order to manage drug release.

In comparison to traditional chemotherapeutics with intravenous administration, injection of a self-healing hydrogels drugs delivery nanosystem to the tumor site not only carries less toxic behaviour for healthy tissue, but also provides superior specific

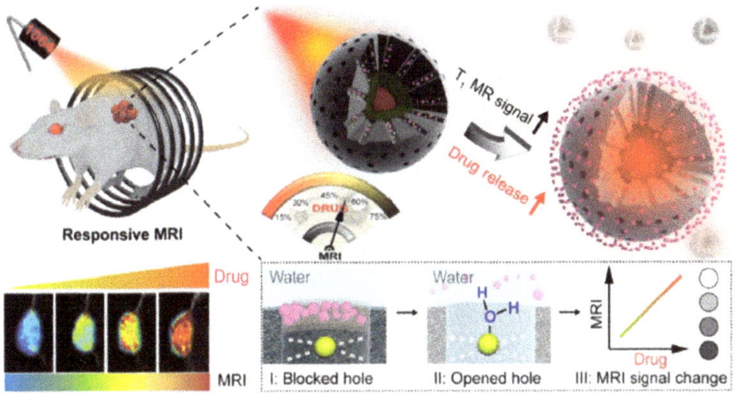

Figure 4.29. Schematical representation of SMART, which has receptive MRI activity for *in situ* reporting drug release activated by NIR-II light (image reproduced with permission from [32], copyright 2019, Tsinghua University Press and Springer-Verlag GmbH Germany, part of Springer Nature, with permission of Springer).

nature for tumor cells on account of fast repair and enhanced retention. Moreover, it is necessary to make introduction of multifunctional nanoscale materials into the self-healing hydrogels loaded with the chemotherapeutics drug to notably improve tumors treatment efficacy. Wang *et al* [33] recently reported rhodamine-B isothiocyanate (RBITC) labeled mesoporous silica nanosphere with Mn–Zn ferrites NPs core with good dispersing in hydrogels systems (MMSN-RBITC). Heat produced in the presence of alternating magnetic field induced the hyperthermic effects for magnetothermal therapies, which also promoted the sensitivity of chemotherapeutics. Hydroxyl radicals were generated by Fenton-like catalyzations after cellular level uptakes of MMSN-RBITC further promoting cell apoptosis by chemodynamic therapies. This nanoplatform also presented excellence in T_2 weighted MRI contrast enhancing. As a result, hydrogel systems were effectually improved and augmented by the introduction of a nanosphere. *In vivo* and *in vitro* outcomes indicated that these strategies of self-healing hydrogels loaded with DOX and MMSN-RBITC may attain tumor diagnosis and proficiently synergistic magnetothermal/chemodynamic therapies. This strategy can motivate researchers to build the most potential platform coupling self-healing hydrogels with multifunctional nanomaterial for effective cancer treatment with resourceful therapeutics method. A schematic of MMSN-RBITC self-healing hydrogels loaded with anti-cancer drugs (DOX) for MRI and synergistic magnetothermal/chemodynamic therapies is shown in figure 4.30. Administrable nanocomposites of self-healing hydrogels with anticancer drugs (DOX) and multifunctional magnetic nanosphere attain enhanced imaging and detection of tumor cells and are recognized as effectual treatments of tumors via newer therapeutic strategies. MRI bioimaging techniques have been explored in clinical level practice with higher spatial resolution and no side effects. T_2 weighted MRI contrast evaluation of MMSN-RBITC@PBS dispersions were estimated with Fe concentrations in the range of 0 to 1.1 mM (figure 4.31(a)). MMSN-RBITC displayed Fe ion concentrations based T_2 weighted MR imaging

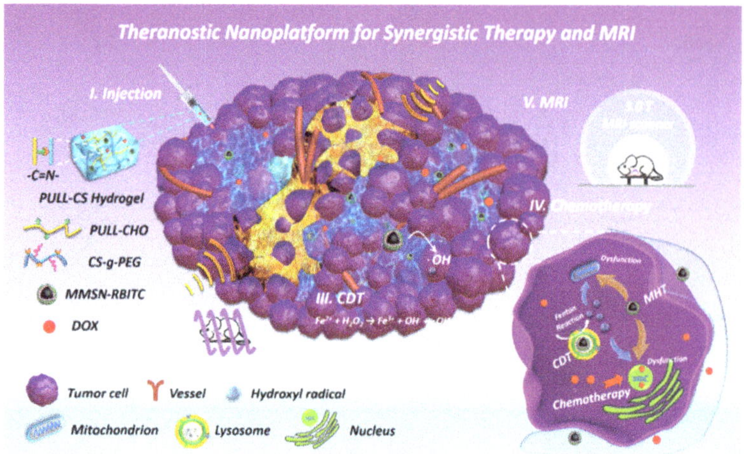

Figure 4.30. Schematical representation of the microstructure of the PULL-CS hydrogel and the theranostics nanoplatforms applying synergistic therapeutics of magnetic hyperthermia, chemodynamic and chemotherapy coupled with MRI for cancer therapeutics (image reproduced from [33], copyright (2020), with permission from Elsevier).

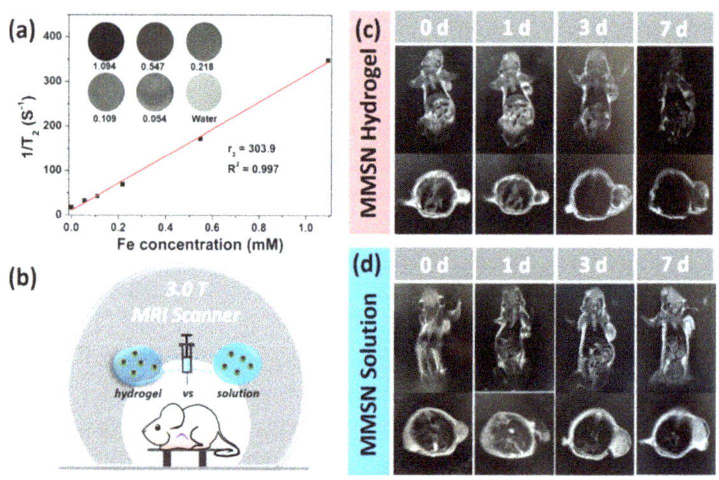

Figure 4.31. (a) T_2-weighted MRI of MMSN-RBITC aqueous dispersions with diverse Fe concentration, and T_2 transverse relaxations rates as a function of Fe concentrations. (b) Schematical representation showing the process of MRI on the difference of the intra-tumoral injections. *In vivo* MRI of a tumor-containing mouse with intra-tumoral injections of (c) MMSN-RBITCs hydrogels and (d) MMSN-RBITCs dispersions (all the images reproduced from [33], copyright (2020), with permission from Elsevier).

intensities. The transverse relaxations rate ($1/T_2$) was incremented with an increase of Fe ion concentration, which yielded a relaxation of 303.9 mM^{-1} s^{-1}. The higher relaxations showed that the nanosphere had the ability to noticeably improve the contrasting effects *in vitro* and *in vivo*. Thus, the *in vivo* MR imaging of the MMSN-SBITCs dispersions and hydrogels were executed by utilizing 3T MRI scanning (figure 4.31(b)). In comparison to imaging in 0 days without interventions, the T_2 weighted tumors image in both the MMSN dispersions and hydrogels groups noticeably becomes darker after intra-tumoral injections. However, the contrasting in hydrogels groups can remain longer, even 7 days so that solution groups due to the hydrogels prolong the retention of the loading nanosphere (figure 4.31(c) and (d)). All the outcomes showed combinational effects of MR imaging and retention effects of self-healing hydrogels. Depending on the effectual therapies of nano-composites hydrogels *in vitro*, their synergistic magnetothermal/chemodynamic therapies efficiency was carried out on breast tumors xenograft models. A mouse with tumor volume more than 100 mm^3 was separated in a random way into the 8 group (n = 5). After a single dose of intra-tumoral injections with diverse formulation, the mouse in the alternating magnetic field treatments group kept in the coil with magnetic field (160 kHz, 328 Oe) each 2 days for a total of four cycles (figure 4.32(a)). The temperature rising in the alternating magnetic field treated group for magnetic hyperthermia therapy was noted by thermal images depicted in figure 4.32(b). The localized temperature at the tumor sites treated with PBS was barely changed, whereas the apparent increment at the tumor regime can be found in the MMSN-RBITC involving groups under similar conditions, showing significant magnetic hyperthermic effects of MMSN-RBITC. Moreover, the temperature of the hydrogels + DOX + MMSN-RBITCs + alternating magnetic field can attain about 44.5 °C after 7 days treatment, then returning to the normal states (38.9 °C) in DOX + MMSN-RBITCs + alternating magnetic field groups. The results showed that, the MMSN-RBITC attianed uniform distribution along with the self-healing hydrogels, which can affirm that each tumor cell receives the same degree of hyperthermic temperature and evades recurrences of breast cancer caused by unfinished treatment. The good and consistent retention effects of the nanosphere loaded in the self-healing hydrogels was proven. The tumors volume was noted for every 2 days, extracted and photographed and weighted at day 15 (figure 4.32(c)).

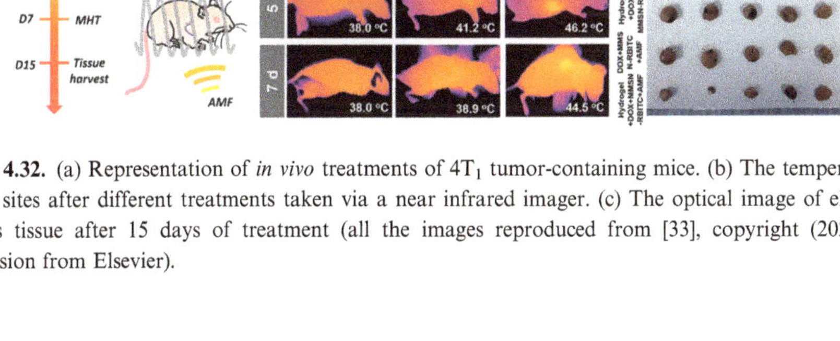

Figure 4.32. (a) Representation of *in vivo* treatments of $4T_1$ tumor-containing mice. (b) The temperatures at tumor sites after different treatments taken via a near infrared imager. (c) The optical image of eliminated tumors tissue after 15 days of treatment (all the images reproduced from [33], copyright (2020), with permission from Elsevier).

Coupling multimodal bioimaging and multiple stimuli-receptive controlled drug release properties inside the singular nanosystem for therapeutic applications is much desired, but there still remain issues to be overcome. Zhou *et al* [34] coated hollow mesoporous silica shells on up-conversion NPs (UCNPs) and coupled pillarene based supramolecular valve onto the surfaces of UCNPs@hm-SiO_2 using amine-coumarin photo-triggers to gain multifunctional NPs. With the benefits from core–shell structured UCNPs, it can serve as a proficient contrasting agent for up-conversion luminescence and T_1 weighted MRI *in vitro* and *in vivo*. For specific anti-cancer applications, the rational employment of both acid and near infrared light can regulate the release amounts and rates of DOX from UCNPs, which accelerates the accretion of DOX in cell nuclei, and thus promotes cancer cells apoptosis, which indicated nanoscale materials have outstanding applications in cancer treatment. These investigations provide novel strategies for building multifunctional UCNPs based nanoplatforms with a multiple stimuli reactive drug release feature, which has greater potentiality in diagnostics and therapeutics of pertinent disease as theranostics nanomedicine. By taking the inspiration from reported results of multi-responsive controlled drugs delivery system, Zhou *et al* designed pillararene based supramolecular valves functionalized UCNPs core–shell mesoporous silica shells, which were effectively employed for up-conversion luminescent (UCL)-MRI and exogenous (near infrared light, electric potential)-endogenous (acids, alkalis, Zn^{2+} etc) stimuli-receptive drug release (figure 4.33). The illustrated design strategies can pave an alternative way to developing diverse nature theranostics nanomedicine with multimodal imaging and multiple stimuli-receptive controlled drug release.

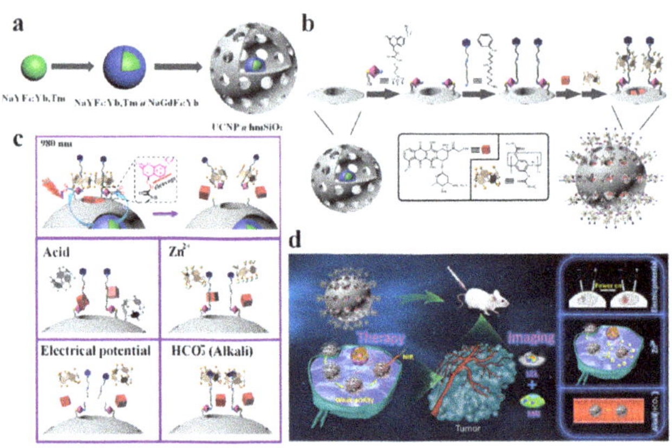

Figure 4.33. (a) Schematical representation of synthesis of UCNPs@hm-SiO_2. (b) Schematical representation of construction of UCNPs@hm-SiO_2-Cou-CysDOX/WP. (c) Quintuple stimuli-responsive release mechanisms of UCNPs@hm-SiO_2-Cou-Cys-DOX/WP. (d) Schematical representation of potential theranostics applications of UCNPs@hm-SiO_2-Cou-Cys-DOX/WP with stimuli-receptive drug release activated by five stimuli and dual-modal imaging (all the images reproduced with permission from [34], copyright (2019) American Chemical Society).

4.4 Image-guided nanomedicine animal models and clinical implications

Multifunctional nanoscale materials having enhanced properties and therapeutics effect are being significantly designed and developed for nanomedicines. However, a tumor's inherent barrier and its heterogeneous nature results in lower *in vivo* therapeutics efficiency. The limited *in vivo* efficacy in passively and actively targeted tumors in nanotherapeutics along with the toxic nature of nanoscale materials have been a major hurdle in nanomedicines. In recent years, image-guided nanomedicines able to transport nanoscale materials in local sites using non-destructive imaging and intervention for ontological methods, have been paid a lot of attention as newer opportunities of nanomedicines.

Different kinds of nanoscale materials with special functionalities not offered in bulk counterparts, can offer opportunities for novel and innovative biomedical applications. Nanomedicines are one of the emerging research fields among the different applications of nanoscale technologies over the last two decades. Cancer is one of the leading diseases, the second most common cause of deaths, and it is rising day by day. Traditional therapeutics has not displayed any notable improvement or results for cancer treatments. Novel innovative techniques are desperately required for effectual cancer treatments. Cancer nanomedicines with extraordinary features of nanoscale materials are desired to offer new opportunities in earlier diagnostics, imaging and treatments of cancer. The smaller size, higher surface areas, uniform solubility, and multifunctionality of nanoscale materials have generated novel biomedical applications. Certainly, the novel features of nanoscale materials have shown the capability to interface with multifaceted cellular functions in newer way. This speedily progressing area, as interdisciplinary research, develops multifunctional nanoscale structures and approaches that can target, diagnose, and treat cancer.

With significant effort, liposomes and lipids based nanoscale materials are being approved by FDA to transport and improve the bioavailability of DOX and other drugs. Micelle and nanoscale complexes have also enhanced the pharmacokinetic profile and biodistributions of hydrophobic drugs molecules. Moreover, carboxymethyl dextran coated iron oxides nanoplatforms are being permitted for Fe supplement in drugs and are tested for MRI contrasting agents in the clinic. Roughly, around 100 nanomedicines products have been commercialized and brought to market. Of other different nanoscale materials, around 800 nanoscale products are in clinical level trial. In pre-clinical test, various nanoscale materials demonstrate very promising properties for cancer imaging and therapeutics. However, few nanoscale materials consisting of Fe, Au, Si, poly-saccharides polymer and natural products are being considered for clinical level practice potentially. Characteristically, iron oxide nanoplatforms, which are one of the components in blood, are being employed for cellular hyperthermic activity and Mei contrasting. The superparamagnetic properties of nanomaterial iron oxides are used for these applications. The magnetic features and functions of nanomedicines are enthusiastically tailor-made for every purpose by varying the size and structure of the nanoscale materials. In recent years, anisotropy and high complex Au nanoscale structures like hyperbranching or dendritic structure are also visualized to be beneficial, as they offer a large number of active sites and surface atoms per unit area in comparison to the sphere type nanomaterials. Differently shaped metal nanoscale materials with specific light absorption properties produce vigorous heat for localized ablations therapy. Higher density metal nanoscale materials allow CT imaging contrasting effects. Disk shaped Au coated magnetic nanomaterials with magnetic spin vortexes can straightforwardly kill cancer cells with magnetomechanical stimulation modulated by external magnetic fields. Temperature sensitized polymer micelles effectually deliver drugs molecules at precise temperatures. A magnetic cluster enhances the MRI properties and at the same time carries many of the drugs with nanoprobes. Further, mesoporous silica nanoscale materials are showing great potentiality as drugs carriers. Up converting nanoscale materials are being developed for stabilized luminescence and multimodal imaging function in pre/intra/post-operative imaging. Those suggested nanomedicines using novel nanoscale materials are attractive for newer approaches to treat cancer.

However, bigger challenges for these nanoscale materials for nanomedicine applications have been of concern during the latest *in vivo* and clinical level translation. The improved permeability and retention (EPR) effects and active targeting using tumor specific molecules are observed to be a notable approach for tumor targeting, but RES sequestrations, tumor inherent barrier and tumors' heterogeneous nature result in extremely low tumor targeting and tumor uptake efficacy. This lower targeted efficacy adversely affects the translations of nanomedicines towards clinical level application. Thus, future cancer nanomedicines powerfully require more local and personal approaches noting the tumors' heterogeneous nature. Many efforts for in- depth understanding of nanoscale nanomaterials and tumor interaction are required. Eventually, nanomedicines will approach the need to be tailor-made and individual based on medical diagnostics and imaging. Medical image-guided intervention for the oncology approach will be one of the significant therapies for future nanomedicines.

Intervention oncology is a special area of intervention radiology that performs diagnostics and treatment of cancer employing targeted non-destructive procedure executed under image supervision. It mainly utilizes x-ray, CT, MRI and ultrasound to assist the guided instrument, e.g. intra-vascular catheter, biopsy needle, ablation electrode etc to permit the targeted and accurate treatments of solid tumor localized in different organs of the human body. Advancements in biomedical imaging and image guiding for the detection, characterization, targeting and therapy of cancer now permits non-invasive image guiding treatment of different solid tumors without the toxic nature of chemotherapeutics and radiation. The image-guided procedure provides results with fewer complications, quick recovery and reduced cost. The broadly utilized procedures are trans-catheter directed therapy with intra-tumoral or intra-arterial deliveries and precutaneous or endoscopic ablative therapy. Biomedical imaging plays an important role in image-guided therapy and intervention procedure. These roles are: (i) pre-procedure arrangement (identification of the tumors volume); (ii) intra-procedure targeting (guided catheter deliveries); (iii) intra-procedure supervision (supervising tumor tissue change caused by therapy); (iv) intra-procedure controlling (doing adjustment); (v) post-procedure evaluation (estimating efficacy and post interventions). Contrasting agents are frequently needed to highlight the targeted sites that are not well highlighted on unimproved scans in pre-procedure, intra-procedure and post-procedure therapy. Although these interventional approaches are chiefly employed for conventional localized therapy like radiotherapy, chemotherapy, laser ablations etc, these traditional interventions of therapeutics are traditionally coupled with multifunctional nanoscale based medicines. In recent years, different image-guided cancer nanomedicines approaches have been tested and have displayed significant outcomes in pre-clinical stages. Improved functioning of nanoscale materials offers higher imaging contrasts effect during the image-guided therapeutics procedure and more tumor specific activated therapeutics at the same time. These characteristics also suggest newer opportunities for nanomedicines that are inactive with lower tumor targeting and toxicity issues for clinical translation. Now, the rising next generation nanomedicines 'image-guided cancer nanomedicines' coupled with the intervention oncology approach fulfils minimum systematic distributions, uniform distributions in the target site, and higer localized delivery of nanomedicines results in enhanced efficiency of cutting edge nanomedicine (figure 4.34). Moreover, the image guiding delivery of nano-medicines will be imperative in future clinical practice (figure 4.34). Firstly, the efficient dose of nanomedicines can be highly localized in the tumor regime with minimum toxicity; secondly, it is achievable to supervise and verify whether nano-scale materials based nanomedicines are appropriately delivered to the tumor sites

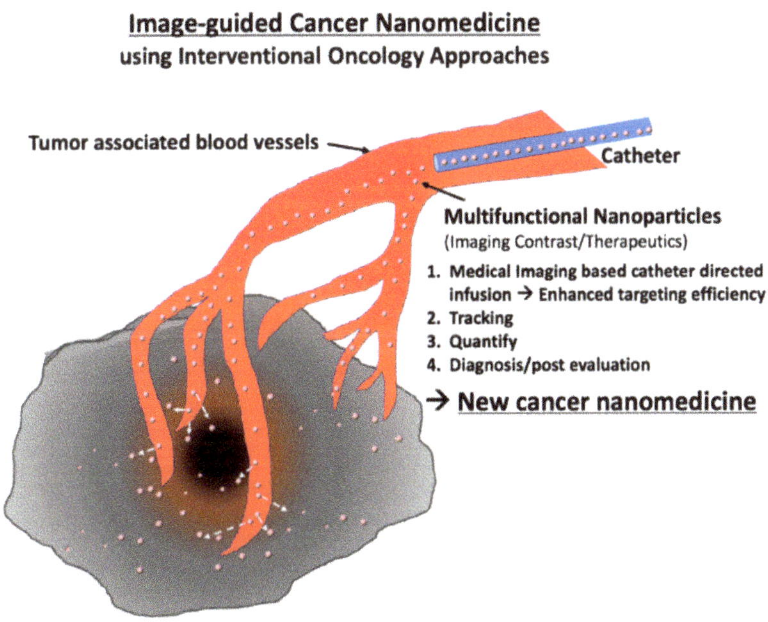

Figure 4.34. Image-guided cancer nanomedicine (image reproduced with permission from [35]).

after the administration (localized infusions and tracking); thirdly, the quantity of the administered nanoscale materials can be quantitatively examined to evaluate the quantity of post-infusions (non-destructive quantifications); finally, the distributions of the administered nanoscale materials inside the body may be supervised for a longer time (diagnostics and post-assessment). The proposed newer image guiding cancer nanomedicines approach can be eventually permitted in patient-specific dosimetry and tumor-specific treatments of cancer for better therapeutics effect in an individualized way. At the same time, it is expected that the use of nanomedicines in intervention oncology will unlock new chapters for extraordinary therapeutics efficacy. It is significant to note that image-guided cancer nanomedicines incorporate newer biomedical imaging techniques, nanomaterials, molecular moiety and a novel class of therapeutics agent as well as existing drugs/therapeutics. Stronger collaborations between multidisciplinary and interdisciplinary teams containing clinicians, basic science scientists and nanotechnologists are needed for advancement of image-guided cancer nanomedicines for clinical translation.

As depicted in figure 4.35, image-guided drug delivery is a speedily emerging field and porphysomes offer good examples of how nanotheranostics can enhance image-guided drug delivery and therapy. Porphysomes can accumulate in a selective manner in the tumor and can be detected by different imaging modalities, such as fluorescent imaging, which can offer specific light radiation of the tumor for improved photothermal and photodynamic therapies. Another example is to employ MRI guided focused ultrasound to heat tumors in a specific manner and activate drug release in localized form. If the thermoresponsive liposomes are loaded with the MRI contrasting agents, the drug release within the tumor can be quantitatively evaluated under MR imaging. These models of treatment consist of multiple feedback loops to target drug delivery and personalized therapy. By incorporation

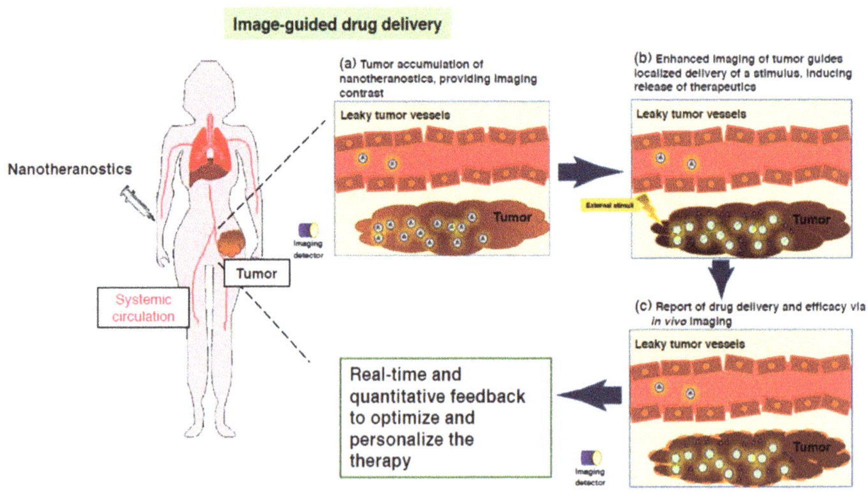

Figure 4.35. Schematic representation of image-guided drugs delivery enabled by nanotheranostics (image reproduced from [36], copyright (2018), with permission from Elsevier).

of various components inside a single nanoscale platform, i.e. making it able to provide multiple functions, the nanoscale particles enhance detection of the tumor under various imaging modalities, report on drug delivery, assist to focus the exterior stimulus to the tumors, release the payload for cancer therapies upon the image-guided stimulus and augment the effects of image-guided treatments like photothermal therapies. This will contribute to the accurate and complete removal of the tumor, individualized adjustment of the doses, specific drug delivery, and synergistically activated cancer therapies.

It is predicted that nanotheranostics will be one of the fast emerging areas in drug delivery and many new systems will be designed, developed and characterized *in vitro* and *in vivo*. New imaging technology or multimodal imaging modality will be designed, developed and included with nanotheranostics. Nanomedicine with theranostics capability will advance into the clinical level path in the upcoming 5–10 years. To prolong the advancements in this field, more nanoscale materials need to be developed for endowment of multiple functionalities to nanoscale materials. For example, new porphyrin was synthesized to integrate large metallic ions to execute theranostics, while holding their photon properties. Newer and targeting chelator agents have been developed for stabilized labeling of radionuclides to nanoscale particles and for precise delivery. Similarly, stabilized drugs encapsulating inside nanoplatforms need to be proficient for improved drug delivery to the tumor and enhanced pharmacokinetic profile in between drugs and delivery systems. Stabilized drug loading to nanoplatforms is mainly accomplished by covalent conjugations, activated loading, and stronger complications between the drugs and the transporters. Newer contrasting agents that can be employed for multimodal imaging are required, and the methodologies for stabilized incorporation of them inside nanoplatforms need to be developed.

The most notable issues in the nanotheranostics field is that, to possess multiple functions, diverse components are included inside a single nanoplatform, making the systems complicated. This poses a notable difficulty for scaling up production and further clinical translation. Nanoscale scientists in this area need to factor this scaling up challenge inside their designs of nanotheranostics systems as early as feasible to alleviate the prospective pitfalls. In comparison, the porphysomes technologies take advantage of the fact that porphyrins, the majority components, are multifunctional and can therefore keep the systems comparatively simple. With many outcomes from nanotheranostics and when newer drug delivery and imaging modalities have been developed, the outlook is optimistic for this area and its clinical level translation can be recognized in the upcoming years to improve cancer therapeutics.

Imaging techniques like MRI, PET, CT, ultrasound, SPECT, x-ray etc offer precious information for diagnostics, stages, and preparative arrangements. However, the excessive cost and sophisticated infrastructure of these imaging modalities limit translation to the operating room. Moreover, the resolution and contrast provided by these imaging modalities do not provide enough sensitivity and specific nature to recognize a surgical margin and localized metastasis.

Image-guided surgeries are capable alternatives for tumor marginal evaluation. Image-guided surgery is defined as surgery guided by real-time imaging feedback. The goal of image-guided surgery is localization of primary tumors, detection of enduring diseases, recognition of lymph node metastases and conservation of the nearby normal cells. Prior to surgery, patients are administered the contrasting agent which accretes in the tumor via passive or active targeting mechanism with rapid clearance from normal tissue, offering a contrast to cancer tissue. With the assistance of imaging systems specifically applied to the types of exogenous probes, surgeons use real-time imaging assistance to resect primary tumors and recognize any remaining cancer in surgical cavities. The surgical tumor imaging method with promising features employs the exogenous probe. Even though there are different imaging modalities and image-guided surgery probes under trial, they usually fulfil similar criteria: images of tumors should be visualized in real time; precise accumulations of the contrasting agents in the tumor site and quick clearance from normal tissue; enabling tumor contrast; the imaging systems and contrasting agents need to recognize the tumor with higher sensitivity and superior resolution, incorporating the detection of lower signals and smaller tumors; image displaying and imaging systems may not interface with the surgical workflows. Presently, different imaging techniques are compatible with tumor resection surgeries. This includes fluorescence, photoacoustic imaging, surface-enhanced Raman spectroscopy, multimodal imaging and theranostics, which couple therapies with imaging. There is superior pace in the applicability of nanoscale platforms for surgical tumor imaging. Figure 4.36 shows the current advancement in the different types of nanoplatforms employed for surgical image guidance.

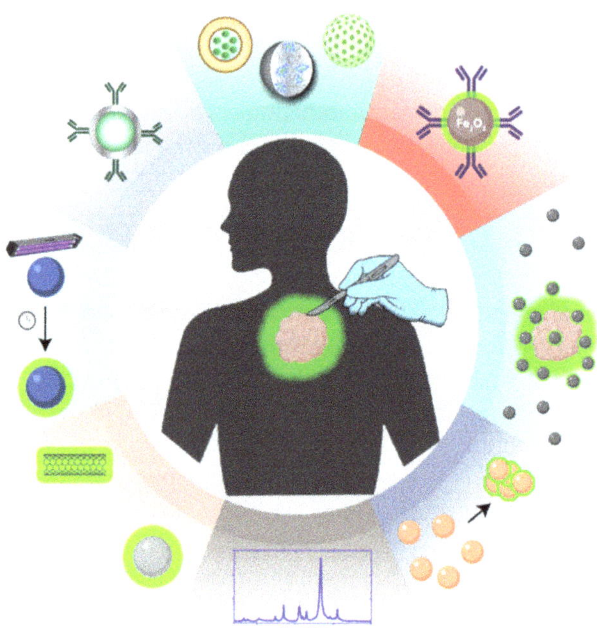

Figure 4.36. Different type of nanoplatforms employed for surgical image guidance (image reproduced with permission from [37], copyright 2020 John Wiley & Sons).

Zheng *et al* [38] investigated the successive use of CF800 for CT based preparative and near infrared fluorescent based intra-operative localizing and visualizing of a primary H and N tumor, malignant lymph nodes and introverted pulmonary nodules (figure 4.37). Endoscopic near infrared fluorescent imaging was employed for intro-operative imaging in both animal models. The long-lasting accretions of liposomes at the tumor site (figure 4.37(a)) make them appropriate for both pre-operative and intra-operative imaging following a single administration. Even though supplementary investigations are required to conclude the reproducibility, sensitivity and specific nature of these liposome agents, the data presented here demonstrated that the surgeon's confidence in tumor localization and malignant lymph nodes recognition can be incremented by the occurrence of intra-operative fluorescent signals provided by liposomes accumulated at this site.

Nanoscale biointerfaces are dynamic, inter-related and tremendously influence the efficiency of nanomedicines. Molecular level imaging modalities like fluorescence are required for understanding nanoscale biointeractions to guide nanomedicine development. With advancements in the dependable labeling of nanoscale particles with fluorophores, integrated Förster resonance energy transfer (FRET) offers receptive fluorescence connected to nanomedicine reliability and functions. For nanoscale medicines created by self-assembly (for example liposomes, polymer micelles, lipoproteins mimetic, nano emulsions, nano bubbles, inorganic nanoparticles with self-assembled coating), structural integrity is significant for maintenance of functionalities. Zhao *et al* [39] recently investigated the influence of integrated FRET for measurements of non-associated kinetic and fates of self-assembled nanomedicine *in vivo*. They have developed NIR-FRET imaging techniques to supervise the stabilities of quantum dots cores self-assembled lipid nanoscale particles, using the NIR quantum dots core as the donor and lipid in the self-assembly of PEGylated lipids coatings as an acceptor (figure 4.38(a)). FRET was substantiated by incrementing the lipids concentration in the nanoparticles formulations and noting the generated FRET with equivalent losses of FD. A key advantage of this FRET design for *in vivo* imaging lies in the larger spectral separations between quantum dots and lipids, making channel cross-talk corrections redundant and permitting imaging of FRET, functional dyspepsia (FD) and fluorescent angiography (FA). Within the tumors, FRET quickly incremented, which indicates faster accretions of the intact nanoscale particles, subsequent to the steady reduction in FRET and analogous increment in FD from 2 h post administration, suggesting nanoparticle dissociation and retention of quantum dots (figure 4.38(b)). As the FA signals decremented during this time, lipids were not retained within the tumors subsequent to the dissociation. The same kind of distribution dynamic was noted in the tumors draining lymph node by *ex vivo* imaging following the pre-tumoral injections (figure 4.38(c)), and was established using intra-vital confocal laser scanning microscopy in a dorsal window chamber model (figure 4.38(d)). Lipid trafficking was further studied using *ex vivo* fluorescent imaging of the clearance organ (figure 4.38(e)). This experiment communally presents an inclusive outlook of the *in vivo* fate of nanoscale particles, involving nanoparticles dissociation within the vasculature, tumors, lymph nodes and liver; lipid association with serum component and trafficking of the kidney; and quantum dots in tumors and lymph node (figure 4.38(f)).

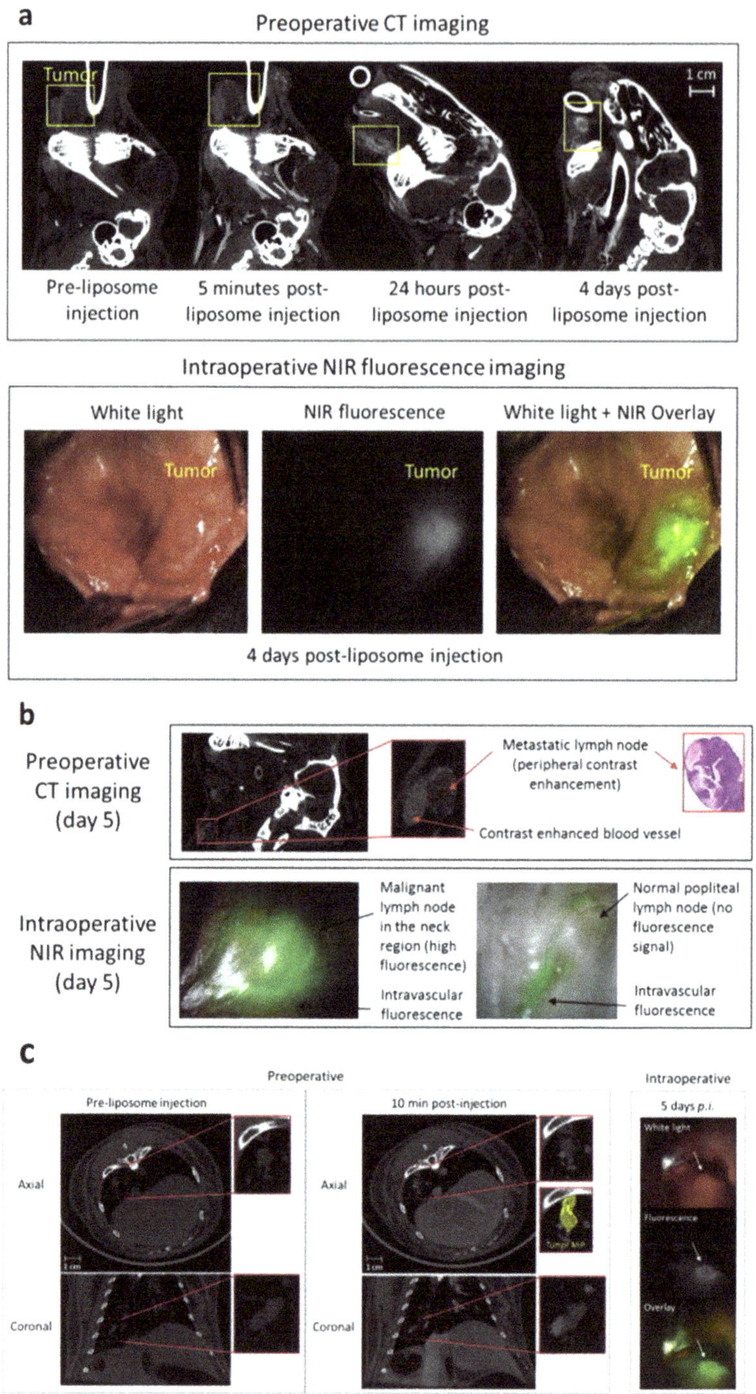

Figure 4.37. Imaging performance in rabbit models of cancer (images reproduced from [38], copyright (2015), with permission from Elsevier).

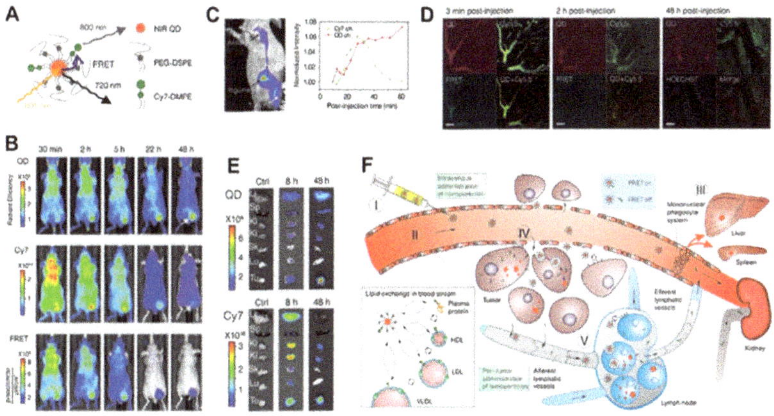

Figure 4.38. Monitoring the *in vivo* dissociation kinetics of self-assembled nanoparticles by integrated Förster resonance energy transfer (FRET) imaging (images reproduced with permission from [39], copyright (2013) American Chemical Society).

Amongst the different studies reported in the literature, representative investigations in which PET was employed to analyze biodistributions of nanomedicines formulation have been reported by Ferrara *et al* [40] who prepared longer circulating PEGylated liposome carrying ^{18}F-containing lipid (figure 4.39(a)). A continuous-bed-motion scan was executed at 1.5 h after intervention injections, to enable PET scanning of the whole animal. Maximum intensities projection was attained, and the biodistributions of free ^{18}F-FDP versus liposomes-incorporated ^{18}F-FD was analyzed. Another investigation representing the appropriate nature of imaging for entire body pharmacokinetics and biodistributions analysis was published by Anfreozzi *et al* [41], who investigated the *in vivo* behaviour of solid lipids nanoscale materials incorporating bovine serum albumin radiolabeled with ^{64}Cu. As depicted in figure 4.39(b), the PET image showed the signal in carotid and heart at 0.5 and 3 h, indicating the presence of solid-lipid nanoparticles in the organized circulation. At a later time point, solid-lipid nanoparticles were cleared from the blood and accreted in theliver, spleen and intestine. Centering on tumor targeting drug delivery, Lee *et al* [42] employed PET to determine the differences between RGD-targeted versus non-targeted nanomedicine. The biodistributions of the construct were estimated in bare mice containing human tumors as shown in figure 4.39(c), the acquired PET images clearly show a dissimilarity in tumor uptake. The higher sensitivity of PET may be beneficial for visualization and identification of the lymph node by employing radio-labeled nanomedicines formulation. An example of this is depicted in figure 4.39(d), showing the mouse containing a high metastatic 4T1-murine breast tumor upon the injection of multimodal ^{64}Cu labeled mesoporous silica nanoparticles.

A good illustration of the suitable nature of SPECT–CT based hybrid imaging for supervising nanomedicines intermediated drug targeting has been reported by Head *et al* [44] who employed synergistic therapeutics approaches, i.e. radio-frequency ablations (RFA) + intravenously injected liposome DOX, to observe and quantify drug delivery to the tumor and analyse the therapeutics effect. RFA treatments were

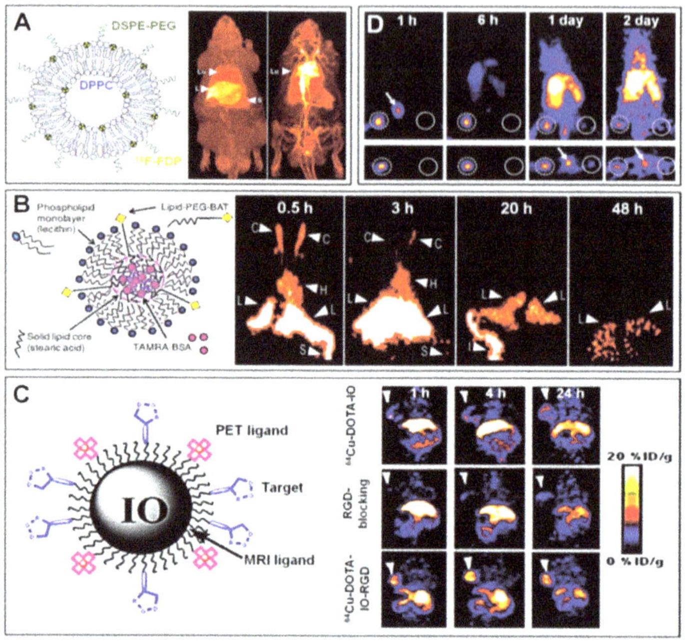

Figure 4.39. Non-invasive imaging of nanomedicines using PET. A reprinted from [40], copyright (2007), with permission from Elsevier; B reprinted with permission from [41], copyright (2011) American Chemical Society; C reprinted with permission from [42], copyright 2008 by Society of Nuclear Medicine; D reprinted from [43], copyright (2012), with permission from Elsevier.

executed 5 m after intravenously injected 99mTc labeled liposome with DOX. One of the two tumors was exposed to the RFA, while the other was employed for intra-individual control. In another investigation, Chrastina *et al* [45] reported the application of hybrid SPECT–CT for non-destructive supervision of nanomedicine based drug targeting to the lung. To this end, generation-5 polymer dendrimer (figure 4.40(A)) was surface functionalized with antibody targeted amino peptides, to mediate the specific lung targeting. By employing the same experimental system, Zhang *et al* [46] utilized SPECT–CT to evaluate the potentiality of targeting of Ephrin B4 receptors for specific targeting of nanomedicine to prostate cancer xenografts. The Ephrin B4 receptors specific peptides (TNYL-RAW) were developed and integrated into the PEGylated and cross-connected polymer micelle (CCPM), which was doubly labeled with ^{111}In and NIR dye Cy7 (figure 4.40(B)).

The imaging of drug release from nanomedicines formulation, as opposed to the supervision of their biodistribution and targeted sites accumulation, is perhaps the most important application for the use of MR imaging and drug delivery research. Since T_1 MRI contrasting agent depends on admittance to a nearby water molecule for producing a signal, its setup and drug release delivery system may be observed and quantified by using MR imaging. This is the main difference from radionuclides, which produce a similar stronger signal prior to and after drug release from the transport material. This special capability of MRI contrasting agent to be employed

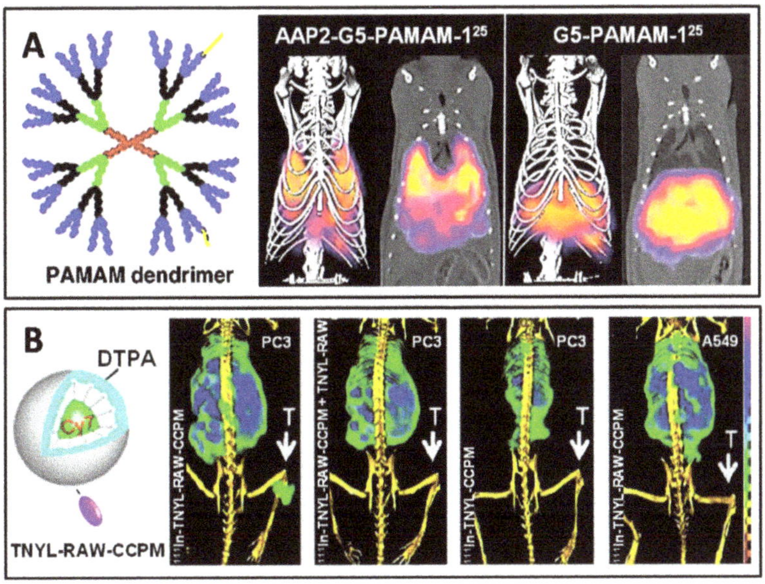

Figure 4.40. Non-invasive imaging of nanomedicines using SPECT. (A) Reprinted with permission from [45], copyright 2011 John Wiley & Sons. (B) Reprinted from [46], copyright (2011), with permission from Elsevier.

for observation and quantification of drug release was neatly investigated by de Smet *et al* [47], who set up the screening content released from temperature sensitive liposomses upon high intensities focusing ultrasound mediated hyperthermic activity (figure 4.41(a)). In this investigation, three animals received a combinational of hyperthermic evaluations and thermosensitive liposomes, and three controlling animals received thermosensitive liposomes without the hyperthermic activity. Onuki *et al* [48] recently formulated similar approaches for simultaneou visualizations of both the drug delivery and drug release by using multifunctional nanomedicine and dual MR imaging. Polymer based NPs containing 5-Fu and Gd-DTPA and SPIONs (figure 4.41(b)) were synthesized, and their properties were estimated in SCID mouse bearing MCF-7 breast cancer xenografts. After the intervention injections, the particles exhibited stronger T_2 contrasting, produced by the accommodated SPIONs, which corresponded to the *in vivo* localizing in the tumor. In a further step, Castelli *et al* [49] supervised and screened both release and intra-tumoral and intra-cellular trafficking of the contrast agents labeled liposomes using MR imaging. They prepared two dissimilar paramagnetic liposomes. The first was employed for the visualization of sub-cellular localizing and releasing using T_1 and T_2 contrasts. By employing both the liposomes formulation and three dissimilar MRI protocols, the authors neatly showed the delicate suitable nature of MRI for analysis of cellular uptake, trafficking, and processing of liposomes (figure 4.41(c)).

Kunjachan *et al* [50] investigated how to evaluate the potentiality of employing functional respiratory imaging (FRI) and FMT for observing biodistribution and targeting site accumulation of near infrared labeled passive targeting tumors

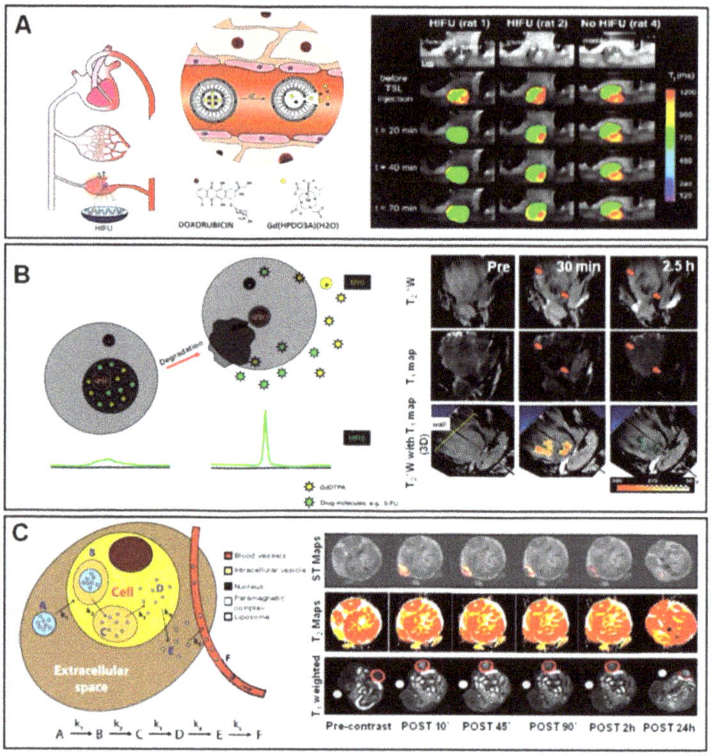

Figure 4.41. Non-invasive imaging of (model) drug release from nanomedicines using MRI. A reproduced from [50], copyright (2011), with permission from Elsevier; B reproduced from [51], copyright (2010), with permission from Elsevier; C reproduced from [52], copyright (2010), with permission from Elsevier.

polymer drug carriers. In their studies, a CD-1 nude mouse containing CT26 colon cancer xenografts was intravenously injected within the co-polymer containing Dy750 (figure 4.42(a)). Two-dimensional FRI was undertaken at different earlier timing points after the intervention injections, displaying localizing in the heart and larger blood vessels, and thus confirming lower circulation properties of the polymer drug delivery system (figure 4.42(b)). In light of the kinetics of EPR mediated tumors targeting, the tumor accumulation of pHPMA-Dy750 was very low at 1 h post injection, but outstanding at 72 h (as shown in figure 4.42(c)). Accordingly, these efforts persuasively demonstrate that combining micro-CT with FMT enables more informative, more practical, and significant optical imaging investigations on the biodistribution of near infrared labeled nanomedicine formulation.

According to the above, combination of drug targeting and imaging may be beneficial for personalizing nanomedicine treatment, and it offers a balanced basis for individual based nanomedicines. A revolutionary study in this view was reported by Harrington *et al* [51], who observed and quantified EPR intermediated passively targeted tumors by ^{111}In labeled PEGylated liposome in a patient suffering from various types of tumor. The liposome was injected into patients with lung

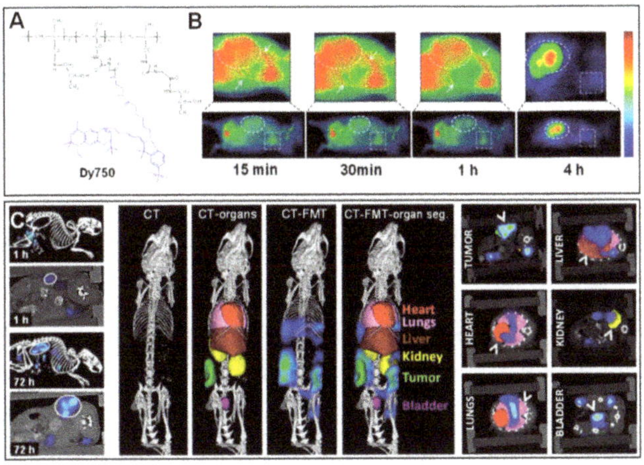

Figure 4.42. Non-invasive optical imaging of nanomedicines (all the images reproduced with permission from [50], copyright (2012) American Chemical Society).

carcinomas, head and neck cancer, and breasts cancer, using whole-body gamma-camera imaging and SPECT. Comparatively proficient passive drug targeting was noted for the previous two malignant tumors.

In addition, Seymour *et al* [52] investigated dynamic nanomedicines intermediated drug targeting in patients. They synthesized polymer drug carriers with functionalization of DOX, radionuclides and receptors, which were over articulated by hepatocytes, and further used gamma-camera and SPECT imaging to supervise the drug targeting to hepato-cellular carcinogenic. The biodistribution of this enthusiastically targeted polymeric drug conjugate, displayed extremely proficient liver targeting. On the other hand, upon imaging the intra-hepatic distributions it was noted that most of the conjugates accumulated in normal tissues more moderately than in the tumor. Recently, Hrkach *et al* [53] fabricated active targeted PLGA based nanoscale particles (TNPs) bearing DTXL and estimated the efficiency of the most optimum formulation *in vitro*, *in vivo* and in patients. DTXL-TNPs were targeted to prostate membrane antigens using targeted ligands and the clinical level efficiency was supervised by contrast enhancing CT imaging. In patients suffering from chalangiocarcinoma with metastatic lung lesions and patients suffering from tonsil cancer, non-destructive imaging offered comparatively earlier insight into the efficiency of the interventions (figure 4.43). This study demonstrates that, alongside supervision nanomedicines biodistributions and targeted site accretion, non-destructive imaging is also extremely beneficial for longitudinal treatment supervision.

The above investigations demonstrate the potentiality of the combination of drug targeting and imaging in clinical situations. By labeling the nanomedicine and by subjecting the patient to gamma cameras, SPECT, and PET imaging, non-destructive and quantitatively observed information on the pharmacokinetics, biodistribution, targeting site accumulation, targeted localizing of the formulation can be gained. This non-destructive imaging information can be employed to choose whether or not to treat the patient with nanomedicine, and it may thus offer a

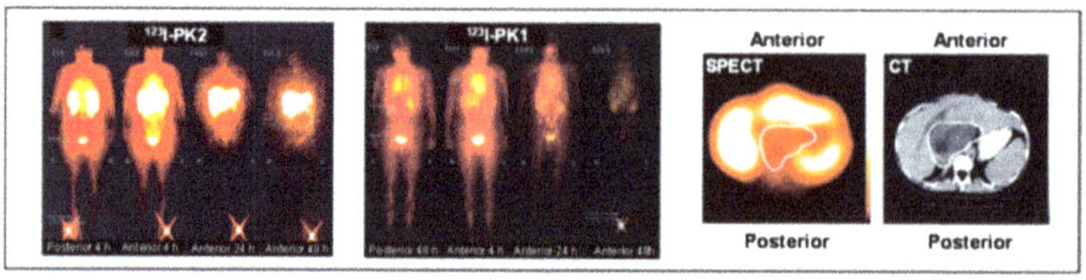

Figure 4.43. Translational imaging of nanomedicines. Reproduced with permission from [51].

framework for individual based nanomedicine cancer testament. It is noteworthy that if the quantity accreting inside the tumor is higher, then targeted treatment will be more proficient than barely any fraction of the intervention injected accumulation at the targeted sites. Moreover, with the combination of the standard imaging based diagnostics procedure during follow-up, significant information on potentiality of the treatment responses can be observed, which can be beneficial for relatively quick decision making with respect to continued nanotherapy. Lastly, it is important to keep in mind that non-destructive imaging may applicable in the case of metastatic diseases. By performing SPECT and PET scan with radionuclides labeled nanomedicine, information can be gained on the accretion of this formulation in both the primary tumor and metastases, and treatment protocol can be personalized consequently. In a similar setup, it looks apparent that if all lesions show noteworthy nanomedicine uptake, then the patient may be treated with nanomedicine formulation. Accordingly, in spite of the fact that it is not much recognized, there is potential for nanomedicine for tumor targeting.

4.5 Conclusions

Current investigations of the nanoscale technologies for cancer therapeutics and diagnostics have displayed their benefits for ontological and inherent limitation. Most iterations have assisted in codification of the current basis, and translation efforts in this area and have shown their extent with multiple emerging fields. From the technology perspective, this area has undergone incredible growth and success. On the other hand, deficient understanding of human cancer biology persists in comparison to application of the nanoplatforms. Although the technical improvements in large-scale imaging modalities like CT–PET or MRI have led to enhancement in pre-operative cancer diagnosis and stages, their utilization is restricted by attainable spatial resolution, sensitivity and practical issues of intra-operative implementation. Moreover, image-guided imaging strategies have conventionally been hindered in surgical practice by the smaller number of presented targeting of near infrared agents, superficial tissue penetration, constrained contrast resolution, quick photo-bleaching and inability to detect multiple cancers or healthy tissue. Noteworthy progress, on the other hand, is being made to tackle the drawbacks, with notable efforts promoted toward development of optically activated and targeted imaging agents, inclusive of particles based probes for clinical level practice. Designed to promote improved sensitivity, specific nature and depth penetrating, these probes promise noticeable improvements in real-time earlier stages molecular level detection and treatment of diseases in conjugations with multi-channel fluorescence camera system with clinical grade precision (figure 4.44). To enhance the chances of pre-clinical nanomedicines to attain clinical trials and to be promoted further towards market product development, we advocate for proficient attitudes toward focusing and endorsement of these nanoscale materials which possess clinical and commercialization potentiality. Figure 4.45 shows the key challenges in

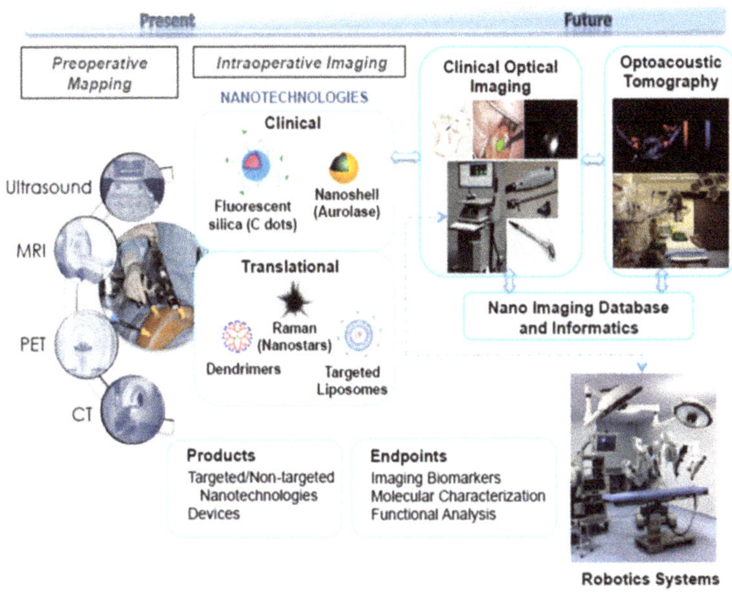

Figure 4.44. Current and upcoming nano-oncology image-guided surgical suites (image reproduced with permission from [55], copyright (2017) American Chemical Society).

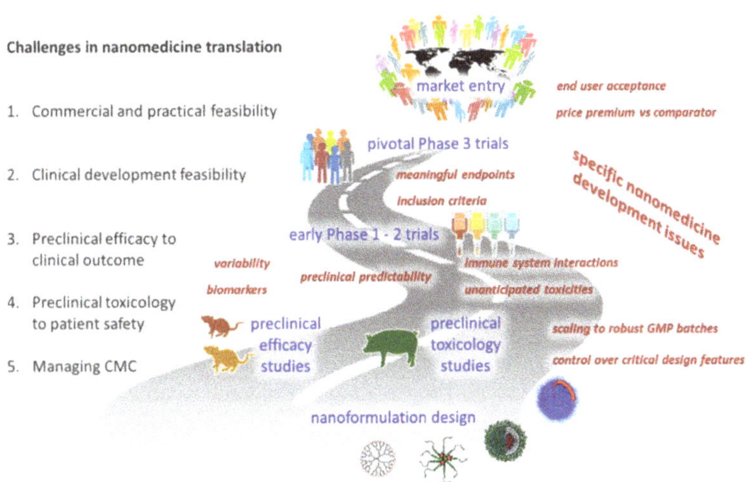

Figure 4.45. Key challenges in nanomedicine translation (image reproduced with permission from [54], copyright 2020, The Authors, with permission of Springer).

nanomedicine translation [54]. Eventually, and in spite of the multiple successive investigations to date, the utilities of the field will only be examined by benefits offered to the cancer patient and their care outcomes. We expect that ongoing research and clinical effort will recognize regimes where nanoscale technologies treatment, diagnostics, and their combinations can make a great difference. We also need to keep in mind that quite a few successful therapeutics took more than 25 years from their initial research to their endorsement and implementation into standard clinical practice.

Conflict of interest

None.

Acknowledgments

Author Sandeep B Somvanshi acknowledges Department of Science and Technology, Government of India for DST-INSPIRE Fellowship (IF170288).

References

[1] Bray F, Ferlay J, Soerjomataram I, Siegel R L, Torre L A and Jemal A 2018 Global cancer statistics 2018: GLOBOCAN estimates of incidence and mortality worldwide for 36 cancers in 185 countries *CA: Cancer J Clin.* **68** 394–424

[2] World Health Organization 2020 WHO report on cancer: setting priorities, investing wisely and providing care for all *Global Report*

[3] Collins I and Workman P 2006 New approaches to molecular cancer therapeutics *Nat. Chem. Biol.* **2** 689–700

[4] Sinha R, Kim G J, Nie S and Shin D M 2006 Nanotechnology in cancer therapeutics: bioconjugated nanoparticles for drug delivery *Mol. Cancer Therap.* **5** 1909–17

[5] Gonzalez-Valdivieso J, Girotti A, Schneider J and Arias F J 2021 Advanced nanomedicine and cancer: challenges and opportunities in clinical translation *Int. J. Pharm.* **599** 120438

[6] Bhushan B, Khanadeev V, Khlebtsov B, Khlebtsov N and Gopinath P 2017 Impact of albumin based approaches in nanomedicine: imaging, targeting and drug delivery *Adv. Colloid Interface Sci.* **246** 13–39

[7] Damasco J A, Ravi S, Perez J D, Hagaman D E and Melancon M P 2020 Understanding nanoparticle toxicity to direct a safe-by-design approach in cancer nanomedicine *Nanomaterials* **10** 2186

[8] Zhou Q, Zhang L and Wu H 2017 Nanomaterials for cancer therapies *Nanotechnol. Rev.* **6** 473–96

[9] Salvioni L, Rizzuto M A, Bertolini J A, Pandolfi L, Colombo M and Prosperi D 2019 Thirty years of cancer nanomedicine: success, frustration, and hope *Cancers* **11** 1855

[10] Tsvetkova Y 2018 Riboflavin-targeted nanomedicines for cancer imaging and drug delivery *PhD Thesis* Universitätsbibliothek der RWTH Aachen

[11] Madamsetty V S, Mukherjee A and Mukherjee S 2019 Recent trends of the bio-inspired nanoparticles in cancer theranostics *Front. Pharmacol.* **10** 1264

[12] Moses W W 2011 Fundamental limits of spatial resolution in PET *Nucl. Instrum. Methods Phys. Res., Sect.* A **648** S236–40

[13] van der Meel R, Sulheim E, Shi Y, Kiessling F, Mulder W J and Lammers T 2019 Smart cancer nanomedicine *Nat. Nanotechnol.* **14** 1007–17

[14] Zeineldin R 2020 Nanotechnology for cancer screening and diagnosis: from innovations to clinical applications *Biomaterials for Cancer Therapeutics* 2nd edn (Cambridge: Elsevier) pp 261–89

[15] Zhang Y, Li M, Gao X, Chen Y and Liu T 2019 Nanotechnology in cancer diagnosis: progress, challenges and opportunities *J. Hematol.Oncol.* **12** 1–13

[16] Zeng J Y, Wang X S, Song W F, Cheng H and Zhang X Z 2019 Metal-organic framework mediated multifunctional nanoplatforms for cancer therapy *Adv. Therap.* **2** 1800100

[17] Zhang C-J, Hu Q, Feng G, Zhang R, Yuan Y, Lu X and Liu B 2015 Image-guided combination chemotherapy and photodynamic therapy using a mitochondria-targeted molecular probe with aggregation-induced emission characteristics *Chem. Sci.* **6** 4580–6

[18] Li M, Luo Z and Zhao Y 2018 Self-assembled hybrid nanostructures: versatile multifunctional nanoplatforms for cancer diagnosis and therapy *Chem. Mater.* **30** 25–53

[19] Li J, Zhen X, Lyu Y, Jiang Y, Huang J and Pu K 2018 Cell membrane coated semiconducting polymer nanoparticles for enhanced multimodal cancer phototheranostics *ACS Nano* **12** 8520–30

[20] Zhang L, Wang D, Yang K, Sheng D, Tan B, Wang Z, Ran H, Yi H, Zhong Y and Lin H 2018 Mitochondria-targeted artificial 'Nano-RBCs' for amplified synergistic cancer phototherapy by a single NIR irradiation, *Adv. Sci.* **5** 1800049

[21] Gao D, Guo X, Zhang X, Chen S, Wang Y, Chen T, Huang G, Gao Y, Tian Z and Yang Z 2020 Multifunctional phototheranostic nanomedicine for cancer imaging and treatment *Mater. Today Bio* **5** 100035

[22] Lu J, Sun J, Li F, Wang J, Liu J, Kim D, Fan C, Hyeon T and Ling D 2018 Highly sensitive diagnosis of small hepatocellular carcinoma using pH-responsive iron oxide nanocluster assemblies *JACS* **140** 10071–4

[23] You H, Shang W, Min X, Weinreb J, Li Q, Leapman M, Wang L and Tian J , 2020 Sight and switch off: nerve density visualization for interventions targeting nerves in prostate cancer *Sci. Adv.* **6** eaax6040

[24] Tay Z W, Chandrasekharan P, Chiu-Lam A, Hensley D W, Dhavalikar R, Zhou X Y, Yu E Y, Goodwill P W, Zheng B and Rinaldi C 2018 Magnetic particle imaging-guided heating *in vivo* using gradient fields for arbitrary localization of magnetic hyperthermia therapy *ACS Nano* **12** 3699–713

[25] Espinosa A, Di Corato R, Kolosnjaj-Tabi J, Flaud P, Pellegrino T and Wilhelm C 2016 Duality of iron oxide nanoparticles in cancer therapy: amplification of heating efficiency by magnetic hyperthermia and photothermal bimodal treatment *ACS Nano* **10** 2436–46

[26] Liu X, Zheng J, Sun W, Zhao X, Li Y, Gong N, Wang Y, Ma X, Zhang T and Zhao L-Y 2019 Ferrimagnetic vortex nanoring-mediated mild magnetic hyperthermia imparts potent immunological effect for treating cancer metastasis *ACS Nano* **13** 8811–25

[27] Nahrendorf M, Zhang H, Hembrador S, Panizzi P, Sosnovik D E, Aikawa E, Libby P, Swirski F K and Weissleder R 2008 Clinical perspective *Circulation* **117** 379–87

[28] Nahrendorf M, Keliher E, Marinelli B, Waterman P, Feruglio P F, Fexon L, Pivovarov M, Swirski F K, Pittet M J and Vinegoni C 2010 Hybrid PET-optical imaging using targeted probes *Proc. Natl. Acad. Sci.* **107** 7910–5

[29] Yoon H Y, Son S, Lee S J, You D G, Yhee J Y, Park J H, Swierczewska M, Lee S, Kwon I C and Kim S H 2014 Glycol chitosan nanoparticles as specialized cancer therapeutic vehicles: sequential delivery of doxorubicin and Bcl-2 siRNA *Sci. Rep.* **4** 1–12

[30] Lammers T, Kiessling F, Hennink W E and Storm G 2010 Nanotheranostics and image-guided drug delivery: current concepts and future directions *Mol. Pharm.* **7** 1899–912

[31] Zhang P, Hu C, Ran W, Meng J, Yin Q and Li Y 2016 Recent progress in light-triggered nanotheranostics for cancer treatment *Theranostics* **6** 948

[32] Ding X, Zhao H, Li C, Wang Q and Jiang J 2019 All-in-one theranostic nanoplatform with controlled drug release and activated MRI tracking functions for synergistic NIR-II hyperthermia-chemotherapy of tumors *Nano Res.* **12** 2971–81

[33] Wang C, Zhao N, Huang Y, He R, Xu S and Yuan W 2020 Coordination of injectable self-healing hydrogel with Mn-Zn ferrite@ mesoporous silica nanospheres for tumor MR imaging and efficient synergistic magnetothermal-chemo-chemodynamic therapy *Chem. Eng. J.* **401** 126100

[34] Zhou S, Ding C, Wang Y, Jiang W and Fu J 2019 Supramolecular valves functionalized rattle-structured UCNPs@hm-SiO_2 nanoparticles with controlled drug release triggered by quintuple stimuli and dual-modality imaging functions: a potential theranostic nanomedicine *ACS Biomater. Sci. Eng.* **5** 6022–35

[35] Dong-Hyun K 2018 Image-guided cancer nanomedicine *J. Imaging* **4** 18

[36] Tang W-L, Tang W-H and Li S-D 2018 Cancer theranostic applications of lipid-based nanoparticles *Drug Discovery Today* **23** 1159–66

[37] Wojtynek N E and Mohs A M 2020 Image-guided tumor surgery: the emerging role of nanotechnology *Wiley Interdiscip. Rev. Nanomed. Nanobiotechnol.* **12** e1624

[38] Zheng J, Muhanna N, De Souza R, Wada H, Chan H, Akens M K, Anayama T, Yasufuku K, Serra S and Irish J 2015 A multimodal nano agent for image-guided cancer surgery *Biomaterials* **67** 160–8

[39] Zhao Y, van Rooy I, Hak S, Fay F, Tang J, Davies C D L, Skobe M, Fisher E A, Radu A and Fayad Z A 2013 Near-infrared fluorescence energy transfer imaging of nanoparticle accumulation and dissociation kinetics in tumor-bearing mice *ACS Nano* **7** 10362–70

[40] Marik J, Tartis M S, Zhang H, Fung J Y, Kheirolomoom A, Sutcliffe J L and Ferrara K W 2007 Long-circulating liposomes radiolabeled with [^{18}F] fluorodipalmitin ([^{18}F] FDP) *Nucl. Med. Biol.* **34** 165–71

[41] Andreozzi E, Seo J W, Ferrara K and Louie A 2011 Novel method to label solid lipid nanoparticles with ^{64}cu for positron emission tomography imaging *Bioconjug. Chem.* **22** 808–18

[42] Lee H-Y, Li Z, Chen K, Hsu A R, Xu C, Xie J, Sun S and Chen X 2008 PET/MRI dual-modality tumor imaging using arginine-glycine-aspartic (RGD)–conjugated radiolabeled iron oxide nanoparticles *J. Nucl. Med.* **49** 1371–9

[43] Huang X, Zhang F, Lee S, Swierczewska M, Kiesewetter D O, Lang L, Zhang G, Zhu L, Gao H and Choi H S 2012 Long-term multimodal imaging of tumor draining sentinel lymph nodes using mesoporous silica-based nanoprobes *Biomaterials* **33** 4370–8

[44] Head H W, Dodd G D III, Bao A, Soundararajan A, Garcia-Rojas X, Prihoda T J, McManus L M, Goins B A, Santoyo C A and Phillips W T 2010 Combination radiofrequency ablation and intravenous radiolabeled liposomal Doxorubicin: imaging and quantification of increased drug delivery to tumors *Radiology* **255** 405–14

[45] Chrastina A, Massey K and Schnitzer J 2011 Overcoming in vivo barriers to targeted nanodelivery *Wiley Interdiscip. Rev. Nanomed. Nanobiotechnol* **3** 421–37

[46] Zhang R, Xiong C, Huang M, Zhou M, Huang Q, Wen X, Liang D and Li C 2011 Peptide-conjugated polymeric micellar nanoparticles for dual SPECT and optical imaging of EphB4 receptors in prostate cancer xenografts *Biomaterials* **32** 5872–9

[47] de Smet M, Heijman E, Langereis S, Hijnen N M and Grüll H 2011 Magnetic resonance imaging of high intensity focused ultrasound mediated drug delivery from temperature-sensitive liposomes: an *in vivo* proof-of-concept study *J. Controlled Release* **150** 102–10

[48] Onuki Y, Jacobs I, Artemov D and Kato Y 2010 Noninvasive visualization of *in vivo* release and intratumoral distribution of surrogate MR contrast agent using the dual MR contrast technique *Biomaterials* **31** 7132–8

[49] Castelli D D, Dastrù W, Terreno E, Cittadino E, Mainini F, Torres E, Spadaro M and Aime S 2010 *In vivo* MRI multicontrast kinetic analysis of the uptake and intracellular trafficking of paramagnetically labeled liposomes *J. Controlled Release* **144** 271–9

[50] Kunjachan S, Gremse F, Theek B, Koczera P, Pola R, Pechar M, Etrych T, Ulbrich K, Storm G and Kiessling F 2013 Noninvasive optical imaging of nanomedicine biodistribution *ACS Nano* **7** 252–62

[51] Harrington K J, Mohammadtaghi S, Uster P S, Glass D, Peters A M, Vile R G and Stewart J S W 2001 Effective targeting of solid tumors in patients with locally advanced cancers by radiolabeled pegylated liposomes *Clin. Cancer Res.* **7** 243–54

[52] Seymour L W, Ferry D R, Anderson D, Hesslewood S, Julyan P J, Poyner R, Doran J, Young A M, Burtles S and Kerr D J 2002 Hepatic drug targeting: phase I evaluation of polymer-bound doxorubicin *J. Clin. Oncol.* **20** 1668–76

[53] Hrkach J, Von Hoff D, Ali M M, Andrianova E, Auer J, Campbell T, De Witt D, Figa M, Figueiredo M and Horhota A 2012 Preclinical development and clinical translation of a PSMA-targeted docetaxel nanoparticle with a differentiated pharmacological profile, *Sci. Transl. Med.,* **4** 128ra139

[54] Metselaar J M and Lammers T 2020 Challenges in nanomedicine clinical translation *Drug Deliv. Transl. Res.* **10** 721–5

[55] Hartshorn C M, Bradbury M S, Lanza G M, Nel A E, Rao J, Wang A Z, Wiesner U B, Yang L and Grodzinski P 2018 Nanotechnology strategies to advance outcomes in clinical cancer care *ACS Nano* **12** 24–43

www.ingramcontent.com/pod-product-compliance
Ingram Content Group UK Ltd.
Pitfield, Milton Keynes, MK11 3LW, UK
UKHW051852100926
8556IPUK00005B/595

9 780750 336734